Headache

in Clinical Practice

Stephen D. Silberstein MD FACP
Thomas Jefferson University Headache Center,
Philadelphia, USA

Richard B. Lipton
Department of Neurology, Montefiore Hospital,
New York, USA

and

Peter J. Goadsby
Institute of Neurology, The National Hospital for
Neurology and Neurosurgery, London, UK

Provided as an educational service by Zeneca
Pharmaceuticals, makers of ZOMIG™ (ZOLMITRIPTAN)

Diane Lee

I S I S
MEDICAL
M E D I A
Oxford

British Library Cataloguing in Publication Data.
A catalogue record for this title is available from the
British Library

ISBN 1 899066 55 1

Silberstein, S D (Stephen)
Headache in Clinical Practice
S D Silberstein, R B Lipton, P J Goadsby (eds)

Always refer to the manufacturer's Prescribing
Information before prescribing drugs cited in this book.

Design and Illustration by
The EDI Partnership, London, UK

Printed and bound by
Book Print Limited, Barcelona, Spain

Distributed in the USA by
Mosby-Year Book, Inc, 11830 Westline Industrial Drive
St Louis MO63145, USA

Distributed in the rest of the world by
Oxford University Press, Saxon Way West, Corby
Northamptonshire NN18 9ES, UK

Contents

Preface

Headache is an almost universal human experience. For some, it is an occasional, episodic nuisance symptom. For others it may be a manifestation of a disabling chronic disease or the first manifestation of a life-threatening condition. The etiology, frequency, severity and life consequences of headache vary widely. To put our current concepts in perspective, the book begins by reviewing the history and epidemiology of headache.

Although headache sufferers differ in their treatment needs, the first step to successful management is a confident, credible, specific diagnosis. Patients often fear that their headaches are symptomatic of a serious underlying disorder. It is important to distinguish a primary headache disorder, such as migraine or tension-type headache, from a secondary headache that is due to a brain mass lesion, infection or metabolic derangement. Individual chapters are devoted to the major primary and secondary headaches. Headache diagnosis and the need and utility of diagnostic studies will be discussed in detail.

In the secondary headache disorders, we have long known that pain can be caused by inflammation, traction or nerve root irritation from intracranial processes. We are beginning to gain insight into the mechanisms of pain for the primary headache disorders. In fact, the molecular basis of one variety of migraine (familial hemiplegic migraine) has been shown to be an abnormality of a calcium channel, suggesting that migraine may be a channelopathy. The book reviews the mechanisms of primary and secondary headache disorders.

Once a specific headache diagnosis is established, the clinician should access the severity and life impact of the disorder. The treatment needs of the patient who has occasional mild headaches are quite different from those of the patient whose attacks are frequent and completely disabling. The goals of treatment should be developed in collaboration with the patient, taking into account his or her needs and preferences.

Our goal is to provide the clinician with a rigorous, accurate yet practical approach to headache. We have devoted our careers to furthering the understanding of the causes of headache and improving the treatment of headache sufferers. We hope to impact some of our enthusiasm to our readers.

Stephen P. Silberstein
Richard B. Lipton
Peter J. Goadsby

Acknowledgements

Richard Lipton thanks Drs Seymour Solomon, Buzz Stewart and Lawrence Newman for their wisdom and friendship and for the creative interchange that leads to new ideas. He also thanks Amy, Justin and Lianna Lipton for their patience and loving support during too many weekends at work instead of play.

Peter Goadsby thanks James Lance for starting him on his headache career and his family for putting up with it.

Stephen Silberstein thanks William Young for covering him at all times he is away, Lynne Kaiser and Linda Kelly for editorial support and Maraha Silberstein for being there.

chapter 1

Historical introduction

Headache has troubled mankind from the dawn of civilization. Trepanation, a sign of neurosurgery, was evident on neolithic skulls dating from 7000 BC.[1] It may have been done to release demons and evil spirits,[1] believed to be the cause of headaches and disorders such as madness and epilepsy, from the head (Figures 1.1 and 1.2).[2] Paul Broca showed that only 30 to 45 minutes were required to remove a slice of bone from the cranium, proving that a patient could survive trepanation.[3] Trepanning was recommended by some 17th century physicians for the treatment of migraine. In 1660, William Harvey recommended trepanation to a patient with intractable migraine.[4] For over millennia, headache triggers, relieving factors, and the signs and symptoms of the migraine complex including headache, aura, prodrome, nausea or vomiting, and familial tendency have been described in the medical and popular literature.[5,6]

References to headache are found as far back as 3000 BC. The earliest published reference is a Sumerian epic poem,[7] an early description of 'the sick headache'.

> The sick-eyed says not
> 'I am sick-eyed'
> The sick-headed not
> 'I am sick-headed.'[8]

The Ebers Papyrus, an ancient Egyptian prescription for headache dating back to about 1200 BC, mentions migraine, neuralgia and shooting head pains, and is said to be based on earlier medical documents from approximately 1550 BC

(Figure 1.3).[9] The Egyptians, like other ancients, believed the gods could cure their ailments and followed the instructions on the Papyrus. A clay crocodile holding grain in its mouth was firmly bound to the head of the patient by means of a strip of linen which bore the names of the gods.[4,8] This may have produced headache relief by compressing and cooling the scalp (Figure 1.4).[4]

Later, from Mesopotamia, comes a description of a headache and an associated visual disturbance, in which '. . . the head is bent with pain gripping his temples . . .

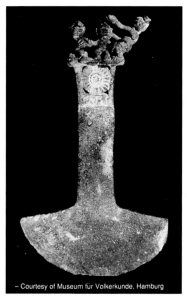

● **Figure 1.2** *Neolithic instrument used for trepanation. (Courtesy of Hamburg Museum of Ethnography.)*

– Courtesy of Museum für Volkerkunde, Hamburg

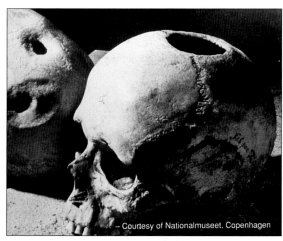

– Courtesy of Nationalmuseet. Copenhagen

● **Figure 1.1** *Neolithic skull showing trepanation hole (c. 7000 BC). (Courtesy of Nationalmuseet, Copenhagen.)*

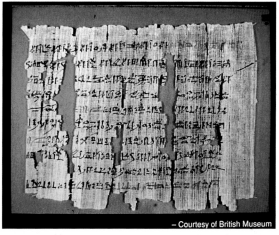

– Courtesy of British Museum

● **Figure 1.3** *An ancient Egyptian headache prescription on papyrus (c.1200 BC). (Courtesy of The British Museum.)*

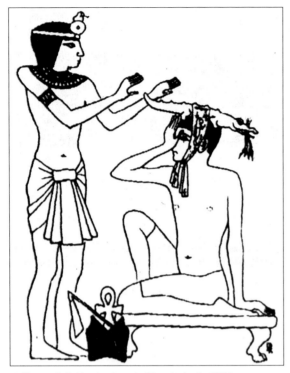

Figure 1.4 *The treatment of headache in 1200 BC.*

and his eyes are afflicted with dimness and cloudiness'. Hippocrates (Figure 1.5), in 400 BC, described the visual aura that can precede the migraine headache and its relief by vomiting.[10] Hippocrates described a shining light, usually in the right eye, followed by violent pain beginning in the temples and eventually reaching the entire head and

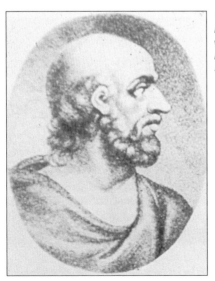

Figure 1.5 *Hippocrates, who described migraine in 400 BC.*

neck area.[4,8] Belief in the cause and trigger of headache is strongly influenced by the medical and intellectual climate. Hippocrates believed that headache could be triggered by exercise and intercourse[8] and that migraine resulted from vapours rising from the stomach to the head and that vomiting could partially relieve the pain of headache.[4,8]

Plato felt that headaches could result from and be triggered by preoccupation with the body:[10]

> 'Yes, indeed,' he said, 'this excessive care for the body that goes beyond simple gymnastics is about the greatest of all obstacles . . . It is troublesome in household affairs and military service and . . . it puts difficulties in the way of any kind of instruction, thinking or private meditation — forever imagining headaches and dizziness and attributing their origins to philosophy . . . It makes the man always fancy himself sick and never cease from anguishing about his body.'

In the Platonic dialogue, *Charmides*, the elements of holistic care are delineated in terms that manage to sound both modern and timeless:[11]

> You must begin by curing the soul . . . The cure . . . has to be effected by use of certain charms, and these charms are fair words, and by them temperance is implanted in the soul, and when temperance comes and stays, there health is speedily imparted . . . This is the great error of our day in the treatment of human beings . . . Men try to be physicians of health and temperance separately.

Celsus (215–300 AD) believed 'drinking wine, or crudity [dyspepsia], or cold, or heat of a fire, or the sun' could trigger migraine. Aretaeus of Cappodocia (2nd century AD), because of his classic descriptions, is credited to be the discoverer of migraine headache. Migraine was well known in the ancient world.[9]

'Migraine' itself is derived from the Greek word hemicrania, introduced by Galen in approximately 200 AD. He mistakenly believed it was caused by the ascent of vapours, either excessive in amount or too hot or too cold. Popular names evolved over the years for this uncomfortable, sometimes disabling, disorder: sick headache, blind headache, and bilious headache.[6,9,12]

In the 12th century, Abbess Hildegarde of Bingen described what has been attributed to her migraine aura in terms that are both mystical and apocalyptic (Figure 1.6):[13]

> I saw a great star, most splendid and beautiful, and with it an exceeding multitude of falling sparks with which the star followed southward . . . and suddenly they were all annihilated, being turned into black coals . . . and cast into the abyss so that I could see them no more.

Timothy Bright tells us in his 1586 essay, *A Treatise of Melancholy*, 'Melancholic humor is . . . settled in the spleane and with his vapour annoyeth the harte and passing up to the brayne, countersetteth terrible objects to the fantasie'.[14]

Thomas Willis in 1683 brilliantly described a woman with severe, periodic, migrainous headache preceded by a prodrome and associated with vomiting.[9]

> . . . beautiful and young woman, imbued with a slender habit of body, and an hot blood, was wont to be afflicted with frequent and wandering fits of headache . . . On the day before the coming of the spontaneous fit of this disease, growing very hungry in the evening, she eat a most plentiful supper, with an hungry, I may say a greedy appetite; presaging by this sign, that the pain of the head would most certainly follow the next morning; and the event never failed this augury . . . she was troubled also with vomiting. . .

Opium and vinegar solutions were widely used as headache remedies in Europe during the 13th century. The vinegar probably allowed opium to be absorbed more quickly through the skin.[4]

Shakespeare discusses headache treatment: Desdemona binds her husband's head with the handkerchief (a remedy still used by many migraineurs) that will later be her undoing:[15]

> OTHELLO: I have a pain upon my forehead here.

> DESDEMONA: Faith, that's with watching; twill away again. Let me but bind it hard, within this hour. It will be well.

In *King John*, a similar remedy is described:[16] 'When your head did but ache, I knit my handkerchief about your brows'. This suggests it was a popular treatment in Elizabethan times.

Migraine was distinguished from common headache by Tisso 1783 who ascribed it to a supraorbital neuralgia,[12] '. . . provoked by reflexes from the stomach, gallbladder, or uterus'. Over the next century DuBois Reymond, Mollendorf and later Eulenburg proposed different vascular

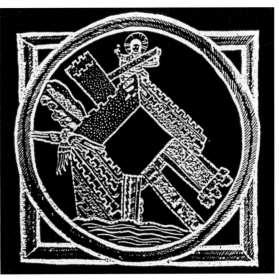

● **Figure 1.6** 'Vision of the Heavenly City' from a manuscript of Hildegard's Scivias *written at Bingen (c. 1180 AD).*

theories for migraine. In the late 1700s, Erasmus Darwin, grandfather of Charles Darwin, suggested treating headache by centrifugation. He believed headaches were caused by vasodilatation, and suggested placing the patient in a centrifuge to force the blood from the head to the feet.[4,8] Fothergill in 1778 introduced the term 'fortification spectra' to describe the typical visual aura of migraine. Fothergill used the term 'fortification'[8] because the visual disturbances resembled a fortified town surrounded with bastions.[6,17]

Airy in 1870 quoted the 19th century poet, Alfred, Lord Tennyson whom he felt depicted a fortification spectra in suitably stately fashion: '. . . as yonder walls rose slowly to a music slowly breathed, a cloud that gathered shape'[18] (Figure 1.7).

In the 18th century, Alexander Pope offers this account of migraine in *The Rape of the Lock*:[19]

> When screen'd in shades from day's detested glare, Spleen sighs forever on her pensive bed, Pain at her side, and megrim at her head.

James Ware (1814) described bouts of visual aura without accompanying headache, which he termed 'muscae volitantes' and which are now called migraine equivalents.[9] Liveing, in 1873, wrote the first monograph[20] on migraine entitled *On Megrim, Sick-headache, and Some Allied Disorders: A Contribution to the Pathology of Nerve-storms* and was the originator of the neural theory of migraine. He ascribed the problem to '. . . disturbances of the autonomic nervous system' which he called 'nerve storms'.[6]

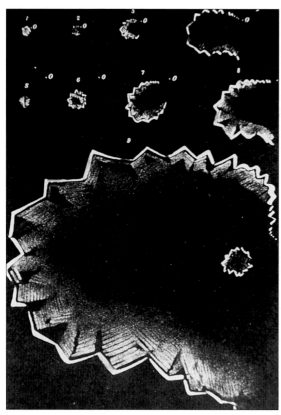

Figure 1.7 *A fortification spectra seen during a migraine aura (as quoted by Airy in 1870 from Tennyson '... as yonder walls rose slowly to a music slowly breathed, a cloud that gathered shape'. (Courtesy of the Royal Society of London.)*

William Gowers, in 1888, published an influential neurology textbook, *A Manual of Disease of the Nervous System*.[17] Gowers emphasized the importance of a healthy lifestyle and advocated using a solution of nitroglycerin 1% in alcohol, combined with other agents, to treat headaches. The remedy later became known as the 'Gowers mixture'. Gowers was also famous for recommending Indian hemp (marijuana) for headache relief.[4,8]

In 1900, Deyl[21] suggested that migraine, including menstrual migraine, resulted from intermittent swelling of the hypophysis with compression of the trigeminal nerve. Spitzer[21] in 1901 suggested that headache was produced by recurrent interventricular foramen blockage causing lateral ventricle dilation.

These theories may sound odd but even Proust tells us of a physician who believes that everything, '. . . whether headache or colic, heart disease or diabetes, was a disease of the nose that had been wrongly diagnosed'.[22] Sinclair Lewis introduces us to Almus Pickerbaugh, a doctor with dubious clinical skills, who says that his wife has 'sick headaches . . . [due to] . . . to early neglect of her diet'.[23,24]

'Yes,' said Mary, beginning to feel faint . . . The pain in her head was setting the room afire. Chairs and tables were developing lurid nimbuses. But she would not give way; not this time. She stared at Willie; he seemed to be standing pale and serene, at the center of a mandala of flame . . .

. . . all morning she had felt as if she might, at any moment, be struck by The Headache, which she feared more than death. When the clamp of fire went round her head, she could not see for the pain and often, she would end up flat on the floor, vomiting from the pain. The Headache, as she always thought of it, to differentiate it from ordinary headaches, had begun many years earlier . . . Her behavior [during an attack] . . . could be . . . like that of a mad woman.

Modern writers often link headache and depression, a connection that has been observed in modern epidemiological studies. Mary Chesnutt, in her Civil War diaries, mentions headaches and being 'nervous and depressed' in the same breath.[25] In *The Razor's Edge*, by Somerset Maugham, Gray Maturin's headaches follow in the wake of severe financial difficulties: 'His frenzied efforts to stave off the disaster that finally overwhelmed him, the burden of anxiety, the humiliation, resulted in a nervous breakdown, and he began to have headaches so severe that he was incapacitated for twenty-four hours and as limp as a wet rag when they ceased'.[26] Gore Vidal, in detailing the agony of Mary Lincoln, describes not only the visual phenomena that can be associated with migraine, but also the attendant pain and behaviour.[27]

Stephen King, the 'horror' novelist, vividly describes the pain, sensory hyperresponsiveness, and feeling of prostration associated with migraine:[28]

The headache would get worse until it was a smashing weight, sending red pain through his head and neck with every pulsebeat. Bright lights would make his eyes water helplessly and send darts of agony into the flesh just behind his eyes. Small noises magnified, ordinary noises as loud as jackhammers, loud noises insupportable. The headache would worsen until it felt as if his head were being crushed inside an inquisitor's lovecap. Then it would even off at that level for six hours. He would be next to helpless.

Stephen King also gives us a contemporary account of exertional headache:[29]

> *Lobsterlike, Richards humped backwards on his knees. His breath came in sharp, doglike gasps. The air was hot, full of the slick taste of oil, uncomfortable to breathe. A headache surfaced within his skull and began to push daggers into the backs of his eyes.*

Lewis Carroll described migrainous phenomena in *Alice in Wonderland* and *Through the Looking Glass*, depicting instances of central scotoma, tunnel vision, phonophobia, vertigo, distortions in body image, dementia and visual hallucinations.

Joan Didion, in her 1968 essay, *In Bed*, describes a mundane reality with which most headache sufferers can probably identify:[30]

> *We have reached a certain understanding my migraine and I. It never comes when I am in real trouble. Tell me that my house is burned down, my husband has left me, that there is gunfighting in the streets and panic in the banks, and I will not respond by getting a headache. It comes when I am fighting not an open but a guerilla war with my own life, during weeks of small household confusions, lost laundry, unhappy help, cancelled appointments, on days when the telephone rings too much and I get no work done and the wind is coming up. On days like that my friend comes uninvited.*

Analgesic overuse is not new. Faulkner's Jason Compson prefers inhaling camphor fumes to more traditional remedies: '. . . there's not a damn thing in that aspirin except flour and water for imaginary invalids'.[31] Caffeine is a popular remedy contained in many over-the-counter analgesics. In *The Woman in White*, Laura Fairlie is dosed with 'restorative tea' for 'that essentially feminine malady, a slight headache'.[32] Many headache sufferers, in literature as in life, have experimented and discovered their own, often bizarre, remedies. Emmett Smith, the Vietnam veteran in Bobbie Ann Mason's *In Country*, is plagued by headaches that his family and friends believe are linked to his exposure to Agent Orange. He is found 'sitting up in bed, his hair crammed into his Pepsi cap, drinking from the Coke can, chasing away that pain in his head'.[33] However, the protagonist of Raymond Carver's *Viewfinder* looks for dietary help: 'I had a headache. I know coffee's no good for it, but sometimes Jello helps'.[6,34]

Ruth Rendell has one of her characters recommend feverfew, only to have the migraine sufferer respond, 'What the hell is feverfew?'[35] A physician in David Williams' *Prescription for Murder* defines it as 'a white flowering hedgerow plant which has substances that may well inhibit the release of natural serotonin in the body'.[6,36]

Emotional well being can effect great change in headache intensity. One dramatic example is found in the *Personal Memoirs of U.S. Grant*. The general describes a 'sick headache' he suffered on 9 August, 1865. He attempts to cure it by 'bathing [his] feet in hot water and mustard and putting mustard plasters on [his] wrists and the back of [his] neck'. He gets complete relief, however, only when he receives word that Robert E. Lee agrees to discuss terms of surrender; '. . . the instant I saw the contents of the note I was cured'.[6,37]

Unfortunately, the most pervasive element running through the appearance of headaches in literature is not a general consensus on causes or treatment, but rather an underlying tone of skepticism. Headache is the Rodney Dangerfield of medical maladies — it gets no respect. Joan Didion puts it most bluntly when discussing the attitudes of those around her:[30] 'For I had no brain tumor, no eyestrain, no high blood pressure, nothing wrong with me at all. I simply had migraine headaches, and migraine headaches were, as everyone who did not have them knew, imaginary'.

In defining the elements of the 'migraine personality', Joan Didion's physician focuses on two areas which are considered, for the most part, to be areas of feminine concern: personal appearance and housework:[6]

> *'You don't look like a migraine personality . . . Your hair's messy. But I suppose you're a compulsive housekeeper.'*

> *Actually my house is kept even more negligently than my hair, but the doctor was right nonetheless; perfectionism can also take the form of spending most of a week writing and rewriting a paragraph.*

> *But not all perfectionists have migraine, and not all migrainous people have migraine personalities.*[30]

In 1938, John Graham and Harold Wolff[38] demonstrated that the drug ergotamine worked by constricting blood vessels, and used this as proof of the vascular theory of migraine.[4] Greek and Roman ancient writings include references to 'blighted grains' and 'blackened bread', and the use of concoctions of powdered barley flower to hasten childbirth. During the Middle Ages, written accounts of ergot poisoning first appeared. Epidemics were described in which the characteristic symptom was gangrene of the feet, legs, hands and arms, often associated with burning sensations in the extremities. The disease was known as 'Ignis Sacer'

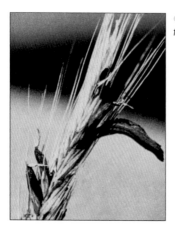

Figure 1.8 Ergot fungus on rye.

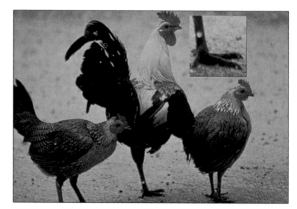

Figure 1.9 Rooster spur which gave ergot its name.

or 'Holy Fire' and, later, as 'St. Anthony's Fire' in honor of the saint at whose shrine relief was obtained. This relief probably resulted from the use of a diet free of contaminated grain during the pilgrimage to the shrine (Figure 1.8).[39]

The term 'ergot' is derived from the French word *argot* meaning 'rooster's spur' (Figure 1.9). It describes the small, banana-shaped sclerotium of the fungus. Louis René Tulasne of Paris in 1853 established that ergot was not a hypertrophied rye seed, but a fungus having three stages in one life cycle and he named it *Claviceps purpurea*. Once infected by the fungus, the rye seed was transformed into a spur-shaped mass of fungal pseudotissue, purple-brown in colour — the resting stage of the fungus, known as the 'sclerotium' (derived from the Greek *skleros* meaning hard).[39]

In 1831, Heinrich Wiggers, a pharmacist of Göttingen, Germany, tested ergot extracts in animals. Among his models was the 'rooster comb test' — a rooster, when fed ergotin, became ataxic, nauseous, acquired a blanched comb, and suffered from severe convulsions, dying days later. The 'rooster comb test' continued to be used into the following century by investigators studying the physiological properties of ergot.[39]

The earliest reports in the medical literature on the use of ergot in the treatment of migraine were those of Eulenberg in Germany in 1883, Thomson in the United States in 1894 and Campbell in England in 1894. Stevens' *Modern Materia Medica* mentioned the use of ergot for the treatment of migraine in 1907.[40]

The first pure ergot alkaloid, ergotamine, was isolated by Stoll in 1918 and used primarily in obstetrics and gynaecology until 1925, when Rothlin successfully treated a case of severe and intractable migraine by a subcutaneous injection of ergotamine tartrate. This indication was pursued vigorously by various researchers over the following decades (Table 1.1) and was reinforced by the belief in a vascular origin for

Table 1.1 A brief history of ergot therapy (E.T.)

Year	Study	Therapy
1883	Eulenberg (Germany)	Injections of ergot extract
1894	Thompson (USA)	Oral ergot extract
1894	Campbell (England)	Mentioned antimigraine effect of ergot in headache book
1918	Stoll (Basel)	Isolated ergotamine and named it Gynergan. Original use OB/GYN
1925	Rothlin (Basel)	First used subcutaneous E.T. for migraine
1926	Maier (Zurich)	Reported use of E.T. at Paris Neurological Society
1927	Tzanck (France)	First systemic study of oral E.T.
1928	Trautman (Germany)	Good results with oral E.T.
1934	Lenox (Boston) Brock, O'Sullivan and Towne (NY) Logan and Allen (Mayo Clinic)	First controlled E.T. studies in USA
1937	Graham and Wolff (NY)	Effect of E.T. on blood vessels. Scientific clinical investigation
1943	Stoll and Hofmann (Basel)	Synthesized DHE
1945	Horton, Peters and Blumenthal (Mayo Clinic)	Used DHE to treat migraine

migraine and the concept that ergotamine tartrate acted as a vasoconstrictor. Lennox in Boston, and others independently, conducted the first controlled studies of ergotamine tartrate in 1934. Graham and Wolff in 1937 demonstrated the effects of ergotamine tartrate on blood vessels.[40]

Dihydroergotamine (DHE) was synthesized by Stoll and Hofmann in 1943 and was used to treat migraine by Horton, Peters and Blumenthal at the Mayo Clinic.[40]

The earliest ergot formulations were simple fluid extracts — some were very potent while others were practically inert, owing to differential extraction of active substances and the instability of the compounds in alkaline solution. The extract was injected or given orally, although the superiority of parenteral administration was noted even then.[40]

The modern approach to the treatment of migraine is exemplified in the development of sumatriptan by Pat Humphrey and his colleagues. Based on the concept that serotonin can relieve headache, they designed a chemical entity that was similar to serotonin, being more stable, however, and with fewer side effects. This development led to the modern clinical trials for acute migraine treatment and to the elucidation of the mechanism of action of what are now called 'selective serotonin agonists'.

We are at the threshold of an explosion in the diagnosis, treatment, and understanding of migraine and other headaches. Many new triptans are in development and many will soon be, or are already, available, including zolmitriptan, naratriptan and rizatriptan.

The gene for familial hemiplegic migraine has been cloned and putative brainstem centres for migraine and cluster have been identified. Let us hope that future headache sufferers will not have to feel this refrain from *Iolanthe*:[41]

> *When you're lying awake with a dismal headache*
> *And repose is taboo'd by anxiety,*
> *I conceive you may use any language you choose*
> *To indulge in without impropriety.*

References

1. Lyons A, Petrucelli RJ. *Medicine: An Illustrated History.* New York: Harry N. Abrams, Inc. Publishers, 1978.
2. Venzmer G. *Five Thousand Years of Medicine.* New York: Taplinger Publishing Co., 1972: 19.
3. Thorwald J. *Science and Secrets of Early Medicine.* London: Thames and Hudson Ltd, 1962: 300–7.
4. Edmeads J. The treatment of headache: a historical perspective. In: Gallagher RM (ed.) *Drug Therapy for Headache.* New York: Marcel Dekker Inc., 1990: 1–8.
5. McHenry LC. *Garrison's History of Neurology.* Charles C. Thomas, Springfield, 1969.
6. Patterson SM, Silberstein SD. Sometimes Jello helps: perceptions of headache etiology, triggers and treatment in literature. *Headache* 1993; 33: 76–81.
7. Alvarez WC. Was there sick headache in 3000 BC? *Gastroenterology* 1945; 5: 524.
8. Lance JW. *Mechanisms and Management of Headache.* 4th edition. London: Butterworth Scientific, 1982: 1–6.
9. Critchley M. Migraine: from Cappadocia to Queen Square. In: Smith R (ed.) *Background to Migraine, Volume 1.* London: Heinemann, 1967.
10. Plato. The Republic. In: Hamilton E, Cairns H (eds). *The Collected Dialogues of Plato.* New York: Pantheon Books, 1961: 651–2.
11. Plato. Charmides. In: Hamilton E, Cairns H (eds). *The Collected Dialogues of Plato.* New York: Pantheon Books, 1961: 103.
12. Sachs O. *Migraine: understanding a common disorder.* Berkeley: University of California Press, 1985.
13. Singer C. The visions of Hildegarde of Bingen. In: *From Magic to Science.* New York: Dover, 1958.
14. Bright T. A treatise of melancholie. In: Ober WB (ed). *Bottoms Up! A pathologist's essays on medicine and the humanities.* Carbondale; South Illinois University Press, 1987: 179.
15. Shakespeare W. Othello, the Moor of Venice (Act III, Scene iii). In: *The Complete Works of William Shakespeare.* Stamford, CT: Longmeadow Press, 1990: 1132.
16. Shakespeare W. King John (Act IV, Scene i). In: *The Complete Works of William Shakespeare.* Stamford, CT: Longmeadow Press, 1990: 1141–2.
17. Raskin NH. Migraine: clinical aspects. In: *Headache.* 2nd edition. New York: Churchill Livingstone 1988: 35–98.

18. Airy H. On a distinct form of transient hemianopsia. *Philos Trans R Soc Lond* 1870;160: 247–70.

19. Pope A. The Rape of the Lock. In: Swallow A (ed.) *The Rinehart Book of Verse.* New York: Holt, Rinehart, and Winston, 1962: 148–9.

20. Liveing E. *On Megrim, Sick Headache, and Some Allied Disorders: A Contribution to the Pathology of Nerve-Storms.* Churchill, 1873.

21. Bille B. Migraine in school children. *Acta Paediatr. Scand.* 1962; 51(suppl. 136): 14–15.

22. Proust M. *The Guermantes Way.* New York: Vintage Books, 1982: 335.

23. Lewis S. *Arrowsmith.* New York: New American Library, 1952.

24. Vidal G. *Lincoln.* New York: Ballentine Books, 1990.

25. Chesnutt M. *Mary Chesnutt's Civil War.* New Haven: Yale University Press, 1981.

26. Maugham WS. *The Razor's Edge.* New York: Penguin Books, 1984.

27. Plant GT. The fortification spectra of migraine. *BMJ* 1986; 293: 1613–17.

28. King S. *Firestarter.* New York: The Viking Press, 1980: 5.

29. King S. *The Running Man.* New York: New American Library, 1982: 78.

30. Didion J. In Bed. In: *The White Album.* New York: Farrar, Straus, and Giroux, 1979.

31. Faulkner W. *The Sound and the Fury.* New York: The Modern Library, 1929.

32. Collins W. *The Woman in White.* New York: Penguin Books, 1985.

33. Mason BA. *In Country.* New York: Harper and Row, 1989: 28.

34. Carver R. *"Viewfinder"* from *What We Talk About When We Talk About Love.* New York: Vintage Books, 1981: 13.

35. Rendell R. *Going Wrong.* New York: The Mysterious Press, 1990.

36. Williams D. *Prescription for Murder.* New York: St. Martin's Press, 1991.

37. Grant US. *Personal Memoirs of U.S. Grant* (E.B. Long, ed.). New York: The DaCapo Press, 1952: 552–3.

38. Graham JR, Wolff HG. Mechanism of migraine headache and action of ergotamine tartrate. *Arch Neurol Psychiat* 1938; 39: 737–63.

39. Bové FJ. *The story of ergot.* Basel, New York: Karger, 1970.

40. Silberstein SD. The pharmacology of ergotamine and dihydroergotamine. *Headache* 1997; 37(Suppl. 1): S15–25.

41. Gilbert WS. *"Love, Unrequited, Robs Me of My Rest (The Nightmare Song)"* from *Iolanthe.*

section 1

Pathophysiology and epidemiology of headache

chapter 2

Classification and diagnosis of headache

Introduction

Headache, like back pain or abdominal pain, is a symptom that can have many causes. The symptom, headache, may occur in relative isolation, as part of an acute symptom complex (i.e. migraine), or as part of an evolving disorder (i.e. brain tumour). Understanding headache classification and diagnosis is a prelude to treatment.

Before 1988, the headache classification systems that were available had no operational rules, and nomenclature was anything but uniform. In 1988 the International Headache Society (IHS) instituted a classification system that has become the standard for headache diagnosis, particularly for clinical research.[1] The system identifies 12 major categories of headache, which can be divided into two broad groups, the primary headache disorders (Categories 1–4) and the secondary headache disorders (Categories 5–12) (Table 2.1). In secondary headache disorders the headache is symptomatic of an underlying condition, such as a brain tumour, stroke or metabolic state. In primary headache disorders there is no underlying cause; the headache itself is the problem. Thus, for the secondary disorders, the IHS provides an aetiological system wherein headaches are classified based on their causes. For the primary headache disorders, the IHS criteria provide a descriptive system wherein headaches are classified based on their symptom profiles. A true aetiological classification is not yet possible for primary headaches because their mechanisms are uncertain and there are no objective diagnostic tests.

The IHS criteria have received broad international support. They have been endorsed by the World Health Organization (WHO), and the principles of the system have been incorporated into the International Classification of Diseases (ICD-10). The criteria have been translated into German, French, Italian, Spanish, Chinese, Greek, Arabic, Turkish, Slovenian, Danish, Swedish, Thai, Japanese and Portuguese. Thus, the IHS criteria have done much to establish uniform terminology and consistent diagnostic criteria for a range of headache disorders. This has facilitated epidemiological studies and the multinational clinical trials that provide the basis for the current research and treatment guidelines including the AHCPR headache guidelines in the United States.[2]

Table 2.1(A) outlines the four major categories of primary headache: migraine, tension-type headache, cluster headache and a miscellaneous group. The eight secondary categories (summarized in Table 2.1(B)) include headache associated with head trauma, vascular disorders, non-vascular disorders, substances, non-cephalic infection, metabolic disorders, disorders of the face and neck, as well as cranial neuralgias. Finally, there is a thirteenth category: headache that is not classifiable elsewhere.

Using the IHS system

Because an individual patient may have more than one headache disorder, the IHS criteria were established to diagnose headache disorders, not patients. If a patient has more than one disorder, each disorder receives its own diagnosis. A careful history is needed to determine how many disorders are present and to characterize each one.[3]

It is not possible or necessary to diagnose each individual headache attack. Single episodes may be difficult to diagnose if the symptoms are poorly recalled, if treatment has attenuated the full expression of symptoms, or if the attack has characteristics that do not fall neatly into a given category. Patients should be asked to describe typical, preferably untreated, attacks and if necessary, keep diary records of attacks. The diagnosis should be based on the pattern of pain, the associated symptoms, and the physical findings and laboratory tests.[4]

The IHS criteria use both clinical features and laboratory tests to provide criteria of inclusion (features needed to establish a particular diagnosis) and exclusion (features that prevent assigning a particular diagnosis). For the primary headaches, the physical examination and laboratory investigations serve to exclude secondary disorders, or they may provide evidence to support the diagnosis of a secondary headache. Thus, the diagnosis of primary headache disorders is based on the patient's report of symptoms of previous attacks, and accurate diagnosis requires explicit rules about the required symptom features. Each major category of primary headache has subtypes that are differentiated based on the symptom profile (migraine with aura versus migraine without aura), the temporal profile, or the attack frequency (episodic versus chronic tension-type headache, episodic versus chronic cluster headache). Details about subtyping are presented in subsequent chapters about each major headache category.

Headaches are subtyped using the principles of classification developed by the American Psychiatric Association. For example, Table 2.2 sets out the criteria for migraine without aura. To diagnose migraine without aura, the requirements under each lettered heading must be met. Some

● **Table 2.1** *The IHS classification system[1]*

A Primary headache disorders	7.3 Intracranial infection
	7.4 Intracranial sarcoidosis and other non-infectious
1 Migraine	inflammatory diseases
1.1 Migraine without aura	7.5 Headache related to intrathecal injections
1.2 Migraine with aura	7.6 Intracranial neoplasm
1.3 Ophthalmoplegic	7.7 Headache associated with other intracranial disorder
1.4 Retinal migraine	
1.5 Childhood periodic syndromes that may be precursors	**8** Headache associated with substances or their withdrawal
to or associated with migraine	8.1 Headache induced by acute substance use or exposure
1.6 Complications of migraine	8.2 Headache induced by chronic substance use or exposure
1.7 Migrainous disorder not fulfilling above criteria	8.3 Headache from substance withdrawal (acute use)
	8.4 Headache from substance withdrawal (chronic use)
2 Tension-type headache	8.5 Headache associated with substances but with uncertain
2.1 Episodic tension-type headache	mechanism
2.2 Chronic tension-type headache	
2.3 Headache of the tension-type not fulfilling above criteria	**9** Headache associated with non-cephalic infection
	9.1 Viral infection
3 Cluster headache and chronic paroxysmal hemicrania	9.2 Bacterial infection
3.1 Cluster headache	9.3 Headache related to other infection
3.1.1 Cluster headache periodicity undetermined	
3.1.2 Episodic cluster headache	**10** Headache associated with metabolic disorder
3.1.3 Chronic cluster headache	10.1 Hypoxia
3.2 Chronic paroxysmal hemicrania	10.2 Hypercapnia
3.3 Cluster headache-like disorder not fulfilling above	10.3 Mixed hypoxia and hypercapnia
criteria	10.4 Hypoglycaemia
	10.5 Dialysis
4 Miscellaneous headaches unassociated with structural lesion	10.6 Headache related to other metabolic abnormality
4.1 Idiopathic stabbing headache	
4.2 External compression headache	**11** Headache or facial pain associated with disorder of cranium,
4.3 Cold stimulus headache	neck, eyes, ears, nose, sinuses, teeth, mouth or other facial
4.4 Benign cough headache	or cranial structures
4.5 Benign exertional headache	11.1 Cranial bone
4.6 Headache associated with sexual activity	11.2 Neck
	11.3 Eyes
B Secondary headache disorders	11.4 Ears
	11.5 Nose and sinuses
5 Headache associated with head trauma	11.6 Teeth, jaws and related structures
5.1 Acute post-traumatic headache	11.7 Temporomandibular joint disease
5.2 Chronic post-traumatic headache	
	12 Cranial neuralgias, nerve trunk pain and deafferentation pain
6 Headache associated with vascular disorders	12.1 Persistent (in contrast to tic-like) pain of cranial nerve origin
6.1 Acute ischaemic cerebrovascular disease	12.2 Trigeminal neuralgia
6.2 Intracranial haematoma	12.2.1 Idiopathic trigeminal neuralgia
6.3 Subarachnoid haemorrhage	12.2.2 Symptomatic trigeminal neuralgia
6.4 Unruptured vascular malformation	12.3 Glossopharyngeal neuralgia
6.5 Arteritis	12.4 Nervus intermedius neuralgia
6.6 Carotid or vertebral artery pain	12.5 Superior laryngeal neuralgia
6.7 Venous thrombosis	12.6 Occipital neuralgia
6.8 Arterial hypertension	12.7 Central causes of head and facial pain other than tic
6.9 Headache associated with other vascular disorder	douloureux
	12.8 Facial pain not fulfilling criteria in groups 11 or 12
7 Headache associated with non-vascular intracranial disorder	
7.1 High cerebrospinal fluid pressure	**13** Headache not classifiable
7.2 Low cerebrospinal fluid pressure	

● **Table 2.2** *Diagnostic criteria for migraine without aura[1]*

A At least five attacks fulfilling B–D	**D** During headache at least one of the following:
	1 Nausea and/or vomiting
B Headache attacks lasting 4 to 72 hours (untreated	2 Photophobia and phonophobia
or unsuccessfully treated)	
	E At least one of the following:
C Headache has at least two of the following characteristics:	1 History, physical and neurological examinations do not
1 Unilateral location	suggest one of the disorders listed in groups 5–11
2 Pulsating quality	2 History and/or physical and/or neurological examinations do
3 Moderate or severe intensity (inhibits or prohibits	suggest such disorder, but it is ruled out by appropriate investigations
daily activities)	3 Such disorder is present, but migraine attacks do not occur
4 Aggravation by walking stairs or similar routine	for the first time in close temporal relation to the disorder
physical activity	

headings (i.e. A and B) have a single mandatory feature. Other headings include several alternative characteristics. For example, in C, only two of four pain features are required. No single 'pain' feature under heading C is absolutely required for diagnosis. The exclusion criteria are provided under category E. They eliminate other headache disorders based on at least one of the history, physical and neurological examinations (E1) or laboratory tests (E2). Alternatively, a secondary headache disorder may be present, if the onset of the primary and secondary disorders are separated in time.

Clinical approach: an overview

In evaluating a headache patient, the first task is to identify or exclude secondary headache based on the history, and the general medical as well as the neurological examinations (Figure 2.1). Important features in the headache history are

summarized in Table 2.3. If suspicious features are present, diagnostic testing may also be necessary. Once secondary headaches are excluded, the task is then to diagnose one (or more than one) specific primary headache disorder. In the initial evaluation, the experienced physician looks for 'headache alarms' that suggest the possibility of a secondary headache disorder. Table 2.4 summarizes some of the

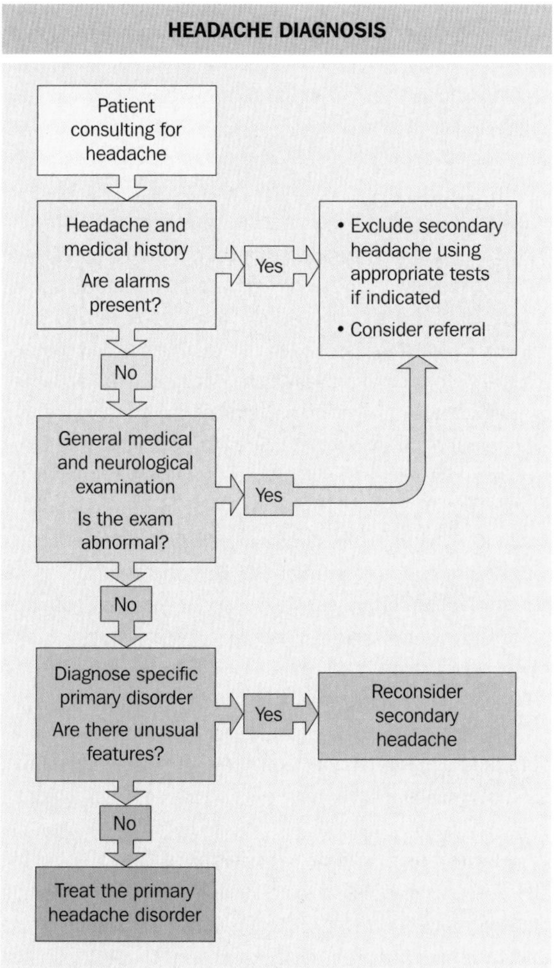

● **Table 2.3** *Headache history*

Attack onset
Pain location
Attack duration
Attack frequency and timing
Pain severity
Pain quality
Associated feature
Aggravating or precipitating factors
Ameliorating factors
Social history
Family history
Past headache history
Headache impact

● **Table 2.4** *Diagnostic alarms in the evaluation of headache disorders*

Headache alarm	Differential diagnosis	Possible work-up
Headache begins after the age of 50 years	Temporal arteritis, mass lesion	Erythrocyte sedimentation rate, neuroimaging
Sudden-onset headache	Subarachnoid haemorrhage, pituitary apoplexy, bleed into a mass or AVM, mass lesion (especially posterior fossa)	Neuroimaging, lumbar puncture
Accelerating pattern of headaches	Mass lesion, subdural haematoma, medication overuse	Neuroimaging, drug screen
New-onset head-ache in a patient with cancer or HIV	Meningitis (chronic or carcinomatous), brain abscess (including toxoplasmosis), metastasis	Neuroimaging, lumbar puncture
Headache with systemic illness (fever, stiff neck, rash)	Meningitis, encep-halitis, Lyme disease, systemic infection, collagen, vascular disease	Neuroimaging, lumbar puncture, blood tests
Focal neurological symptoms or signs of disease (other than typical aura)	Mass lesion, arteriovenous malfunction, stroke, collagen vascular disease (including antiphospholipid antibodies)	Neuroimaging, collagen vascular evaluation
Papilloedema	Mass lesion, pseudotumour, meningitis	Neuroimaging, lumbar puncture

HEADACHE DIAGNOSIS

● **Figure 2.1** *Core algorithm for headache diagnosis.*

alarming features, a partial differential diagnosis, and some considerations in the work-up.

Recent studies have demonstrated that computed tomography (CT) and magnetic resonance imaging (MRI) of the head have extremely low yields in headache patients in the absence of 'alarms'. If patients do not fit neatly into the IHS diagnostic categories or if response to treatment is atypical, the issue of secondary headache should be revisited.[5]

Headache history

Overview

The majority of headache patients have normal medical and neurological examinations. A comprehensive history is therefore usually the most important tool for accurate diagnosis. The headache history should yield a comprehensive view of the patient's headaches and the associated conditions and problems that might influence diagnosis or treatment (Table 2.3).

The headache history also provides an opportunity to establish a rapport that will serve as a basis for an ongoing relationship. It is not uncommon for headache sufferers to fear that they are afflicted with some terrible malady. We generally let patients give an unstructured account of their problem ('Tell me about your headaches') and then systematically explore various features. Many patients have more than one type of headache or a change in headache pattern over time. We begin with the headache that is the greatest concern to the patient, the one that motivated the person to seek care. We then explore other current headache patterns and their evolution. Wherever possible, patients complete a self-administered questionnaire prior to the consultation. This tool helps patients to focus on their symptomatology and course, improving the reliability and efficiency of the history.

Headache onset

Details of headache onset are important for diagnosis. The age of headache onset is significant, since primary headaches usually begin in childhood or early adult life. When headaches begin after the age of 55 years, serious disorders such as mass lesions or giant cell arteritis are much more likely. The hypnic headache syndrome is a benign form of headache that begins after the age of 60 years. Events associated with the headache onset may also give clues to diagnosis. A headache that begins after a head injury suggests a post-concussive headache disorder or intracranial pathology (however, both migraine and cluster may be triggered by head trauma.) Headaches occurring in the peripartum period may be due to cortical vein or sagittal sinus thromboses. Fever in association with headache

onset suggests an infectious aetiology. Exertion (i.e. weight lifting) may precipitate subarachnoid haemorrhage or benign exertional headache.

Location and duration of pain

Localization of pain at onset and the pattern of spread may be important. A unilateral, hemicranial headache usually suggests migraine or cluster headache. In many migraineurs, the pain changes sides from attack to attack, although there is often a predilection for one side. Cluster headaches are almost always unilateral, with the pain centered in or around the eye, temple, cheek or adjacent areas. In contrast to migraine, only 10–15% of cluster patients note a change in the side of pain from one bout of cluster to another. Tension-type headache pain is typically bilateral.

Localized pain may also occur with organic diseases. The trigeminal nerve is the major source of innervation to the pain-producing structures in the supratentorial space. Infratentorial pain-producing structures receive innervation from the upper cervical, glossopharyngeal and vagus nerves. Supratentorial lesions often cause frontal headaches, while infratentorial tensions often produce pain in the occipital region although overlap in the distribution of neurons projecting to the trigeminocervical complex leads to referral outside this strict pattern (see Chapter 5). When headache is strictly limited to the periorbital region, ocular pathology should be excluded. Trigeminal neuralgia may cause pain in any area of the face innervated by the trigeminal nerve. Over half of patients with brain tumours complain of headache, and in 80% the site of pain is on the same side as the tumour. Headaches associated with cerebrovascular disease may be global or lateralized. When lateralized, the headaches are ipsilateral to the lesion only half of the time.

Pain duration can provide clues to diagnosis. Migraines typically last from 4 to 72 hours. When they persist for more than 72 hours, the term 'status migrainosus' is applied. Cluster headaches usually last an average of 15–180 minutes; they may, however, be as short as 10 minutes or as long as several hours. The headaches of paroxysmal hemicrania typically last 5–20 minutes, with a range from 1 to 120 minutes. Episodic tension-type headaches tend to last from 30 minutes to 7 days. Headaches of organic origin do not have a characteristic duration; progression of attack duration suggests the need for a diagnostic evaluation.

Frequency and timing of attacks

The frequency and timing of headaches help determine both diagnosis and treatment. If there is no temporal pattern, we ask patients how often their attacks occur. We also ask them what is the longest headache-free period they have had in the last six months. Migraine attacks may occur at random, in association with the menstrual cycle, or with specific temporal patterns (on weekends, on vacation, or upon relaxing after stress). Episodic cluster headaches typically occur in a regular pattern. During the cluster period, which usually lasts between 2 weeks and 6 months, headaches may occur as rarely as once every other day or as often as 8 times a day. The attacks tend to recur at similar times of the day or night, often waking the patient during rapid eye-movement (REM) sleep. Episodic tension-type headaches recur less than 15 times a month or are classified as chronic tension-type headache. Headache patterns may suggest useful preventive strategies. For example, menstrual migraines may respond to perimenstrual non-steroidal anti-inflammatory medications. Nocturnal cluster attacks may be prevented by administering ergotamine at bedtime. Organic headaches may be episodic or daily and continuous. Headaches that are organic in origin do not occur with any set pattern and may mimic the known primary headaches, but if the frequency of headache increases, diagnostic evaluation is needed.

Pain severity and quality

The severity of the pain and the rapidity of onset and resolution are diagnostically important. We advise using a 1 to 10 scale, where 1 represents minimal discomfort and 10 the most excruciating pain the patient can imagine. While these numbers may not be completely comparable across patients, they are very useful for charting individual improvements. As most headaches vary in intensity during an attack and across different attacks, it is also useful to inquire about the range of pain experienced during a headache. Headaches of very sudden onset are worrisome. The headache of subarachnoid haemorrhage (SAH) typically has a sudden, explosive onset.

The quality of the pain also provides diagnostic clues. The pain of migraine is characteristically throbbing or pulsatile, but it often begins as a dull, steady ache that slowly evolves; it may not acquire a throbbing quality until the pain becomes moderate or severe in intensity. The pain of cluster headaches is usually deep, boring or piercing. It is sometimes likened to having a red-hot poker thrust into an eye. A dull, band-like or vice-like sensation is often used by patients to describe their tension-type headaches. The characteristic headache of a brain tumour resembles tension-type headache. The headache from a rupture of an aneurysm or arteriovenous malformation is most often a continuous, intense, aching or throbbing pain.

Associated features

Associated symptoms may occur prior to, concurrent with, or following the headache. The associated features of each headache disorder are discussed in appropriate subsequent chapters. We highlight a few points about history-taking here. We generally ask: 'When you get this headache, are there other features that come before, during, or after the pain? Is there anything else you note?' If the patient does not volunteer cardinal features, the physician should inquire, taking care not to elicit false-positive responses. It is important to distinguish symptoms associated with the disorder from symptoms that are chronically present. For example, if someone is always sensitive to light and the sensitivity does not change during the headache, then this is not an associated feature of the headache. Headache-associated photophobia refers to an unusual or heightened sensitivity to light during a headache attack.

Neurological deficits may accompany the headache of organic disease, depending upon the localization of the lesion. Intracranial mass lesions are associated with nausea and vomiting or vomiting without nausea (projectile) in half the cases. Giant cell arteritis may be associated with localized scalp tenderness, malaise, arthralgias or myalgias (polymyalgia rheumatica), low-grade fevers, depression or other constitutional symptoms, and visual disturbances or stroke. Jaw claudication, if present, is virtually pathognomonic for giant cell arteritis.

Aggravating or precipitating factors

Identifying factors that precipitate or aggravate headache attacks is useful in establishing a diagnosis and implementing a treatment programme. Recognizing triggers helps patients avoid precipitants.

The pain of migraine can be worsened or triggered by myriad internal or external factors. The most frequently reported triggers include menstruation, stress, relaxation after stress, fatigue, too much or too little sleep, skipping a meal, weather changes, high humidity, high altitude, exposure to glare or flickering lights, loud noises, perfumes or chemical fumes, postural changes, physical activity, or coughing. Food triggers occur in approximately 10% of migraineurs and most often include chocolate, cheeses, alcoholic beverages (especially red wine), citrus fruits, and foods containing monosodium glutamate, nitrates and aspartate. Cocaine use and cocaine withdrawal may also trigger a migraine-like headache. Cluster headaches are triggered by ingesting alcohol during a cluster period, usually within 30 minutes after imbibing. During the remission phase of a cluster headache, alcohol may be consumed without precipitating an attack. The pain of cluster headaches is often aggravated by lying down. Tension-type headaches are said to be aggravated by the stresses of everyday life and so are worse at the end of the day. Patients with trigeminal neuralgia have trigger points on the face and mucous membranes of the mouth. Slight stimulation of these trigger points by eating, speaking, exposure to cold air, brushing the teeth, stroking, shaving, or washing the face may provoke an attack.

Headaches caused by brain tumours are intensified by exertion, postural changes, bending over or coughing. Aneurysmal rupture may be precipitated by exertion associated with increased blood pressure, such as seen with sexual activity.

Ameliorating factors

Identifying the factors that ameliorate the discomfort of both the headache and the associated symptoms may provide useful diagnostic and therapeutic information. This includes both non-pharmacological and pharmacological factors. Migraineurs commonly volunteer that they must retire to a dark, quiet room and lie motionless to obtain relief; many patients find that sleep will clear their attacks. Not infrequently, pressing on the superficial temporal artery brings relief, but only during the period of compression. Hot or cold compresses are often applied. Migraine frequency and severity often decreases during the last two trimesters of pregnancy or with the onset of menopause and this is probably also true of cluster headache. Cluster headache patients note that sitting upright, rocking in a chair, pacing to and fro, or engaging in vigorous movement seems to lessen the pain. Tension-type headache may be alleviated by relaxation, rest or sleep.

If medications have been used, determine their dosage, frequency, efficacy and side effects. Inquire how long the prescription has been used. The patient may be using the drug erroneously, either taking a subtherapeutic dosage or taking the medication too infrequently. Conversely, they may be overusing or abusing the medications. Often patients will not recognize how much analgesic they are using until you ask 'How long does a bottle of 100 pills last?'

Social history

Social factors may play a significant role in headache. The examiner should explore the patient's marital and family status, education, occupation, outside interests and friendships. Are any of these areas a source of stress? Has the patient recently had a major life change such as marriage, divorce, separation, new job, retirement, or death in the family? Is work satisfying or merely drudgery? Is there conflict in the workplace? What is the patient's employment? Exposure to drugs or toxins in the workplace may trigger headaches. Workers in munitions factories may develop nitroglycerin headaches or have migraine triggered. Carbon monoxide exposure can occur in either the workplace or home due to poor ventilation. Inquire about other habits, such as the use of alcohol, tobacco, caffeine or illicit drugs.

A history of homosexual or bisexual activities should prompt a search for a potential infectious cause of the headache. Sleep habits may be significant. Sleep apnoea is not uncommon in middle-aged obese men and may cause morning headache. Depression may be manifested by difficulty in falling asleep, difficulty staying asleep or early morning awakening. Likewise, trouble falling asleep may occur with anxiety. Careful questioning about the above possible stressors may uncover a source of conflict or a psychological component to the headache.

Family history

As some headache disorders are familial, it is useful to obtain a family history. Attempt to get a description of the headache and associated features, rather than accepting the patient's diagnosis of the relative's headache. It would be ideal to get a brief description of the headache from the affected relative, as third-party reports of symptoms are often unreliable. Approximately 50–60% of migraineurs have a parent with the disorder and up to 80% have at least one first-degree relative with migraine. Cluster headaches rarely occur within the same family. Forty percent of patients with tension-type headaches have family members with similar headaches.

Familial headaches do not necessarily imply a genetic basis although this seems to be the case in migraine sufferers. Shared environmental exposures may also cause familial headaches. For example, a leaky furnace may cause familial headaches induced by carbon monoxide.

Past headache history

A history of the medications previously prescribed and the dosages in which they were given is useful for many reasons. First, treatment response may support a diagnosis. Second, a detailed history may help explain past treatment failures. Unsuccessful treatment is often the result of incorrect dosing strategies or not allowing enough time to obtain a potential benefit (e.g. discontinuing a beta-blocker after only a 1-week trial). Third, the history of benefits and side effects will narrow the future treatment plan. For each past and current medication, ascertain its benefits or side effects and the reason for its discontinuation. Inquire about the use and efficacy of prior non-drug therapies such as psychotherapy, biofeedback, acupuncture or chiropracty.

The patient's current approach to headache treatment should be reviewed. Many headache sufferers overuse medications, willingly or unwittingly. Many over-the-counter pain relievers contain caffeine with acetaminophen (paracetamol) or aspirin. Excessive use of these agents as well as narcotics, barbiturates and ergots can produce withdrawal or rebound headaches. Again, determine the dosages and the frequency of drug use. If subtherapeutic regimens are being employed, correction may lead to better headache control. Conversely, abuse or overuse of medications must be addressed and may require hospitalization for detoxification.

Many patients with long-standing headaches have had a multitude of diagnostic procedures and have taken a variety of medications. Every reasonable effort should be made to verify prior test results. Obtain a copy of the test report or, better still, a copy of the test itself.

Impact of headache

Diagnosis alone does not provide enough information about the primary headache disorders to optimize therapy. Within a diagnostic category, headaches differ in severity. Some patients seek help primarily out of a concern that the headache is symptomatic of a serious underlying disease. For these patients, reassurance may be the most important intervention. Other patients have severe pain and disability and require a programme of care for improving their lives. If is therefore important to ask patients how their headaches effect their lives and what they were hoping for in seeking care.

THE IMPACT OF HEADACHE	
Question	**Response**
1. On how many days in the last 3 months have you had a headache?	1.
2. How would you rate the pain from your headaches on a scale from 0 to 10? (0 is "no pain at all" and 10 is "pain as bad as it can be".)	2.
3. How many days in the last 3 months have you been kept away from work activities (work or school) for at least half of the day because of your headaches?	3.
4. When you have a headache while you work (work or school), how much is your ability to work reduced? (0% is "not reduced at all" and 100% is "unable to work".)	4.
5. How many days in the last 3 months have you been kept from doing housework or chores for at least half of the day because of your headaches?	5.
6. How much is your ability to do housework or chores reduced? (0% is "not reduced at all" and 100% is "unable to work".)	6.
7. How many days in the last 3 months have you been kept from non-work activities (family, social, or recreational) because of your headaches?	7.
8. How much is your ability to engage in non-work activities (family, social or recreational) reduced? (0% is "not reduced at all" and 100% is "unable to do activities".)	8.

● *Figure 2.2 Patient self-assessment form.*

More formal approaches to assessing headache severity are being developed. Figure 2.2 contains a working version of a self-administered instrument currently in development. The questions provide information about functional limitations in various domains. It can help doctors and patients focus on how headache affects a patient's life. Formal validation studies of several disability questionnaires are underway.

Physical and neurological examinations

A thorough examination should include vital signs, examination of the heart and lungs, and auscultation of the eyes and the carotid and vertebral arteries for bruits. Palpate the head and neck, looking for trigger points, other tender areas, masses, bruises or thickened blood vessels. Examine the temporomandibular joint for tenderness, decreased mobility, asymmetry, or 'clicking'.

A few key signs on the neurological examination bear emphasis. Evidence of papilloedema suggests increased intracranial pressure and warrants an imaging procedure to rule out a mass lesion. Nuchal rigidity due to meningeal irritation is seen with meningitis, intracerebral mass lesions, and intraparenchymal or subarachnoid haemorrhages, and prompts a rapid work-up. Focal neurological deficits may indicate structural brain disease and likewise require neuroimaging. A thickened or nodular temporal artery, diminished or absent temporal artery pulsations, reddened, tender scalp nodules, or necrotic lesions of the scalp or tongue indicate giant cell arteritis. Horner's syndrome may be seen with cluster headaches, chronic paroxysmal hemicrania, or intracranial lesions.[6]

While most patients with a chief complaint of headache will have an entirely normal examination, this portion of the consultation must not be overlooked, for it will help guide subsequent diagnostic and treatment strategies.

History after the initial visit

On occasion, a diagnosis may not be established on the first visit, or the initial assessment may be incorrect. It is useful to ask the patient to keep a headache diary for both diagnostic and treatment purposes. The frequency, severity and duration of the headaches are logged, as are the medications that were used and the possible headache triggers. On subsequent visits, reviewing the diary may uncover previously unrecognized patterns that can provide clues in diagnosis. The headache triggers that are identified may suggest behavioural interventions.

● **Table 2.5** *Differential diagnosis of selected headache disorders*

Headache type	Age of onset (years)	Location	Duration	Frequency/ timing	Severity	Quality	Associated Features
Migraine	10–40	Hemicranial	Several hours to 3 days	Variable	Moderate –severe	Throbbing > steady ache	Nausea, vomiting, photo/phono/ osmophobia, scotomata, neurological deficits
Tension type	20–50	Bilateral	30 min to 7 days +	Variable	Dull ache may wax/ wane	Vise-like, band-like pressure	Generally none
Cluster	15–40	Unilateral peri/retro-orbital	30–120 min	1–8 times per day, nocturnal attacks	Excruciating	Boring piercing	Ipsilateral conjunctival injection, lacrimation, nasal congestion, rhinorrhea, miosis, facial sweating
Mass lesion	Any	Any	Variable	Intermittent, nocturnal, upon arising	Moderate	Dull steady/ throbbing	Vomiting, nuchal rigidity, neurological deficits
Subarachnoid haemorrhage	Adult	Global, often occipitonuchal	Variable	Not applicable	Excruciating	Explosive	Nausea, vomiting, nuchal rigidity, loss of consciousness, neurological deficits
Trigeminal neuralgia	50–70	2nd–3rd > 1st division's trigeminal nerve	Seconds, occur in volleys	Paroxysmal	Excruciating	Electric shock-like	Facial trigger facial points, spasm of muscles ipsilaterally (Tic)
Giant cell arteritis	>55	Temporal, any region	Intermittent, then contin-uous	Constant, ? worse at night	Variable	Variable	Tender scalp arteries, polymyalgia rhematica, jaw claudication

Conclusions

Obtaining a complete and accurate history is an art that takes practice. Though taking a headache history can be time consuming and frustrating, time invested at the initial assessment facilitates diagnosis and is a good opportunity to establish a relationship with the patient. The use of diaries and other patient-completed questionnaires can improve the accuracy of the history and save time in the long run. Table 2.5 summarizes features of the various headache disorders discussed in this chapter and throughout the text.

References

1. Headache Classification Committee of the International Headache Society. Classification and diagnostic criteria for headache disorders, cranial neuralgia, and facial pain. *Cephalalgia* 1988; 8(Suppl. 7): 1–96.
2. Prysé-Phillips WEM, Dodick DW, Edmeads JG et al. Guidelines for the diagnosis of migraine in clinical practice. *Can Med Assoc J* 1997; 156(9): 1273–87.
3. Silberstein SD. Evaluation and emergency treatment of headache. *Headache* 1992; 32: 396–407.
4. Dalessio DJ, Silberstein SD. Diagnosis and classification of headache. In: *Wolff's Headache and Other Head Pain*. 6th edition. New York: Oxford University Press, 1993: 3–18.
5. Quality Standards Subcommittee of the American Academy of Neurology. Practice parameter: the utility of neuroimaging in the evaluation of headache in patients with normal neurologic examinations (summary statement). *Neurology* 1994; 44: 1353–4.
6. Edmeads J. Emergency management of headache. *Headache* 1988; 28: 675–9.

chapter 3

Epidemiology and impact of headache disorders

Introduction

Epidemiology has important implications for the diagnosis and treatment of headache disorders. Headache's scope and distribution and its impact on individuals and on society need to be addressed. Examination of sociodemographic, familial and environmental risk factors helps identify those groups at highest risk for headache and may ultimately provide clues to preventive strategies or disease mechanisms. Epidemiological studies have identified a number of conditions that are comorbid (that is, occurring at a higher frequency than would be expected) with migraine; comorbidity must be considered in formulating treatment plans and may provide insights into the mechanisms of disease.[3,4]

Epidemiological studies evaluate individuals in the population, whether or not they are seeking care, to identify their headache disorders. This is important since only 15–30% of active migraine sufferers actually see a doctor each year,[5,6] and consultation rates are even lower for tension-type headache. As a consequence, there is substantial selection bias in clinic-based studies, where factors that predispose individuals to consult may be mistaken for attributes of the disease.

Recent studies have employed the criteria of the International Headache Society (IHS), which are more complete, explicit and rigorous than the criteria that were used in past studies.[1,2,13] In this chapter, we will review the epidemiology of headache, emphasizing the population-based studies of primary headache disorders that use the IHS criteria.

Epidemiology

Epidemiologic principles (Table 3.1)

For clinical practice and epidemiological research, it is important to have precise definitions to enable reliable and valid diagnosis. There is no true diagnostic gold standard for the primary headache disorders, which makes it difficult to study validity. Validity is supported by creating a surrogate diagnostic gold standard by using groups of headache patients with common risk factors, natural history, treatment responses, profiles and biological markers. Epidemiological studies often focus on prevalence or incidence. Prevalence increases as the period selected for study increases and is an important measure of the burden of disease. Prevalence is determined by the product of average incidence and average duration of

disease. Migraine prevalence may increase because either incidence or duration of disease is increasing.

It is difficult to define diagnostic boundaries for symptom-based conditions. In headache, the most difficult boundary is the one between migraine and tension-type headache. While some view these disorders as distinct entities, others favour the 'spectrum' or 'continuum' concept, the idea that migraine and tension-type headache exist as polar ends on a continuum of severity, varying more in degree than in kind.[15–17] For example, Waters examined the associations among his key migraine features (warning, unilateral pain, nausea or vomiting) in women between the ages of 20 and 64 years and found that as headache intensity increased, migrainous symptoms occurred together more frequently.[17,18] He concluded: 'The distribution of the headache severity extends as a continuous spectrum from mild attacks, which usually have neither unilateral distribution nor warning nor nausea, to severe headaches which are frequently accompanied by the three migraine features'. Other authors have provided empirical support for the continuum concept.[15,19]

There is ongoing debate regarding the relationship between migraine and tension-type headache.[12,15,17] In our view, the available data do not distinguish the opposing models. Much of the epidemiological work assumes that migraine is a distinct disorder. If the continuum concept is correct, the current literature describes the epidemiology of the upper tail of a distribution of severity rather than the epidemiology of a distinct disorder.

Table 3.1 Definitions of epidemiological terms

Reliability:	That independent diagnostic evaluations yield consistent diagnostic results.
Validity:	The assigned diagnosis is related to the underlying biology of the disorder.
Prevalence:	The proportion of a given population that has a disorder over a defined period of time.
Lifetime prevalence:	The proportion of individuals who have ever had the condition.
Period prevalence:	The proportion of individuals who have had at least one attack within a defined interval, usually within one year of the time of ascertainment.
Incidence:	The onset of new cases of a disease in a defined population over a given period of time

● **Table 3.2** *Lifetime prevalence of headache*

Type	Prevalence (%)
Primary headache	
Tension-type headache	78
Migraine	16
Secondary headache	
Fasting	19
Nose/sinus disease	15
Head trauma	4
Non-vascular intracranial disease (including brain tumor)	0.5
After Rasmussen et al.[8]	

Epidemiology of primary and secondary headache

Rasmussen's group examined the population distribution of all headache disorders using in-person clinical assessment in a large, representative community sample in the greater Copenhagen area using the IHS criteria. The lifetime prevalence of various headache disorders is summarized in Table 3.2.

Tension-type headache was a far more common primary headache than migraine. Of the secondary headaches, fasting headache (a headache precipitated by hunger) was the most common, followed by the headache of nose/sinus disease and head trauma. Non-vascular intracranial disease, which includes infections and brain tumours, is extremely rare. The rest of the chapter will focus on migraine, tension-type headache and cluster headache.

Migraine incidence studies

Though migraine incidence is best evaluated in longitudinal studies of persons at risk for migraine, cross-sectional data can be used to derive incidence estimates. Stewart *et al.* estimated migraine incidence using prevalence data[20] (Figure 3.1). In men, the incidence of migraine with aura peaked around 5 years of age at 6.6/1000 person-years; the peak for migraine without aura was 10/1000 person-years between 10 and 11 years. New cases of migraine were uncommon in men in their twenties. In women, the incidence of migraine with aura peaked between ages 12 and 13 (14.1/1000 person-years); migraine without aura peaked between ages 14 and 17 (18.9/1000 person-years). Thus, migraine begins earlier in men than in women and migraine with aura begins earlier than does migraine without aura.

Stang *et al.*[21] used the linked medical records system in Olmstead County, Minnesota to identify migraine sufferers who sought medical care for headaches. Their incidence was lower (probably because many people with migraine do not consult doctors or receive a medical diagnosis[5–7,22]) and their peaks later than those identified by Stewart's group (because medical diagnosis may occur long after the age of onset).

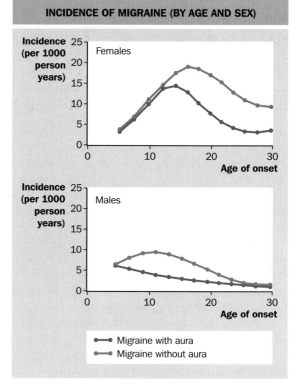

INCIDENCE OF MIGRAINE (BY AGE AND SEX)

● **Figure 3.1** *Age- and sex-specific incidence of migraine (from reference 20).*

Migraine prevalence studies

The published estimates of migraine prevalence have varied widely.[1,2,23] Twenty-four studies that met inclusion criteria were subjected to a meta-analysis.[23] Most (70%) of the variation in estimated prevalence is accounted for by differences in the definitions of migraine, as well as by the age and gender distribution of the study samples.[23] Rasmussen *et al.* conducted the first epidemiological study using the operational diagnostic criteria of the IHS[8] in Copenhagen. For men, the lifetime prevalences were 93% for any kind of headache, 8% for migraine and 69% for tension-type headache. For women, the lifetime prevalences were 99% for all headache, 25% for migraine and 88% for tension-type headache. The 1-year period prevalence of migraine was 6% in men and 15% in women; the 1-year period prevalence of tension-type headache was 63% and 86% respectively.

In the American Migraine Study, questionnaires were mailed to 15 000 households representative of the US population.[9] Migraine diagnosis differed from the IHS criteria in that the headache duration and the lifetime number of previous migraine attacks were not considered. Migraine prevalence was 17.6% for women and 6% for men, closely paralleling the estimates of Rasmussen *et al.*

In France, Henry and coworkers reported that the prevalence of IHS migraine was 11.9% in women and 4.0% in men.[10] In this study, diagnoses were assigned based on lay interviews using a validated algorithm. For the group that included 'borderline migraine', prevalence estimates were 17.6% for females and 6.1% for males, remarkably close to the findings of Stewart *et al*. A number of other recent studies in Western Europe and the United States have examined the prevalence of migraine.[2,11,24–26]

Sociodemographic variables

Migraine prevalence varies by age and gender. Before puberty, migraine prevalence is higher in boys than in girls; prevalence then increases more rapidly in girls than in boys as adolescence approaches.[14,28–33] Prevalence increases until approximately age 40, after which it declines (Figure 3.2).[9,23,27] These dramatic age effects account for some of the variation in previous studies.

The gender ratio (ratio of migraine prevalence in females over the prevalence in males) also varies with age (Figure 3.3).[9,27] Cyclical hormonal changes associated with menses may account for some aspects of the migraine prevalence ratio.[34] However, hormonal factors cannot account for all of the gender differences; prevalence remains substantially higher in women than men, even at the age of 70 years, well beyond the time that cyclical hormonal changes can be considered a factor.

Physician- and clinic-based studies have suggested that migraine is associated with high intelligence and social class. Bille did not demonstrate an association between migraine prevalence and intelligence in school children.[14,28]

Epidemiological studies in adults using intelligence testing and occupation as measures of socioeconomic status do not confirm a direct relationship between migraine and social class or intelligence.[35] In the American Migraine Study, migraine prevalence was inversely related to income[9] (i.e. migraine prevalence fell as household income increased) (Figure 3.4). The National Health Interview Study confirmed that migraine prevalence is highest in low-income groups;[36] prevalence was lowest for middle-income groups and began to rise in the high-income group. Since this study relied on self-reported migraine, and migraine awareness rises with income, differential ascertainment by income may account for this relationship in higher income groups. A population-based study in Kentucky[25] and a managed care-based study[36] have confirmed this inverse relationship in the USA.

Individuals from high income groups were much more likely to report a medical diagnosis of migraine than were those with lower income.[22] Migraine appears to be a disease of high income in the doctor's office, but not in the community. As Waters suggested, people from higher income households are more likely to consult physicians and are therefore disproportionately included in clinic-based studies.[43]

The higher migraine prevalence in the lower socioeconomic groups may be a consequence of a circumstance associated with low income and migraine, such as poor diet, poor medical care, or stress.[9] It may also reflect social selection; that is, migraineurs may have lower incomes because migraine interferes with educational and occupational function, causing a loss of income or the ability to rise from a low-income group. The relationship of migraine and socioeconomic status requires further study. It may be influenced by patterns of medical consulting behaviour and access to medical care in different countries, since the relationship between migraine prevalence and social class has not been found in some European studies.[1,8,11,17,18,37]

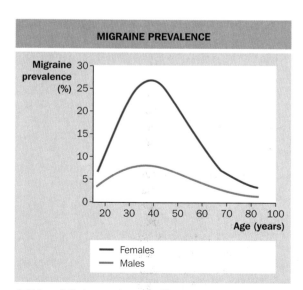

Figure 3.2 *Age- and sex-specific prevalence of migraine (from reference 44).*

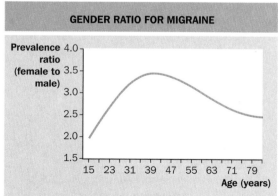

Figure 3.3 *Female-to-male prevalence ratio of migraine by age (from reference 27).*

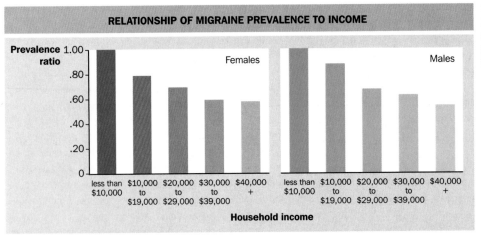

Is migraine prevalence increasing?

Migraine prevalence may be increasing.[38] According to the Centers for Disease Control, self-diagnosed migraine prevalence in the United States increased 60%, from 25.8/1000 to 41/1000 persons, between 1981 and 1989. Improved recognition of migraine could have produced this result; however, migraine prevalence increased in Rochester, Minnesota, during an earlier observation period,[21] and migraine prevalence in school children in Finland appears to be rising.[33] We are not aware of any major changes in migraine awareness or in patterns of diagnosis in the 1980s that could account for these findings. The apparent rise in migraine prevalence internationally could result from an increasing incidence of disease, an increasing duration of disease, or both. It will be important to identify internationally distributed risk factors that contribute to this increase in migraine prevalence.

Comorbidity of migraine

Why study comorbidity?

Originally coined by Feinstein,[39] the term 'comorbidity' is now used to refer to the greater than coincidental association of two conditions in the same individual.[4] Migraine is comorbid with a number of neurological and psychiatric disorders, including stroke, epilepsy, depression and anxiety disorders. Understanding the comorbidity of migraine is potentially important from a number of different perspectives.[4]

First, the occurrence of comorbidity has implications for headache diagnosis. Migraine has substantial symptomatic overlap with several of the conditions comorbid with it. For example, both migraine and epilepsy can cause transient alterations of consciousness as well as headache. This problem of differential diagnosis is well recognized. Less well rec-

ognized is the problem of concomitant diagnosis. When two conditions are comorbid, the presence of migraine should increase, not reduce, the index of suspicion for epilepsy, depression and anxiety disorders. Second, comorbidity has important implications for treatment. Comorbid conditions may impose therapeutic limitations, but may also create therapeutic opportunities. For example, when migraine and depression occur together, an antidepressant may successfully treat both conditions. The anti-migraine, anti-epileptic agent, divalproex sodium, may prevent attacks of both migraine and epilepsy. Finally, the study of comorbidity may provide epidemiological clues to the fundamental mechanisms of migraine.

Migraine and stroke

Both migraine and stroke are chronic neurological disorders associated with focal neurological deficits, alterations in cerebral blood flow and headache. The relationships between migraine and stroke are complex. Headaches have been associated with stroke as ictal, pre-ictal or post-ictal phenomena.[40] The association between migraine and stroke appears more often for migraine with aura and for stroke within the posterior circulation.[42–44] Migraine aura, if prolonged, may give rise to stroke a condition termed 'true migrainous infarction'.[12,40]

A number of hospital series have attempted to estimate the proportion of all stroke attributable to migraine using case-by-case clinical review. In patients under 50 years of age, 1–17% of strokes were attributed to migraine.[40–42] Bougousslavsky et al. (1988) reported that among patients with stroke, if the stroke occurred during the migraine attack, only 9% had arterial lesions; if the stroke was remote from the migraine attack, 91% had an arterial lesion.[45] Mechanisms other than traditional arterial disease may underlie migrainous infarction.

A number of case-control studies have examined migraine as a risk factor for stroke. The Collaborative Group for the Study of Stroke in Young Women compared hospitalized stroke patients with both hospital-based and community controls.[46] There was a twofold increase in the risk of stroke for women with migraine when compared with community controls but not relative to hospital controls.[46] Henrich and Horowitz found an association between migraine and stroke in a hospital-based case-control study, but differences disappeared after adjusting for stroke risk factors.[47]

Tzourio et al.[48,49] reported that migraine was associated with a fourfold increased risk of stroke in women under 45 years of age, with an even greater risk in women who smoked. These studies did not examine the relationship between migraine and stroke at the time of the attack, making inferences about causal mechanisms difficult.

In a longitudinal study, Henrich et al. estimated that the incidence of cerebral migrainous infarction was 3.36/100 000; if subjects with other stroke risk factors are excluded, estimates fall to 1.44/100 000.[50] Overall rates of ischaemic stroke in the population under age 50 years range from 6.5/100 000 to 22.8/100 000.[51] To interpret these data, we need to estimate the relative risk in migrainous and non-migrainous populations, stratified by migraine type (with and without aura) and adjusting for potential confounders.

To better understand the relationship between migraine and stroke, Welch has proposed a classification system that recognizes four types of relationships between migraine and stroke: coexistent stroke and migraine, stroke with clinical features of migraine, migraine-induced stroke and uncertain classification (Table 3.3).[40]

For stroke and migraine to be coexistent, '... a clearly defined stroke syndrome must occur remotely in time from a typical migraine attack'.[40] It may be not be possible to establish the presence or absence of a causal relationship in an individual case. At least some cases may be coincidentally related. Some cases may be linked by underlying risk factors, such as mitral valve prolapse or an antiphospholipid antibody syndrome.

In stroke with clinical features of migraine, Welch[40] indicates that '... a structural lesion that is unrelated to migraine pathogenesis presents with clinical features of a migraine attack'. He identifies two subtypes: symptomatic and migraine mimics. In the symptomatic group, an established structural disease causes episodes typical of migraine with aura, an example of which is an arteriovenous malformation that masquerades as migraine. For migraine mimic, stroke is accompanied by headache and other neurological symptoms and signs that resemble migraine.

In migraine-induced stroke, the neurological deficit of the stroke must be identical to the neurological symptoms of prior migraine attacks. In addition, the stroke must occur in the course of a typical migraine attack and other causes of stroke must be excluded.

In the group with uncertain classification, migraine and stroke appear related but causal attribution is difficult. For example, a patient may have a typical migraine with aura, take a vasoactive drug such as ergotamine, and then have a cerebral infarction. When this rare sequence occurs, it is not clear if the stroke is a consequence of the migraine itself, the treatment, or an interaction of the two. To clarify the causal mechanisms, we would need to compare the rates of stroke in close proximity to migraine with aura with and without vasoactive treatment. Migraine-like headaches and stroke may be associated with systemic vasculitides, antiphospholipid antibody syndrome, mitochondrial encephalopathies and oral contraceptive use. The classification of stroke and migraine in these settings may be difficult.

Migraine and epilepsy

Migraine and epilepsy are comorbid. Andermann and Andermann[52] reported a median epilepsy prevalence of 5.9% (range: 1–17%) in migraineurs, which greatly exceeds the population prevalence of 0.5%.[53] The reported migraine prevalence in epileptics ranges from 8 to 23%.[52] Methodology problems make these studies difficult to interpret.[52]

Ottman and Lipton[54–56] explored the comorbidity of migraine and epilepsy using Columbia University's Epilepsy Family Study. Among the subjects with epilepsy (probands), the prevalence of a migraine history was 24%. Among relatives with epilepsy, 26% had a history of migraine. In the control relatives without epilepsy, the prevalence of a migraine history was 15%. Epilepsy increases the relative risk of migraine by 2.4, both in probands and their epileptic relatives (Figure 3.5).

Migraine risk was not related to age of epilepsy onset, but was higher in patients with partial and generalized seizures and was highest in post-traumatic epileptics (relative risk = 4.1).

Migraine risk is elevated in both before and after seizure onset; therefore it cannot be accounted for solely as a cause or solely as a consequence of epilepsy. Because migraine

● **Table 3.3** *Classification of migraine-related stroke*

Category	Feature
I	Coexisting stroke and migraine
II	Stroke with clinical features of migraine A Symptomatic migraine B Migraine mimic
III	Migraine-induced stroke A Without risk factors B With risk factors
IV	Uncertain

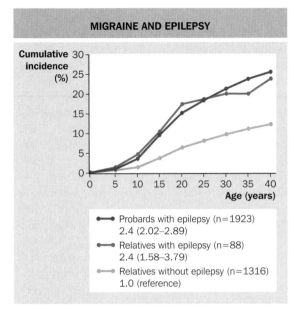

MIGRAINE AND EPILEPSY

Cumulative incidence (%)

- Probards with epilepsy (n=1923)
  2.4 (2.02–2.89)
- Relatives with epilepsy (n=88)
  2.4 (1.58–3.79)
- Relatives without epilepsy (n=1316)
  1.0 (reference)

● **Figure 3.5** *Cumalitive incidence of migraine headache by age, in probands with epilepsy, relatives with epilepsy and relatives without epilepsy.*

risk is elevated post-traumatic epileptics, and head injury is also a risk factor for both disorders, shared environmental risk factors may contribute to their comorbidity.[57,58] However, known environmental risk factors cannot fully account for this comorbidity, because migraine risk is also elevated in individuals with idiopathic epilepsy. Shared genetic risk factors cannot completely account for comorbidity, as migraine risk is elevated in probands with and without a positive family history of epilepsy.

Perhaps an altered brain state increases the risk of both migraine and epilepsy and thus accounts for the comorbidity of these disorders.[54] Genetic or environmental risk factors may increase neuronal excitability or decrease the threshold to both types of attack. A reduction in brain magnesium[60] or alterations in neurotransmitters provide plausible potential substrates for this alteration in neuronal excitability.[59–61]

The association between migraine and epilepsy has implications for clinical practice. When treating patients for one disorder, it is important to maintain a heightened index of suspicion for the other disorder. Differentiating migraine and epilepsy can be difficult,[52,62] as both conditions are characterized by episodes of neurological dysfunction. Headache without other neurological features is rare as a manifestation of epilepsy. The most difficult diagnostic issue is differentiating migraine with aura from partial complex seizure. If the aura is brief (< 5 min) and associated with alteration of consciousness, automatisms and other positive motor features

(tonic–clonic movements), epilepsy is more likely. If the aura is of long duration (> 5 min) and has a mix of positive (scintillations, tingling) and negative features (visual loss, numbness), migraine is more likely.

Treatment strategies for patients with comorbid migraine and epilepsy should be governed by the presence of comorbid disease. For example, in the treatment of migraine, drugs that lower seizure threshold should be used cautiously. Examples of such drugs include the tricyclic antidepressants, the selective serotonin re-uptake inhibitors and neuroleptics. On the other hand, it is sometimes advantageous to treat both migraine and epilepsy with a single drug. Divalproex sodium has well established efficacy in this setting.[63]

Migraine, major affective disorders and anxiety

Several population-based studies have examined the comorbidity of migraine, major depression, panic disorder and other psychiatric disorders.[24,65–68] Stewart *et al.* reported on the relationships of migraine with panic disorder and panic attacks.[66] Migraine headache in the one-week period prior to a telephone interview was higher in persons with a history of panic disorder. The relative risk was 7.0 for men and 3.7 in women.

Stewart *et al.*[67] found that 14.2% of women and 5.8% of men with a headache in the previous 12 months had consulted a doctor for headache. An unexpectedly high proportion of those who had consulted a physician for headache had a history of panic disorder. Of those who had recently seen a physician, 15% of women and 12.8% of men between the ages of 24 and 29 years had panic disorder. Comorbid psychiatric disease is apparently associated with seeking care for headache disorders.

In Zurich, Switzerland, Merikangas *et al.*[65] found that anxiety and affective disorders were more common in migraineurs. The odds ratios were 2.2 for depression, 2.9 for bipolar spectrum disorders, 2.7 for generalized anxiety disorder, 3.3 for panic disorder, 2.4 for simple phobia and 3.4 for social phobia. Major depression and anxiety disorders were commonly found together. In persons with all three disorders, the onset of anxiety generally precedes the onset of migraine, whereas the onset of major depression usually follows the onset of migraine.

Breslau and coworkers[24,69–71] studied the psychiatric comorbidity of IHS-defined migraine in young adults in southeast Michigan. Lifetime rates of affective and anxiety disorders were elevated in migraineurs. After adjusting for sex, the odds ratios were 4.5 for major depression, 6.0 for manic episode, 3.2 for any anxiety disorder and 6.6 for panic disorder. Migraine with aura was more strongly associated with the various psychiatric disorders than was migraine without aura.

Breslau *et al.*[71] also prospectively studied migraine and major depression. Comparing subjects with and without migraine, the relative risk for the first onset of major depression during the follow-up period was 4.1. Comparing subjects with and without major depression, the relative risk for the first onset of migraine during the follow-up period was 3.3. This bidirectional influence of each condition on the risk for the other is incompatible with simple unidirectional causal models.[71] Migraine is neither simply a cause nor simply a consequence of depression.

In summary, recent population-based studies demonstrate an association between migraine and major depression. The longitudinal studies show a bidirectional influence, from migraine to subsequent onset of major depression and from major depression to first migraine attack. Furthermore, these epidemiological studies indicate that migraineurs have increased prevalence of bipolar disorder, panic disorder and anxiety disorders.[64]

Migraine and personality characteristics

The relationships between migraine and personality characteristics have been discussed far more often than they have been systematically studied.[64] The idea of a migraine personality first grew out of clinical observations of the highly selected patients seen in subspecialty clinics. Many early authors have described migraineurs as perfectionistic, rigid, competitive, frustrated and overly sensitive.[72,73]

Many investigators use personality scales such as the Minnesota Multiphasic Personality Inventory (MMPI) or the Eysenck Personality Questionnaire (EPQ) to study migraine and personality characteristics.[74–77] These studies have been limited by several factors.[66,67] Most have used historical norms instead of concurrent controls. Many have not used explicit diagnostic criteria for migraine. Because the MMPI studies are usually clinic-based, their findings are of limited generalizability and subject to selection bias. Despite these limitations, most studies show elevation of the neurotic triad, although this is often not statistically significant (Figure 3.6).[64]

In the first population-based case-control study of personality in migraine, Brandt *et al.*[78] used the EPQ in the Washington County Migraine Prevalence Study sample. The EPQ is a well-standardized measure that includes four scales: psychoticism (P), extroversion (E), neuroticism (N) and lie (L). Migraineurs had higher scores than controls on

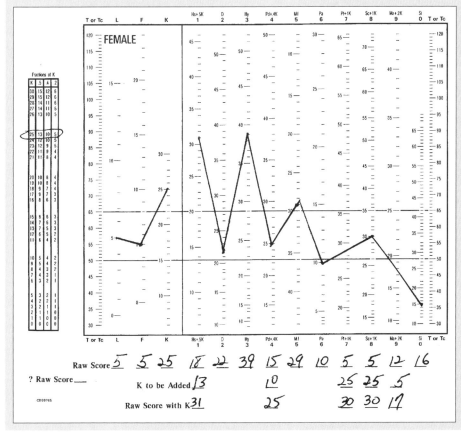

● **Figure 3.6** *MMPI showing conversion-V. (© 1989 Regents of the University of Minnesota.)*

the EPQ N scale, indicating that they were more tense, anxious and depressed than the control group. Women with migraine scored significantly higher than controls on the P scale, indicating that they were more hostile, less interpersonally sensitive, and out of step with their peers.

Merikangas et al.[68] investigated the cross-sectional association between personality, symptoms, and headache subtypes as part of a prospective longitudinal study of 19- and 20-year olds in Zurich, Switzerland. Migraineurs scored higher on neuroticism indicators than did non-migraine subjects.

Even the population-based studies of migraine and personality have generally not controlled for drug use, headache frequency and headache-related disability. Nor have they controlled for major psychiatric disorders (such as major depression or panic disorder), which, as discussed above, occur more commonly in migraineurs. Because major psychiatric disorders are associated with both migraine and personality disorders, confounding may alter the measured associations between these disorders and migraine.[64]

Breslau and Andreski[72] assessed the association between migraine and personality, adjusting for the co-occurrence of psychiatric disorders, using their epidemiological study of young adults in Detroit. They reported an association between migraine and neuroticism, which remained significant after controlling for sex and history of major depression and anxiety disorders. Differences between migraine sufferers and controls cannot be accounted for by *prior* depression and anxiety.

Impact of migraine

Migraine is a public health problem of enormous scope that has an impact on both the individual sufferer and on society.[79] The American Migraine Study estimates that 23 million US residents have severe migraine headaches.[9] Twenty-five percent of women experience four or more severe attacks a month; 35% experience one to four severe attacks a month; 40% experience one, or less than one, severe attack a month. Similar frequency patterns were observed for men.

In the American Migraine Study, more than 85% of women and more than 82% of men with severe migraine had some headache-related disability. About one-third were severely disabled or needed bedrest. In addition to the attack-related disability, many migraineurs live in fear, knowing that at any time an attack could disrupt their ability to work, care for their families or meet social obligations.

Migraine has an enormous impact on society. An American survey of 40 000 households (112 000 persons) found that 5.5 days of restricted activity per 100 person-years were due to headache.[80] In the Washington County study, 8% of males and 14% of females missed all or part of a day of work or

school in the 4-week period prior to the interview.[6] In the US, annual lost productivity due to migraine costs over $1 billion a year[36] and may cost as much as $17 billion a year.[81]

Migraine's impact on healthcare utilization is marked as well. The National Ambulatory Medical Care Survey, conducted from 1976 to 1977, found that 4% of all visits to physicians' offices (over 10 million visits a year) were for headache.[82] Migraine also results in major utilization of emergency rooms and urgent care centres.[83] Vast amounts of prescription and over-the-counter medications are taken for headache disorders.

Migraine is a lifelong disorder. Bille followed a cohort of children with severe migraine for up to 37 years.[14,27] As young adults, 62% were migraine-free for more than 2 years, but only 40% continued to be migraine-free after 30 years, suggesting that migraine is often a lifelong disorder. Hockaday reported similar long-term remissions.[84] For 15 years, Fry collected information on migraine patients in his general practice in Kent.[85] His data showed a tendency for the severity and frequency of attacks to decrease as the patients got older. After 15 years, 32% of the men and 42% of the women no longer had migraine attacks. Waters noted a similar decrease in migraine prevalence.[17,35]

There is a subgroup of migraine sufferers afflicted with a syndrome variously called chronic daily headache evolving from migraine, transformed migraine or malignant migraine, in which attacks increase in frequency over a number of years until a pattern of daily headache evolves.[34,86-88] In subspecialty clinics, about 80% of patients with this disorder are overusing acute headache medication. Medication overuse is believed to contribute to the accelerating pattern of pain through a mechanism that has been termed 'rebound headache'. When the cycle of medication overuse is broken, the headaches often improve.[89] However, in subspecialty clinics, this process of acceleration occurs without medication overuse in about 20% of patients, suggesting that there is a subgroup of migraine sufferers with a progressive condition.

Genetics of migraine

Introduction
The familial aggregation of migraine was first noted by Tissot in 1790.[90] Since then, numerous studies have examined the transmission of migraine within families, the concordance for migraine among twins, and the linkage of migraine to particular chromosomal loci (for reviews see references[91-93]). With the demonstration of a genetic locus for familial hemiplegic migraine (FHM) on chromosome 19[94] and the discovery of a candidate gene product from that locus,[95] the study of migraine genetics has truly entered the molecular era.

Studies of familial aggregation

Many studies have examined the risk of migraine among relatives of migraine probands and non-migrainous controls.[92,93] The controlled studies show an increased family risk of migraine among the relatives of migraine probands.[92,93] In the early studies, relative risks ranged from 1.5 to 19.3.[92] Variation in the family relative risk in the early studies is accounted for, at least in part, by methodological differences among studies.

The recent population-based migraine family studies avoid many of the limitations of earlier studies. Russell and Olesen (1995) used IHS criteria and directly interviewed first-degree relatives by telephone to determine migraine status.[96] First-degree relatives of probands who had migraine with aura had a fourfold increased risk of migraine with aura. The relatives of probands who had migraine without aura had a 1.9-fold increased risk of migraine without aura. Transmission of migraine type within families appears to be specific.

The familial studies strongly support the familial aggregation of migraine. Unfortunately, the evidence from segregation analysis does not provide consistent evidence for any single mode of inheritance.[97–99] The inconsistent results may reflect the genetic heterogeneity of migraine. Some families show apparent autosomal dominant transmission while others show autosomal recessive transmission with incomplete penetrance.

Twin studies

Clinic-based twin studies have consistently shown that monozygotic (MZ) twins are more concordant for migraine than are dizygotic (DZ) twins,[93] a finding that supports an aetiological role for genetic factors. Three recent studies conducted in population-based twin registries also support a genetic basis for migraine in Australia,[100] Finland[101] and Sweden.[102]

In the Australian study of 5844 twins,[100] proband-wise concordance for female same-sex twins was 0.44 for MZ twins and 0.24 for DZ twins. In males, the MZ concordance rate was 0.31 and the DZ concordance rate was 0.18. In all three studies, about half of the variation in migraine prevalence was attributable to the additive effect of genetic factors. Thus, the twin studies support the importance of genetic as well as risk factors for migraine. These data also demonstrate that non-genetic factors must play a role as the MZ concordance rate was well below 1.0. If genetic factors fully accounted for migraine, MZ twins would be fully concordant (i.e. both twins would always have migraine or always be free of the approximal chromosal locations of pathogenic genes).

Linkage studies

Linkage studies are under way for migraine both with and without aura. Familial hemiplegic migraine (FHM) (a rare autosomal dominant disorder with hemiplegia as one component of the aura) is linked to chromosome 19[99] in many,[103,104] but not all, unrelated families. Thus, even this autosomal dominant, relatively stereotyped disorder is genetically heterogeneous. Some non-chromosome 19 FHM has been linked to chromosome 19. The Dutch group has identified a neuronal calcium channel protein believed to be the product of the pathogenic gene on chromosome 19.[100] It is possible that the gene or genes involved in non-chromosome 19 FHM may code for a functionally related protein (see chapter 5).

The relationship between this chromosome 19 linkage marker/gene product and more common types of migraine is not clear. One group found an association between the chromosome 19 marker and migraine both with and without aura in a study of 28 families.[100] Another group did not find an association in a small number of families.[105] The chromosome 19 marker may be associated with migraine in a small percentage of the population. The heterogeneity of FHM underscores the likely heterogeneity of the more common types of migraine.

Tension-type headache

Estimates of the prevalence of tension-type headache have varied widely. In Western countries, one year period prevalence ranges from 28 to 63% in men and 34 to 86% in women.[8,11,26] This variation is explained, in part, by differences in case definition, sampling methods, and the procedures that were used to elicit histories. Few tension-type headache studies have been conducted outside the Western world. Wong *et al.*[106] found very low prevalences in a study he conducted in mainland China. A study of Nigerian college students found a prevalence of 42%. Rasmussen *et al.*[107] reported a prevalence of about 3% for chronic tension-type headache.

Tension-type headache is more common in women, with gender ratios ranging from 1.04 to 1.4. Prevalence peaks between the ages of 20 and 50 years and then declines. No association has been found between tension-type headache prevalence and education. Pryse-Phillips[26] reported an increased prevalence in higher income groups, although the results were not consistent.

Tension-type headaches often interfere with activities of daily living. Eighteen percent of tension-type headache sufferers had to discontinue normal activity, while 44% experienced some limitation of function. Attacks occur with a mean frequency of 2.9 days a month or 35 days a year: most sufferers have less than one attack a month and about one-third have two or more attacks a month.

Like migraine, tension-type headache is a disorder of middle life, striking individuals early in life and continuing to affect them through their peak productive years. All migraineurs, and 60% of tension-type headache patients, have a diminished capacity for work or other activities. Despite prominent disability, nearly 50% of migraineurs and more than 80% of tension-type headache patients had never consulted their general practitioner because of headache.

In a Danish study, 43% of employed migraineurs and 12% of employed tension-type headache sufferers missed one or more days of work because of headache. Migraine caused at least one day of missed work in 5% while tension-type headache caused a day of missed work in 9%. Annually, per 1000 employed persons, 270 lost work days were due to migraine and 820 were due to tension-type headache.

Individuals with frequent episodic tension-type headache may be at increased risk for chronic tension-type headache. When migraine and tension-type headache coexist, tension-type headache may be more frequent and more severe. The process whereby headache frequency increases and an episodic disorder becomes chronic is sometimes referred to as transformation. Overuse of ergotamine and/or analgesics is the most common factor leading to transformation. If analgesics are not withdrawn,

these patients may be refractory to prophylactic therapy and have a very poor prognosis.

Conclusion

Using the IHS criteria, large population-based epidemiological studies in Denmark, the United States, France, Canada and elsewhere, have shed light on the descriptive epidemiology of migraine. While migraine is a remarkably common cause of temporary disability, many migraineurs, even those with disabling headache, have never consulted a physician for the problem. Prevalence is highest in women, in persons between the ages of 25 and 55 years, and, at least in the United States, in individuals from low-income households. Nonetheless, prevalence is high in groups other than these high-risk groups. Migraine prevalence may be increasing in the United States, but this has not been proven. Longitudinal studies are required to better determine the incidence and natural history of migraine as well as the life course of comorbid conditions.

References

1. Lipton RB, Silberstein SD, Stewart WF. An update on the epidemiology of migraine. *Headache* 1994; 34: 319–28.
2. Rasmussen BK. Epidemiology of headache. *Cephalalgia* 1995; 15: 45–68.
3. Lipton RB, Amatniek JC, Ferrari MD et al. Migraine: identifying and removing barriers to care. *Neurology* 1994; 44(Suppl 6): 56–62.
4. Lipton RB, Silberstein SD. Why study the comorbidity of migraine. *Neurology* 1994; 44(7): 4–5.
5. Lipton RB, Stewart WF. Medical consultation for migraine. *Neurology* 1994; 44(Suppl 4): 199.
6. Stang PE, Osterhaus JT, Celentano DD. Migraine: patterns of health care use. *Neurology* 1994; 44(Suppl 4): 47–55.
7. Linet MS, Stewart WF, Celentano DD, Siegler D, Sprecher M. An epidemiologic study of headache among adolescents and young adults. *JAMA* 1989; 261: 2211–16.
8. Rasmussen BK, Jensen R, Schroll M, Olesen J. Epidemiology of headache in a general population - a prevalence study. *J Clin Epidemiol* 1991; 44: 1147–57.
9. Stewart WF, Lipton RB, Celentano DD, Reed ML. Prevalence of migraine

headache in the United States. *JAMA* 1992; 267: 64–9.
10. Henry P, Michel P, Brochet B et al. A nationwide survey of migraine in France: prevalence and clinical features in adults. *Cephalalgia* 1992;12: 229–37.
11. Gobels H, Petersen - Braun M, Soyka D. The epidemiology of headache in Germany: a nationwide survey of a representative sample on the basis of the headache classification of the International Headache Society. *Cephalalgia* 1994; 14: 97–106.
12. Headache Classification Committee of the International Headache Society. Classification and diagnostic criteria for headache disorders, cranial neuralgias, and facial pain. *Cephalalgia* 1988; 8(Suppl 7): 1–96.
13. Friedman AP, Finley KH, Graham JR. Classification of headache. *Arch Neurol* 1962; 6:173–6.
14. Bille B. Migraine in school children. *Acta Paediatr Scand* 1962; 51(Suppl 136): 1–151.
15. Featherstone HJ. Migraine and muscle contraction headaches: a continuum. *Headache* 1985; 24:194–8.
16. Raskin NH. *Headache* (2nd Edition). New York, Churchill-Livingstone, 1988.

17. Waters WE. *Headache* (Series in Clinical Epidemiology). Littleton, MA, PSG Co. Inc., 1986.
18. Waters WE. *Headache and Migraine in General Practitioners, the Migraine Headache and Dixarit. Proceedings of a symposium held at Churchill College.* Cambridge: Boehringer Ingelheim Brachnell, 1972.
19. Celentano DD, Stewart WF, Linet MS. The relationship of headache symptoms with severity and duration of attacks. *J Clin Epidemiol* 1990; 43: 983–94.
20. Stewart WF, Linet MS, Celentano DD, Van Natta M, Ziegler D. Age and sex-specific incidence rates of migraine with and without visual aura. *Am J Epidemiol* 1993; 34: 1111–20.
21. Stang PE, Yanagihara T, Swanson JW et al. Incidence of migraine headaches: A population-based study in Olmstead County, Minnesota. *Neurology* 1992; 42: 1657–62.
22. Lipton RB, Stewart WF, Celentano DD, Reed ML. Undiagnosed migraine: a comparison of symptom-based and self-reported physician diagnosis. *Arch Int Med* 1992; 152: 1273–8.

23. Stewart WF, Simon D, Schechter A, Lipton RB. Population variation in migraine prevalence: a meta-analysis. *J Clin Epidemiol* 1995; 48: 269–80.

24. Breslau N, Davis GC, Andreski P. Migraine, psychiatric disorders and suicide attempts: an epidemiological study of young adults. *Psychiatry Res* 1991; 37: 11–23.

25. Kryst S, Scherl E. A population-based survey of the social and personal impact of headache. *Headache* 1994; 34: 344–50.

26. Pryse-Phillips W, Findlay H, Tugwell P *et al.* A Canadian population survey on the clinical epidemiologic and societal impact of migraine and tension-type headache. *Can J Neurol Sci* 1992; 19: 333–9.

27. Lipton RB, Stewart WF. Migraine in the United States: epidemiology and health care use. *Neurology* 1993; 43(Suppl 3): 6–10.

28. Bille B. Migraine in children: prevalence, clinical features, and a 30-year follow up. In: Ferrari MD and Lataste X (eds.) *Migraine and other headaches.* New Jersey: Parthenon, 1989.

29. Sillanpaa M. Prevalence of migraine and other headache in Finnish children starting school. *Headache* 1976; 15: 288–90.

30. Sillanpaa M. Prevalence of headache in prepuberty. *Headache* 1983; 23:10–14.

31. Sillanpaa M. Changes in the prevalence of migraine and other headaches during the first seven school years. *Headache* 1983; 23:15–19.

32. Sillanpaa M, Piekkala P, Kero P. Prevalence of headache at preschool age in an unselected child population. *Cephalalgia* 1991; 11: 239–42.

33. Sillanpaa M. Headache in children. In: Olesen J (ed.). *Headache Classification and Epidemiology.* New York, Raven Press 1994; 273–81.

34. Silberstein SD, Silberstein JR. Chronic daily headache: long-term prognosis following inpatient treatment with repetitive IV DHE. *Headache* 1992; 32: 439–45.

35. Waters WE. Migraine: intelligence, social class, and familial prevalence. *Br Med J* 1971; 2:77–81.

36. Stang PE, Sternfeld B, Sidney S. Migraine headache in a pre-paid health plan: ascertainment, demographics, physiological and behavioral factors. *Headache* 1996; 36: 69–76.

37. D'Alessandro R, Benassi G, Lenzi PL et al. Epidemiology of headache in the Republic of San Marino. *J Neurol Neurosurg Psychiatry* 1988; 51 :21–7.

38. MMWR. Prevalence of chronic migraine headaches — United States, 1980–89. *MMWR* 1991; 40: 331–8.

39. Feinstein AR. The pretherapeutic classification of comorbidity in chronic disease. *J Chronic Dis* 1970; 23: 455–68.

40. Welch KMA. Relationship of stroke and migraine. *Neurology* 1994; 44(Suppl 7): 33–6.

41. Alvarez J, Matias-Guiu J, Sumalla J *et al.* Ischemic stroke in young adults, I: analysis of etiological subgroups. *Acta Neurol Scand* 1989; 80: 29–34.

42. Tatemichi TK, Mohr JP. Migraine and stroke. In: Barnett HJM, Stein BM, Mohr JP, Yarsu FM (eds.). *Stroke: Pathophysiology, Diagnosis and Management.* New York: Churchill Livingstone, 1986, pp. 845–63.

43. Bougousslavsky J, Regli F. Ischemic stroke in adults younger than 30 years of age: cause and prognosis. *Arch Neurol* 1987; 44: 479–82.

44. Rothrock J, North J, Madden K et al. Migraine and migrainous stroke: risk factors and prognosis. *Neurology* 1993; 43: 2473–6.

45. Bougousslavsky J, Regli F, Van Melle G *et al.* Migraine stroke. *Neurology* 1988; 38: 223–27.

46. Collaborative Group for the Study of Stroke in Young Women. Oral contraceptives and stroke in young women. *JAMA* 1975; 281: 718–22.

47. Henrich JB, Horowitz RI. A controlled study of ischemic stroke risk in migraine patients. *J Clin Epidemiol* 1989; 42: 773–80.

48. Tzourio C, Tehindrazanarivelo A, Iglesias S et al. Case-control study of migraine and risk of ischaemic stroke. *Br Med J* 1993; 307: 289–92.

49. Tzourio C, Tehindrazanarivelo A, Iglesias S *et al.* Case-control study of migraine and risk of ischaemic stroke in young women. *Br Med J* 1995; 310: 830–3.

50. Henrich JB, Sandercock PAG, Warlow CP, Jones LN. Stroke and migraine in the Oxfordshire Community Stroke Project. *J Neurol* 1986; 233: 257–62.

51. Kittner SJ, McCarer RJ, Sherwin RW et al. Black–white differences in stroke risk among young adults. *Stroke* 1993; 24(Suppl 1): 113–115.

52. Andermann E, Andermann FA. Migraine–epilepsy relationships: epidemiological and genetic aspects. In: Andermann FA, Lugaresi E, (eds.). *Migraine and Epilepsy.* Boston: Butterworths, 1987, pp. 281–91.

53. Hauser WA, Annegers JF, Kurland LT. Prevalence of epilepsy in Rochester, Minnesota: 1940–1980. *Epilepsia* 1991; 32: 429–45.

54. Ottman R, Lipton RB. Comorbidity of migraine and epilepsy. *Neurology* 1994; 44: 2105–10.

55. Lipton RB, Ottman R, Ehrenberg BL, Hauser WA. Comorbidity of migraine: the connection between migraine and epilepsy. *Neurology* 1994; 44(Suppl 7): 28–32.

56. Ottman R, Lipton RB. Is the comorbidity of epilepsy and migraine due to a shared genetic susceptibility? *Neurology* 1997, In press.

57. Schechter A, Stewart WF, Celentano DD *et al.* An epidemiologic study of migraine and head injury (abstract). *Neurology* 1990; 40(Suppl 1): 345.

58. Annegers JF, Grabow JD, Groover RV et al. Seizures after head trauma: a population study. *Neurology* 1980; 30: 683–9.

59. Welch KMA. Migraine: a behavioral disorder. *Arch Neurol* 1987; 44: 323–7.

60. Welch KMA, Barkley GL, Tepley N, D'Andrea G. Magnetoencephalographic studies of migraine: evidence for central neuronal hyperexcitability. In: Rose, FC (ed.). *New Advances in Headache Research, Volume 2.* London: Smith Gordon, 1991, pp.127–30.

61. Olesen J. Synthesis of migraine mechanisms. In: Olesen J, Tfelt-Hansen P, Welch KMA (eds.). *The Headaches.* New York: Raven Press, 1993, pp. 247–53.

62. Marks DA, Ehrenberg BL. Migraine-related seizures in adults with epilepsy, with EEG correlation. *Neurology* 1993; 43: 2476–83.

63. Jensen R, Brinck T, Olesen J. Sodium valproate has a prophylactic effect in migraine without aura. *Neurology* 1994; 44: 647–51.

64. Silberstein SD, Lipton RB, Breslau N. Migraine: association with personality characteristics and psychopathology. *Cephalalgia* 1995; 15: 1–15.

65. Merikangas KR, Angst J, Isler H. Migraine and psychopathology. Results of the Zurich cohort study of young adults. *Arch Gen Psychiatry* 1990; 47: 849–53.

66. Stewart WF, Linet MS, Celentano DD. Migraine headaches and panic attacks. *Psychosom Med* 1989; 51: 559–69.

67. Stewart WF, Schechter A, Liberman J. Physician consultation for headache pain and history of panic: results from a population-based study. *Am J Med* 1992; 92: 35–40.

68. Merikangas KR, Stevens DE, Angst J. Headache and personality: results of a community sample of young adults. *J Psychiat Res* 1993; 27:187–96.

69. Breslau N, Davis GC. Migraine, major depression and panic disorder: a prospective epidemiologic study of young adults. *Cephalalgia* 1992; 12: 85–9.

70. Breslau N, Davis GC. Migraine, physical health and psychiatric disorders: a prospective epidemiologic study of young adults. *J Psychiatric Res* 1993; 27(2): 211–21.

71. Breslau N, Davis GC, Schultz LR et al. Migraine and major depression: a longitudinal study. *Headache* 1994; 7: 387–93.

72. Breslau N, Andreski P. Migraine, personality, and psychiatric comorbidity. *Headache*, In press.

73. Wolff HG. Personality features and reactions of subjects with migraine. *Arch Neurol Psychiat* 1937; 37: 895–921.

74. Sternbach RA, Dalessio DJ, Junzel M et al. MMPI patterns in common headache disorders. *Headache* 1980; 20: 311–15.

75. Kudrow L, Sutkus GJ. MMPI pattern specificity in primary headache disorders. *Headache* 1979; 19: 18–24.

76. Weeks R, Baskin S, Sheftell F et al. A comparison of MMPI personality data and frontalis electromyographic readings in migraine and combination headache patients. *Headache* 1983; 23: 75–82.

77. Invernizzi G, Gala C, Buono M et al. Neurotic traits and disease duration in headache patients. *Cephalalgia* 1989; 9: 173–8.

78. Brandt J, Celentano D, Stewart WF et al. Personality and emotional disorder in a community sample of migraine headache sufferers. *Am J Psychiatry* 1990; 147: 303–8.

79. Ziegler DK. Headache: public health importance. *Neurol Clin* 1990; 8(4): 781–91.

80. Black ER. *Acute conditions: incidence and associated disability: United States, July 1976—June 1977*. Vital and Health Statistics, Series 10, No. 125, D.H.E.W. Publication No. 78-1553. Washington, DC: U.S. Government Printing Office, 1978.

81. Osterhaus JT, Gutterman DL, Plachetka JR. Health care resources and lost labor costs of migraine headaches in the United States. *Pharmacoeconomics* 1992; 2: 67–76.

82. National Center for Health Statistics. *Vital and Health Statistics of the United States*. D.H.E.W., PHS Publication No. 53. Advance data. Hyattsville, MD. National Center for Health Statistics, 1979.

83. Celentano DD, Stewart WF, Lipton RB, Reed ML. Medication use and disability among migraineurs: a national probability sample. *Headache* 1992; 32: 223–8.

84. Hockaday JM. Definitions, clinical features, and diagnosis of childhood migraine. In Hockaday JM, (ed.). *Migraine in Children*. London, Butterworth 1988, pp. 5–24.

85. Fry J. *Profiles of Disease*. Edinburgh, Livingstone 1966.

86. Mathew NT, Stubits E, Nigam MP. Transformation of episodic migraine into daily headache: analysis of factors. *Headache* 1982; 22: 66–8.

87. Mathew NT, Reuveni U, Perez F. Transformed or evolutive migraine. *Headache* 1987; 27:102–6.

88. Silberstein SD, Lipton RB, Solomon S, Mathew NT. Classification of daily and near daily headaches. Proposed revisions to the IHS criteria. *Headache* 1994; 34: 1–7.

89. Silberstein SD, Silberstein JR. Chronic daily headache: long-term prognosis following inpatient treatment with repetitive IV DHE. *Headache* 1992; 32: 439–45.

90. Tissot S. Nervous traits and diseases [in French]. In: *The Works of M.Tissot, vol. 13,* Lausanne, 1790, pp. 92–3.

91. Ziegler DK. Genetics of migraine. In: Rose FC (ed.). *Headache*. New York:Elsevier Science Publishers, 1986, pp. 28–30.

92. Merikangas KR. Genetic epidemiology of migraine. In: Sandler M, Collins GM (eds.). *Migraine: A Spectrum of Ideas*. Oxford: Oxford University Press, 1990, pp. 40–7.

93. Merikangas KR. Genetics of migraine and other headaches. *Current Opinion in Neurology* 1996;9(3):202–5.

94. Joutel A, Bousser MG, Biousee V et al. A gene for familial hemiplegic migraine maps to chromosome 19. *Nature Genetics* 1993; 5: 40–5.

95. May, A, Ophoff RA, Terwindt GM et al. Familial hemiplegic migraine locus on 19p13 is involved in the common forms of migraine with and without aura. *Hum Genet* 1995; 96: 604–8.

96. Russell MB, Olesen J. Increased familial risk and evidence of genetic factor in migraine. *BMJ* 1995; 311: 541–4.

97. Devoto M, Lozito A, Staffa G et al. Segregation analysis of migraine in 128 families. *Cephalalgia* 1986; 6: 101–105.

98. D'Amico D, Leone M, Macciardi F, Valentini S, Bussone G. Genetic transmission of migraine without aura: a study of 68 families. *Ital J Neurol Sci* 1991; 12: 581–4.

99. Mochi M, Sangiorgi S, Cortelli P et al. Genetic transmission of migraine without aura: a study of 68 families. *Ital J Neurol Sci* 1991; 12: 581–4.

100. Merikangas KR, Tierney C, Martin NG, Heath AC, Risch N. Genetics of migraine in the Australian Twin Registry. In: Rose CF (ed.). *New Advances in Headache Research 4*. London: Smith-Gordon, 1994, pp. 27–8.

101. Honkasalo ML, Kaprio J, Winter T et al. Migraine and concomitant symptoms among 8167 adult twin pairs. *Headache* 1995; 35: 70–8.

102. Larsson B, Bille B, Pederson N. Genetic influence in headaches: a Swedish twin study. *Headache* 1995; 35: 513–19.

103. Joutel A, Ducros A, Vahedi K et al. Genetic heterogeneity of familial hemiplegic migraine. *Am J Hum Genet* 1994; 55: 1166–72.

104. Ophoff RA, Van Eijk R, Sandkuijl LA et al. Genetic heterogeneity of familial hemiplegic migraine. *Genomics* 1994; 22: 21–6.

105. Hovatta I, Kallea M, Farkkila M, Peltonen L. Familial migraine: exclusion of the susceptibility gene from the reported locus of familial hemiplegic migraine on 19p. *Genomics* 1994; 23: 707–9.

106. Wong TW, Wong KS, Yu TS, Kay R. Prevalence of migraine and other headaches in Hong Kong. *Neuroepidemiology* 1995; 14: 82–91.

107. Rasmussen BK, Jensen R, Olessen J. Impact of headache on sickness absence and utilization of medical services: a Danish population study. *J Epidemiol Comm Health* 1992; 46: 443–6.

chapter 4

Diagnostic testing and ominous causes of headache

Headache diagnosis is based on a complete and thorough history supplemented by the general physical and neurological examinations (see Chapter 2). Testing (see Table 4.1) serves to:

- exclude organic causes of headache
- rule out comorbid diseases which could complicate headache and its treatment
- establish a baseline for and exclude contraindications to drug treatment, and
- measure drug levels to determine compliance, absorption or medication overuse.

Diagnostic testing is often recommended for other reasons. These include:

- the quest for diagnostic certainty
- in busy practices, a shortcut for a thorough evaluation
- patient expectations
- financial incentives
- professional peer pressure where tests are expected, and
- medicolegal issues.

The attitudes and demands of patients and families and the practice of defensive medicine are especially important.[1]

● **Table 4.1** Why do headache studies?

Study*	Diagnosis	Baseline	Compliance/toxicity
Complete blood cell count, differentiation	✓	✓	✓
Sedimentation rate	✓		
Chemistry profile	✓	✓	✓
Electrocardiogram		✓	✓
Blood gases	✓		
Drug screen	✓		✓
Drug level			✓
Lyme disease, HIV, VDRL	✓		
ANA, lupus anticoagulant, anticardiolipin antibodies	✓		

*HIV = human immunodeficiency virus;
VDRL = venereal disease research laboratory;
ANA = antinuclear antibody.

The selection of appropriate headache studies is hindered by the lack of controlled trials. Managed care systems often dictate which studies can be performed on their members, based often on economic, not medical, considerations. Omitting a test for economic reasons can have grave consequences for the patient and the physician. Lack of funds and underinsurance continue to be barriers for appropriate diagnostic testing for many patients.[1,2,3] Therefore, the cost–benefit ratio of performing a study must be considered, as must the medical/legal implications of omitting it.

Few guidelines exist for headache (particularly migraine) investigation.[1,2] One expert[4] states that '. . . magnetic resonance imaging (MRI) should be reserved for those patients in whom the diagnosis of migraine cannot be made unequivocally on clinical grounds', and another[5] says that '. . . in practice the recurrent pattern of migraine is so characteristic that it is rarely necessary to undertake any investigation'. We do not know if the diagnosis of migraine is always valid if it satisfies the criteria established by the International Headache Society (IHS),[6] nor do we know how many 'migraine mimics' are falsely diagnosed.

Validity depends on the sensitivity and the specificity of the diagnostic test:

- *Sensitivity* is defined as the ability of a test to identify correctly those who have the disease (high sensitivity will have few false-negatives).
- *Specificity* is defined as the ability of a test to identify correctly those who do *not* have the disease (high specificity will have few false-positives).

Additional indicators of benign migraine might include:

- regular or near-regular perimenstrual or periovulatory timing of the headache
- its appearance after *sustained* exertion
- its abatement with sleep, and
- acquisition of food-, odour-, or weather-change-induced headache occurring concurrently with unprovoked headache.

These criteria have not been tested and have not been used to screen patients to improve the yield of diagnostic testing. For example, the IHS criteria for migraine require exclusion of secondary organic causes of headache. It is uncertain how specific the IHS criteria are and how many 'migraine mimics' meet the IHS criteria. This is the fundamental problem. Most studies performed to investigate organic disease (neuroimaging or electroencephalography (EEG)) used the more imprecise ad hoc criteria or even more vague headache definitions, which makes the studies very difficult to interpret. If the prevalence of the suspected organic disorder increases (by using additional indications of benign and malignant headache), the diagnostic test yield improves. Thus, the presence of any atypical feature increases the yield of organic diagnostic testing.

Studies establishing a cost–benefit analysis in the area of headache diagnosis are just beginning. In a typical healthy migraineur, laboratory tests may not be necessary for diagnosis, but are often recommended prior to treatment, as, for example, an electrocardiogram in the older migraineur prior to the use of sumatriptan, dihydroergotamine or ergotamine.

Refractory headache patients who attend tertiary referral centres usually undergo a greater number of studies than do those patients seen in specialists' or primary care physicians' offices. Since secondary causes of headache frequently are not apparent on physical examination, laboratory tests are performed routinely on the initial visit to facilitate their diagnosis. A complete blood count and differential may rule out anaemia or infection. The antinuclear antibody test screens for autoimmune conditions. A sedimentation rate not only acts as a screen for serious diseases such as a malignancy or collagen vascular disease, but it can also establish the diagnosis of temporal arteritis, a cause of headache in the elderly. Thyroid function studies are performed to rule out thyroid disease such as thyrotoxicosis, a condition that may exacerbate headache and is a relative contraindication to ergot administration. Unexpected or overused medication that has a direct impact on headache and its treatment can be identified by a drug screen and toxicology studies. Specific studies (such as electrolytes and liver or kidney function studies) may be needed before starting drug treatment.

Methods of investigation

Electroencephalography (EEG)

The EEG is a non-invasive and relatively low-cost study. It lacks specificity and sensitivity, however, and while it reveals different rates of abnormality in headache subtypes, it is not helpful in distinguishing between subtypes (Figure 4.1). Between 12–15% of healthy adults who have no history of head injury, seizures, headaches, or other neurological diseases have non-specific EEG abnormalities.[7] Older studies have reported EEG abnormalities in migraine. Slater[8] found posterior quadrant, bilateral but asymmetric, slow-wave

abnormalities in 82 of 184 migraine patients. He also observed abnormal responses to photic stimulation and hyperventilation. He concluded that migraine causes a disorder of cerebral functioning that produces EEG changes. Smyth and Winter[9] found that 43% of 202 migraineurs had abnormal interictal records, with slowing in either the theta or delta range. The incidence of delta rhythm was related to headache severity, disease duration and a positive family history of migraine. Lauritzen et al.[10] found no EEG abnormalities on hyperventilation or photic stimulation, during attacks or interictally, in 11 patients with migraine without aura or in 8 of 10 patients with migraine with aura. Two patients who had migraine with aura had frontal slowing between and during attacks. While the interictal EEG may reveal diffuse or focal abnormalities to be more common in migraineurs, there is no migraine-specific pattern.

The American Academy of Neurology (AAN) has reviewed the use of EEG in headache diagnosis and found that many studies suffer from major flaws.[11] These include referral bias

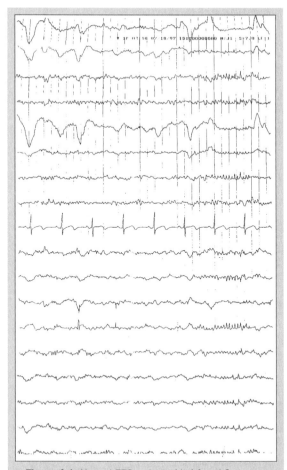

● **Figure 4.1** *Normal EEG variant with 14 and 6 positive spikes.*

(studies not population-based) and poor controls (studies usually uncontrolled and, when controlled, not age- or sex-matched). The studies are frequently non-blinded and have high intraobserver variability. In addition, archaic criteria for normalcy are employed (patterns originally considered abnormal are now considered normal, e.g. posterior slow waves of youth).

Studies designed to determine if headache patients have an increased prevalence of EEG abnormalities give conflicting results. In migraineurs, prominent photic driving at high flash frequencies (H-response) is the most consistently reported difference between headache patients and controls. The reported sensitivity of the H-response varied from 26–100%, the specificity from 80–91% (Figure 4.2).

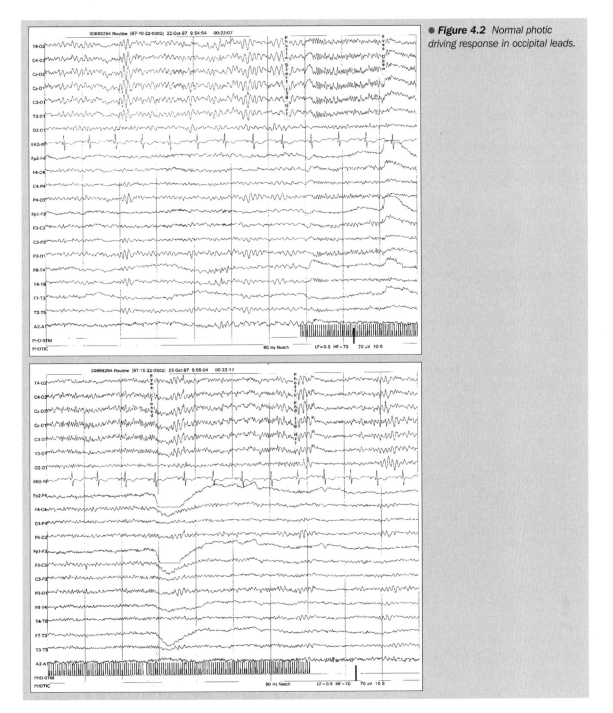

● **Figure 4.2** *Normal photic driving response in occipital leads.*

Literature addressing the question of whether or not EEG can identify a structural cause for headache is scarce, suggesting that the EEG does not effectively identify or screen out underlying lesions in headache patients.

Since the EEG does not identify headache subtypes, nor does it screen for structural causes of headache, the AAN has concluded that EEG is not useful in the evaluation of *routine* patients presenting with headache. Indications for performing an EEG are outlined in Table 4.2.

Computed tomography (CT) and magnetic resonance imaging (MRI)

Mitchell *et al.*[12] used computed tomography (CT) scanning with contrast enhancement to evaluate 350 headache patients. Patients were included in the study regardless of the presence or absence of physical or neurological signs or findings. Seven patients (2%) had CT findings that were felt to be clinically significant, including multiple metastases, epidural abscesses, frontal meningiomas and subdural haematomas. Three of these patients (1%) had abnormalities on physical or neurological examination. Another four patients (1%) had unusual clinical symptoms in addition to headache. Twenty-five (7%) had scans that were interpreted as abnormal but incidental to the headache complaint (e.g. atrophy, sinus disease and arachnoid cysts). Mitchell *et al.* concluded that routine CT has a low likelihood of uncovering significant intracranial disease in headache patients with normal physical and neurological examinations.

Cala and Mastaglia[13] studied 46 patients who exhibited increasing headache frequency or severity or whose headaches were associated with neurological symptoms. Abnormal CT scans were found in 37 (80%). Abnormalities included:

- mild white-matter oedema in one or both hemispheres, thought to be due to increased fluid content on the basis of regional cerebral ischaemia due to vasospasm or alternatively due to reduced cerebral blood flow, 17 (45%)
- cerebral atrophy, 8 (17%)
- occipital infarctions, 6 (9%), of whom four had homonymous hemianopsia, and
- unexpected tumours, 2 (4%), both of whom had abnormal neurological examinations.

Dorfman[14] described 4 migraineurs who had cerebral infarct: 2 had persistent neurological defects and 1 had transient weakness associated with the headache.

Kaplan and Solomon[15] suggested that MRI may be superior to CT scanning in headache evaluation. Nine patients

● **Table 4.2** Indications for ordering EEG

- Alteration or loss of consciousness
- Transient neurological symptoms without ensuing headache
- Suspected encephalopathy
- Residual persisting neurological defects
- Baseline EEG prior to the institution of medicines or procedures which could induce seizures

with different headache types had both CT and MRI. In 5 patients with a normal CT, MRI demonstrated cerebral infarction in 2 cases, and in 1 case, a 24-year-old woman with a diagnosis of 'migraine equivalent', a high-intensity signal focus in the medulla that proved to be an astrocytoma.

Robbins and Friedman[16] compared the MRI of 46 migraineurs to sex-matched controls. Thirteen percent of the migraineurs had white-matter lesions, compared to 4% of the controls. This finding may not be clinically significant.

Igarashi[17] found that 36 of 91 (31%) migraineurs had small foci of high intensity, predominantly in the centrum semiovale and frontal white matter, on T2-weighted MRI and proton density-weighted images. This was significantly more than the 11% seen in the age-matched controls. There was no correlation between MRI abnormalities and migraine type, ergotamine consumption, or frequency, duration or intensity of headaches. These abnormalities may be a consequence of migraine (Figure 4.3).

Forsyth and Posner[18] identified 111 patients with primary and metastatic brain tumours, and headache was found in 48%. The features of the headache were similar to tension-type headache in 77%, to migraine in 9%, and to other types of headache in 9%. The 'classic' presentation of early morning headache was seen in only 14%. Patients with a history of prior headache were more likely

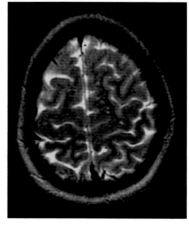

● **Figure 4.3** MRI abnormalities that may be a consequence of migraine.

to have headache associated with brain tumours than were those with no previous history. Thirty-six percent of these patients with severe headache had pain identical to previous headache, but it was associated with seizures, confusion, prolonged nausea, hemiparesis, or other abnormal neurological signs. The authors conclude that a change in headache symptoms is an indication for neuroimaging, but did not specify criteria for imaging.

The AAN has reviewed the role of neuroimaging in evaluating a headache patient whose neurologic examination is normal. The AAN position paper, based on an analysis of 16 CT and MRI studies, most of which were retrospective case reports, concluded that CT and MRI are not likely to produce substantial benefit and their routine use is not warranted in patients whose headaches fit a broad definition of recurrent migraine and who have had no recent change in headache pattern, no history of seizures, and no focal neurological findings.[19] Indications for CT or MRI in headache investigation are outlined in Table 4.3.

In patients in whom an aneurysmal subarachnoid haemorrhage (SAH) is suspected, both CT and MRI have been utilized.[1] MRI is not as reliable as CT in detecting an acute SAH in the first 24 hours. Since CT scan without contrast provides a rather high initial sensitivity, it is the neuroimaging study of choice in the detection of acute SAH. In a co-operative series of 3521 patients, findings on the first CT scan after rupture of a saccular aneurysm were as follows: normal, 8.3%; decreased density, 1.1%; mass effect, 6.1%; aneurysm, 5%; hydrocephalus, 15.2%; intraventricular haematoma, 16.7%; intracerebral haematoma, 17.4%; subdural haematoma, 1.3%; and SAH, 85.2%. CT scan detected aneurysmal SAH in 92% of patients on day 0, decreasing to 58% on day 5. The percentage of scans that were normal on day 0 was 3.3%; on day 1, 7.2%; and on day 5, 27.3% (Table 4.4).[20,21] In detecting a SAH, MRI is not the equal of CT during the first 24 hours. From 24 to 72 hours, MRI was slightly superior to CT and from 3 to 14 days MRI was superior to CT.[22]

Cerebral angiography

Unless aneurysm, vasculitis, or arteriovenous malformation (AVM) is suspected, there is little reason to perform angiography in a patient who has a normal neurological examination, a normal CT or MRI, and a history consistent with a benign primary headache disorder.[23] Older case reports suggest that complications may occur when angiography is performed in migraineurs, particularly during an attack.[24,25] However, Schuaib and Hachinsky have concluded that migraine does not increase the risk of complication, even if performed during the attack. Transient neurological symptoms, however, are not infrequent, especially in patients with migraine with aura.[26]

Magnetic resonance angiography

Although magnetic resonance angiography (MRA) allows for detection of aneurysms as small as 3–4 mm in the vicinity of the circle of Willis, this study has limitations:

- small aneurysms may be better visualized than larger, thrombosed aneurysms, and
- a high signal intensity thrombus within an aneurysm could be mistaken for slow blood flow.

As with conventional arteriography, vasospasm (with its diminished blood flow) may result in poor visualization of the aneurysm. If SAH is detected on CT, one should proceed to conventional angiography. Aneurysms that occur in the supraclinoid internal carotid artery (ICA) or the parasellar area, or outside the circle of Willis, are more difficult to detect. If an acute SAH is suspected, CT scan would be the imaging method of choice.

In spite of its limitations, MRA is a safe and non-invasive tool that is particularly useful for screening for a suspected aneurysm or AVM in patients who have not had an SAH.[27,28]

● **Table 4.3** *Indications for neuroimaging*

- The first or worst headache of the patient's life, particularly if it is of rapid onset (thunderclap headache)
- A change in the frequency, severity or clinical features of the headache attack
- An abnormal neurological examination
- A progressive or new daily persistent headache
- Neurological symptoms that do not meet the criteria of migraine with typical aura or that themselves warrant investigation
- Persistent neurological defects
- Definite EEG evidence of a focal cerebral lesion
- Perhaps hemicrania that is always on the same side and associated with contralateral neurological symptoms
- If routine therapy has not led to the anticipated improvement

● **Table 4.4** *Approximate probability of recognizing an aneurysmal hemorrhage on computed tomographic scan after the initial event*[20,21]

Time post-initial event	Probability (%)
Day 0	95
Day 3	74
One week	50
Two weeks	30
Three weeks	Almost 0

Lumbar puncture

The lumbar puncture (LP) is crucial in four distinct clinical situations. These include the patient who presents with:

- the first or worst headache of his life
- a severe, rapid-onset, recurrent headache
- a progressive headache, and
- an atypical chronic intractable headache.[29]

An LP should be performed if neuroimaging is normal, non-diagnostic or suggestive of a disorder that can only be diagnosed by measuring cerebrospinal fluid (CSF) pressure, cell count and chemistries. It should be performed first if imaging is not available and meningitis is suspected.

Patients who present with the sudden onset of a 'first-or-worst' headache must always be considered to have an acute neurological event, even though migraine can present in this manner. Focal neurological signs or symptoms or a change in consciousness or mental status suggest an intracranial process. It is almost impossible to differentiate between severe, acute-onset migraine (thunderclap headache) and SAH.[30] A brain image should be performed, if possible, prior to LP.

The best way to detect xanthochromia is spectrophotometry, since it cannot be detected by the naked eye about half the time.[31] The probability of detecting xanthochromia by spectrophotometry at various times after SAH is: 12 hours, 100%; 1 week, 100%; 2 weeks, 100%; 3 weeks, > 70%; and after 4 weeks, > 40% (Table 4.5). Other causes of xanthochromia include: jaundice, usually with a total plasma bilirubin of 10–15 mg/dl; CSF protein > 150 mg/dl; dietary hypercarotenaemia; malignant melanomatosis; and oral intake of rifampin.[32]

An LP is crucial to rule out an intracranial infection in the patient who presents with a confusional state, fever or meningeal signs (with or without headache). If CT is readily available, it should be performed first. However, if an imaging procedure is not readily available, an LP should be performed when there is a strong suspicion of meningitis. Delaying the LP and thus the diagnosis may lead to increased morbidity and mortality. If the headache has the characteristics of a postural (orthostatic) headache and there is no obvious cause, an LP will establish the diagnosis of CSF hypotension.

Many disorders are associated with the syndrome of increased intracranial pressure. Patients who have papilloedema and are suspected of having increased intracranial pressure should have an initial neuroimaging procedure (MRI or CT) to rule out a mass lesion. If these studies are normal, a tentative diagnosis of idiopathic intracranial hypertension can be made. Identical symptoms can be caused by chronic meningitis, however, so it is crucial to perform an LP to document increased intracranial pressure, rule out chronic meningitis (particularly in patients who are immunosuppressed), and ascertain the therapeutic effect of drugs given to decrease intracranial pressure.

Patients with intractable chronic daily headache commonly fail to respond to the usual treatment modalities, and it is often assumed that their problems are not organic in origin. A frequently overlooked cause of head pain is increased intracranial pressure without papilloedema. An LP is necessary to make the diagnosis.

Patients with daily headaches of subacute onset can also have a chronic fungal meningitis (particularly those who are immunosuppressed), the meningitis of Lyme disease or carcinomatous meningitis, all of which require an LP to diagnose.

Unless a diagnosis of meningitis, SAH, or high- or low-pressure syndrome is suspected, there is no reason to perform a spinal tap during a headache.[33] CSF pleocytosis may occur; it is rare, however, in migraine with or without aura and is more frequently seen in complicated migraine.[34]

Thermography

Abnormal thermograms have been described in headache patients. Temperature asymmetry is the most prominent finding in migraineurs. In patients with cluster headache and chronic paroxysmal hemicrania, a cold spot along the supraorbital area, or the inner orbit and canthus, is noted. The Therapeutics and Technology Assessment Subcommittee of the AAN reviewed the use of thermography in headache in 1990 and concluded that it had not been shown to provide sufficiently reliable information to be useful as a diagnostic test.[35]

Electromyography (EMG)

Increased activity in the neck and scalp muscles occurs in some patients with migraine and tension-type headache, but there is no correlation between increased EMG activity and pain or tenderness. Relaxation of these muscles does not relieve headache. Sophisticated EMG studies measuring reflex muscular contraction in response to painful electrical stimulation of the face demonstrate changes in some patients with frequent headache, but EMG abnormalities do not have sufficient sensitivity or specificity for diagnostic testing.

● **Table 4.5** *The probability of detecting xanthochromia with spectrophotometry in the cerebrospinal fluid at various times after a subarachnoid haemorrhage*[32]

Time post-haemorrhage	Probability (%)
12 hours	100
One week	100
Two weeks	100
Three weeks	>70
Four weeks	>40

Investigating specific headache types

Migrainous infarction and migraine with prolonged or atypical aura

Migrainous infarction always warrants investigation. When a migraineur presents with weakness, numbness, speech difficulty, or a persistent visual field defect, investigation for an organic aetiology such as stroke, tumour, subdural haematoma, or AVM should be undertaken. If there is a strong suspicion of carotid disease, vasculitis, or large artery dissection, MRA or arteriography should be performed promptly. Carotid duplex scanning, transcranial Doppler, electrocardiogram and Holter monitoring may be necessary. Antiphospholipid antibodies, protein S, protein C and occasionally antithrombin III levels may need to be determined in younger patients (under 55 years). Without an obvious cause of stroke a more thorough diagnostic evaluation including clotting factor analysis should be undertaken.

Basilar migraine

Basilar migraine should be suspected in the presence of syncope, diplopia, vertigo, ataxia, change in mental state and confusion. EEG should be performed to see if epileptiform activity is present and MRI or CT should be performed to exclude brainstem AVM or a space occupying lesion. Where vertebrobasilar disease is suspected, especially in older patients, MRA and transcranial Doppler may be necessary. If there is uncertainty about vascular disease, an angiogram may be necessary.

Migraine aura without headache[7]

The disorder that was previously known as 'acephalic migraine' is now called 'migraine aura without headache'; in the elderly, it is known as 'late-life migraine accompaniment'.[36] Diagnostic criteria for migraine aura without headache are outlined in Table 4.6.

The headaches are either totally absent or mild if present at all. Neuroimaging and arteriogram, if performed, are normal. Cerebral thrombosis, embolism, dissection, subclavian steal syndrome, epilepsy, thrombocytopenia, polycythemia, hyperviscosity syndrome and antiphospholipid antibody must be excluded.[37]

Warlow and Morris[38] defined transient ischaemic attacks (TIA) as the acute loss of focal cerebral or monocular function with symptoms lasting less than 24 hours, which, after adequate investigation, is presumed to be embolic or thrombotic vascular disease. Dennis and Warlow[37] compared a group of patients with migraine aura without headache to a group with TIA, and found that 98% of the patients with migraine aura without headache had visual symptoms. These visual symptoms were binocular in 71%. Seventy-one percent described positive visual features, and 30% had other aura symptoms, including sensory disturbances, aphasia or dysarthria. Patients who had migraine aura without headache had longer attacks than did those with TIA. Symptoms lasted between 15 minutes and 1 hour in 74% of patients with migraine aura without headache.

The manifestations of migraine aura without headache are variable in extent, duration, severity and quality. Diagnosis is more difficult when the condition occurs for the first time in a patient over the age of 40 years. The diagnosis should still be made by exclusion unless the symptoms are 'classic' (e.g. scintillating scotoma lasting 30 minutes).

Headache of sudden onset

Headache of sudden onset and extended duration may indicate an SAH or a sentinel headache without haemorrhage. More benign causes of this condition include migraine of sudden onset and coital cephalalgia (Table 4.7).

Thunderclap headache and subarachnoid haemorrhage

Thunderclap headache is the sudden onset of a severe headache that reaches maximum intensity within one minute. It can be further defined by the absence of an SAH.

The first or worst attack of migraine may be very difficult to differentiate from an SAH, particularly if the pain is acute in onset. The classical presentation of an aneurysmal SAH is an acute-onset, severe headache associated with a stiff neck, photophobia, nausea, vomiting and perhaps obtundation or

---

● **Table 4.6** *Late-life migrainous equivalents*

- The gradual appearance of focal neurological symptoms, spreading or intensifying over a period of minutes, not seconds
- Positive visual symptoms characteristic of 'classic' migraine, even if these come on abruptly, specifically fortification spectra (scintillating scotoma), flashing lights, dazzles, or a 'march' of paraesthesias
- Previous similar symptoms associated with 'classic' migraine or a more severe headache
- Serial progression from one accompaniment to another, such as a visual aura progressing to an aura with paraesthesias
- The occurrence of two or more identical spells
- A duration of 15–25 minutes (transient ischaemic attacks, TIAs, usually last less than 15 minutes)
- The occurrence of a 'flurry' of accompaniments (these generally occur in the 50–60-year-old age group)
- A generally benign course without permanent sequelae

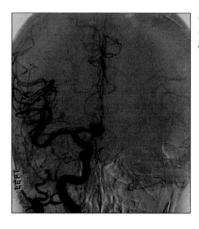

● Figure 4.4
Unruptured aneurysms.

● Table 4.7 *Headache of sudden onset*

Primary headache disorders
- Crash migraine
- Cluster
- Benign exertional headache
- Benign orgasmic cephalgia

Secondary headache disorders
- Associated with vascular disorders
  Unruptured saccular aneurysm
  Subarachnoid haemorrhage
  Internal carotid artery dissection
  Cerebral venous thrombosis
  Acute hypertension
    pressor response
    phaeochromocytoma
- Associated with non-vascular intracranial disorders
  Intermittent hydrocephalus
  Benign intracranial hypertension
  Pituitary apoplexy
  Cephalic infection
    meningoencephalitis
    acute sinusitis
  Acute mountain sickness
  Disorders of eyes
    acute optic neuritis
    acute glaucoma

woman who presented with the acute onset of the worst headache of her life. Examination, CT and LP were normal. An angiogram showed a distal right ICA aneurysm. Raps et al.[45] looked at the clinical spectrum of unruptured intracranial aneurysms. Acute, severe thunderclap headache, comparable to SAH but without nuchal rigidity, was seen in 7 of 111 patients (6.3%) with unruptured aneurysms, most of which were located in the anterior circle of Willis. Since the true frequency of unruptured aneurysm among patients with thunderclap headache is unknown, all patients in whom unruptured aneurysm is a possibility should undergo at least an MRA. The routine use of cerebral angiography is proscribed by the risk of permanent (0.1%) and transient (1.2%) deficits in this low-yield population (Figure 4.4).[46]

coma; it is easily differentiated from migraine. This catastrophic presentation is often preceded by a minor haemorrhage that can signal the likelihood of a major rupture.

An extensive neurological evaluation, including CT and LP, is indicated in patients presenting with their first or worst headache, particularly one associated with focal neurological signs, stiff neck or changes in cognition. Computed tomography, which would be performed by most physicians under these clinical circumstances, can miss subarachnoid blood in as many as 25% of cases, particularly if it is not performed until days after the onset of headache.[20] An MRI may be more sensitive after 24 hours, but only with the LP can one unerringly diagnose SAH.

Day and Raskin[39] have stated that all patients presenting with severe, sudden-onset headache should be evaluated for an aneurysm with angiography, even if CT, MRI and LP do not show evidence of SAH.[40] Several prospective studies[41,42] suggested that thunderclap headache is usually benign and angiography probably not necessary if neurological examination, CSF examination, and CT or MRI are normal. However, Hughes[43] reported two cases of thunderclap headache due to unruptured aneurysms. Ng and Pulst[44] reported a 53-year-old

Coital headache (Table 4.8)

The coital headache, which usually begins at or shortly before orgasm, is of high intensity, is frontal or occipital in location, is explosive or throbbing in nature, and persists for a few minutes to 48 hours.[47] A second, less ominous type of headache begins earlier in intercourse, is occipital or diffuse in location, is characterized as dull and aching, and is most severe at orgasm. For a coital headache of sudden onset, a CT scan should be performed and even if this is negative, an LP should be obtained. The question of whether to carry out angiography, even when the CSF is bloodless, is controversial; Raskin[39] however, advocates angiography. Aneurysm without rupture has presented as coital headache. Again, MRA may be a reasonable alternative.

Exertional and cough headaches

Originally described by Tinel[48] in 1932 ('la céphalée a l'effort') and later by Symond,[49] exertional headache mainly affects middle-aged men; it runs its course over a few years and is uncommon in the clinic. Transient, severe head pain upon coughing, sneezing, lifting, bending, straining at stool, or stooping defines exertional headache. MRI must be performed to

● **Table 4.8** *International Headache Society diagnostic criteria for coital headache*

4.6 Headache associated with sexual activity

A   Precipitated by sexual excitement

B   Bilateral in onset

C   Prevented or eased by ceasing sexual activity before orgasm

D   Not associated with an intracranial disorder such as aneurysm

● **Table 4.9** *Headache of sudden onset*

Bilateral	Unilateral
Idiopathic, stabbing headache	Idiopathic stabbing headache
Benign cough and exertional headache	Trigeminal neuralgia
Coital headache	SUNCT
Headaches due to structural disease	Chronic and episodic paroxysmal hemicrania
Colloid cyst of IIIrd ventricle and other IIIrd ventricular tumours	Cluster headache
Pineal region tumours and masses	
Arnold–Chiari malformation	
Platybasia/basilar impression	
Phaeochromocytoma	

SUNCT = short-lasting unilateral neuralgiform headache with conjunctival injection and tearing.

rule out hindbrain abnormalities, which include Arnold–Chiari malformation, posterior fossa meningioma, midbrain cyst, basilar impression and acoustic neurinoma (Figure 4.5). Other causes of brief severe headache are listed in Table 4.9.

Spontaneous internal carotid artery dissection

Spontaneous ICA dissection is an uncommon but not altogether rare cause of headache and acute neurological deficit in younger patients. Headache, the most common symptom, is often unilateral and located in the orbital, periorbital and frontal regions. It may be accompanied by neck pain. The pain is usually moderate to severe and steady or throbbing in nature. A bruit or Horner's syndrome is often present. Focal cerebral symptoms such as TIA or stroke may either precede the headache or follow it by up to 2 weeks. The gold standard test for dissection is arteriography. A promising modality for demonstrating carotid dissection is high-resolution MRI and MRA, which, especially in the axial planes, can demonstrate the vessel lumina and changes in the arterial wall (Figure 4.6).

Summary

In adult patients with recurrent headaches that have been defined as migraine with no recent change, no history of seizures, and no other focal neurological signs or symptoms, the routine use of neuroimaging and other diagnostic testing is not warranted. Some testing is appropriate prior to beginning treatment or if there are clinical features that suggest an organic aetiology for the disorder. In patients with atypical headache patterns, such as chronic daily headache, or a history of seizures or focal neurological signs or symptoms, additional testing, including CT or MRI, is often indicated.

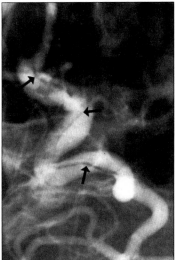

● **Figure 4.6**
*Internal carotid artery dissection.
(Reproduced with permission from Mokri B et al. Headache in spontaneous carotid and vertebral artery dissections. In: Goadsby PJ, Silberstein SD (eds). Headache. Boston: Butterworth–Heinemann 1997, pp. 327–54.)*

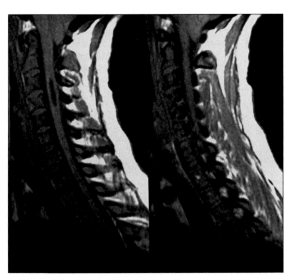

● **Figure 4.5** *Arnold–Chiari malformation seen at MRI showing low-lying cerebellar tonsils and associated syrinx.*

References

1. Evans RW. Diagnostic testing for the evaluation of headaches. *Neurologic Clinics* 1996; 14: 1–26.
2. Adams RD, Victor M (eds.). *Principles of Neurology.* New York: McGraw-Hill, 1989: 718–54.
3. Ziegler DK, Friedman AP. Intermittent or paroxysmal disorders, Migraine. In: Rowland LP (ed.). *Merritt's Textbook of Neurology.* New York: McGraw-Hill, 1993: 773–80.
4. Raskin NH. Migraine: clinical aspects. In: *Headache.* New York: Churchill-Livingstone, 1988: 35–98.
5. Lance JW (ed.). *Mechanism and Management of Headache.* London: Butterworth Scientific, 1993: 68–90.
6. Headache Classification Committee of the International Headache Society. Classification and diagnostic criteria for headache disorders, cranial neuralgia and facial pain. *Cephalalgia* 1988; 8(7): 56–7.
7. Selby G. Assessment and investigation of the patient with migraine. In: *Migraine and its Variants.* Australia: Adis Press, 1983: 74–93.
8. Slater KH. Some clinical and EEG findings in patients with migraine. *Brain* 1968; 91: 85–98.
9. Smyth VOG, Winter AL. The EEG in migraine. *Electroenceph Clin Neurophysiol* 1964; 16: 194–202.
10. Lauritzen M, Trojaborg, Olesen J. The EEG in common and classic migraine attacks. In: Rose FC (ed.). *Advances in Migraine Research and Therapy.* New York: Raven Press, 1982: 79–84.
11. Report of the Quality Standards Subcommittee of the American Academy of Neurology. Practice parameter: the electroencephalogram in the evaluation of headache (summary statement). *Neurology* 1995; 45: 1411–13.
12. Mitchell CS, Osborn RE, Grosskreutz SR. Computed tomography in the headache patient: is routine evaluation really necessary? *Headache* 1993; 33: 82–6.
13. Cala LA, Mastaglia FL. Computerized axial tomography findings in a group of patients with migrainous headaches. In: *Proceedings of the Australian Association of Neurologists* 1976: 35–41.
14. Dorfman LJ, Marshall WH, Enzmann DR. Cerebral infarction and migraine: clinical and radiological correlations. *Neurology* 1979; 29: 317–22.
15. Kaplan RD, Soloman GD, Diamond S, Freitag FG. The role of MRI in the evaluation of a migraine population: preliminary data. *Headache* 1987; 27: 315–18.
16. Robbins L, Friedman H. MRI in migraineurs. *Headache* 1992; 32: 507–8.

17. Igarashi H, Sakai F, Kan S, Okada J, Tazaki Y. Magnetic resonance imaging of the brain in patients with migraine. *Cephalalgia* 1991; 11: 69–74.
18. Forsyth PA, Posner JB. Headaches in patients with brain tumours: a study of 111 patients. *Neurology* 1993; 43: 1678–83.
19. Frishberg BM. The utility of neuroimaging in the evaluation of headache in patients with normal neurologic examinations. *Neurology* 1944; 44: 1191–7.
20. Adams HP, Kassell NF, Torner JC, Sahs AL. CT and clinical correlations in recent aneurysmal subarachnoid hemorrhage: a preliminary report of the cooperative aneurysm study. *Neurology* 1983; 33: 981–8.
21. VanGijn J, VanDongen KG. The time course of aneurysmal hemorrhage on computed tomograms. *Neuroradiology* 1982; 23: 153–6.
22. Ogawa T, Inugami A, Shimosegawa E *et al.* Subarachnoid hemorrhage: evaluation with MR imaging. *Radiology* 1993; 186: 345–51.
23. Silberstein SD, Saper JR. Migraine: diagnosis and treatment. In: Dalessio DJ, Silberstein SD (eds.). *Wolff's Headache and Other Head Pain.* New York: Oxford University Press, 1993: 97–170.
24. Kwentus J, Kattah J, Koppicar M, Potolicchio SJ. Complicated migraine and cerebral angiography: a report of an unusual adverse reaction. *Headache* 1985; 25: 240–5.
25. Dalessio DJ. Migraine. In: Dalessio DJ (ed.). *Wolff's Headache and Other Head Pain.* New York: Oxford University Press, 1980; 56–130.
26. Schuaib A, Hachinsky VC. Migraine and the risks from angiography. *Arch Neurol* 1988; 45: 911–12.
27. Glicklich M, Ross JS. MR angiography: clinical applications. *Appl Radiol* 1992; 10: 77–83.
28. Bosmans H, Marchal G, Van Hecke P, Vanhoenacker P. MRA review. *Clin Imaging* 1992; 16: 152–67.
29. Silberstein SD, Corbett JJ. The forgotten lumbar puncture. *Cephalalgia* 1993; 13: 212–13.
30. Silberstein SD. Evaluation and emergency treatment of headache. *Headache* 1992; 32(8): 396–407.
31. Vermeulen M, VanGijn J. The diagnosis of subarachnoid hemorrhage. *J Neurol Neurosurg Psychiatry* 1990; 53: 365–72.
32. Vermeulen M, Hasan D, Blijenberg BG *et al.* Xanthochromia after subarachnoid hemorrhage needs no revisitation. *J Neurol Neurosurg Psychiatry* 1989; 52: 826–8.

33. Kovács K, Bors L, Tóthfalusi L, Jelencsik I *et al.* Cerebrospinal fluid (CSF) investigations in migraine. *Cephalalgia* 1989; 9: 53–7.
34. Schraeder PL, Burns RA. Hemiplegic migraine associated with an aseptic meningeal reaction. *Arch Neurol* 1980; 37: 377–9.
35. Report of the Therapeutics and Technology Assessment Subcommittee of the American Academy of Neurology. Assessment: thermography in neurologic practice. *Neurology* 1990; 40: 523–5.
36. Fisher CM. Late-life migraine accompaniments — further experience. *Stroke* 1986; 17: 1033–42.
37. Dennis M, Warlow C. Migraine aura without headache: transient ischemic attach or not? *J Neurol Neurosurg Psychiatry* 1992; 55: 437–40.
38. Warlow CP, Morris PJ. Introduction. In: Warlow CP, Morris PJ (eds). *Transient Ischemic Attacks.* New York: Dekker, 1982: vii–xi.
39. Day JW, Raskin NH. Thunderclap headache: symptom of unruptured cerebral aneurysm. *Lancet* 1986; 2: 1247–8.
40. Kassell NF, Torner JC, Haley EC *et al.* The international cooperative study on the timing of aneurysm surgery. Part I: Overall management results. *J Neurosurg* 1990; 73: 18–36.
41. Wijdicks EFM, Kerkhoff H, Van Gijn J. Long-term follow-up of 71 patients with thunderclap headache mimicking subarachnoid hemorrhage. *Lancet* 1988; 2: 68–70.
42. Harling DW, Peatfield RC, Van Hille PT, Abbott RJ. Thunderclap headache: is it migraine? *Cephalalgia* 1989; 9: 87–90.
43. Hughes RL. Identification and treatment of cerebral aneurysms after sentinel headache. *Neurology* 1992; 42: 118–19.
44. Ng PK, Pulst S-M. Not so benign 'thunderclap headache'. *Neurology* 1992; 260(3): 42.
45. Raps EC, Rogers JD, Galetta SL *et al.* The clinical spectrum of unruptured intracranial aneurysms. *Arch Neurol* 1993; 50: 265–8.
46. Leow K, Murie JA. New information on several painful conditions: thunderclap headache mimicking subarachnoid hemorrhage. *Neurology Alert* 1988; 75–6.
47. Johns DR. Benign sexual headache within a family. *Arch Neurol* 1986; 43: 1158–60.
48. Tinel J. Un syndrome d'algie veineuse intracranienne. La cephalee a l'effort. *Prat Med Fr* 1932; 13: 113–19.
49. Symonds C. Cough headache. *Brain* 1956; 79: 557–68.

chapter 5

The pathophysiology of primary headache

Headache is a common human experience, diverse in its expression, complex in its manifestation, and difficult to understand in any simple mechanistic way. While the biology may seem daunting there are some important common threads that can illuminate the darker areas of understanding. The basic anatomy of the pathways responsible for head pain applies to most manifestations of the problem independent of cause. Pain control systems modulate headache of all causes and may be primarily involved in some headache syndromes. In this chapter we shall present common themes as illustrated by migraine in detail. Much of the fundamental anatomy and physiology has implications for all primary headaches.

Headache genetics: the predisposition

Migraine is predominantly an affliction of young people. The strong familial association and early onset of the disorder suggest that there is a important genetic component. Migraine is a feature of some of the mitochondrial disorders, such as MELAS. This association helped to draw attention to the possible genetic basis for migraine. The first genetic locus for a migrainous disease was found on chromosome 19p13 for familial hemiplegic migraine (FHM).[1] This was the beginning of a large effort to unravel the fundamental defect(s) that leads to migraine. The gene for FHM has been mapped to chromosome 19p13 in some, but not all, families (Figure 5.1). This region may also be involved in more common forms of migraine.[2] The defect in FHM has been found to be due, in five families, to four different missense mutations in a brain-specific P/Q Ca^{2+} channel α_1-subunit gene CACNL1A4 covering 300 kb with 47 exons.[3] This is the same gene associated with episodic ataxia with cerebellar vermal atrophy. [4,5]

P-type neuronal Ca^{2+} channels mediate 5-hydroxytryptamine (5-HT) release. Dysfunction of these channels may impair 5-HT release and predispose patients to migraine attacks or impair their self-aborting mechanism. Magnesium deficiency occurs in the cortex of migraineurs[6] and magnesium interacts with Ca^{2+} channels. Ca^{2+} channels are important in spreading depression, which may initiate the migraine aura. Impaired function may predispose to more frequent and severe attacks. This suggests that migraine may be part

of the spectrum of channelopathies. FHM can be compared to other so-called channelopathies, such as hyperkalaemic periodic paralysis, paramyotonia congenita, hypokalaemic periodic paralysis, myotonia congenita and episodic ataxia with myokymia.[7] In some of these episodic disorders patients are normal between attacks yet may have profound disability during the attack. To account for a further 15% of families with FHM a recent locus on chromosome 1 has been identified.[8,161] A headache sufferer probably inherits a diathesis or constitution that makes them liable to headache. Triggers can bring on an attack due to the individual's increased susceptibility which involves the basic neurobiology of migraine. The female predominance and the association with menstruation does not assist in differentiating the site of the problem, since the hormonal changes described[9] could affect either neural or vascular structures and probably act to further lower the threshold to migraine. However, linkage in some families to the X chromosome may explain in part the female preponderance. Thus far candidate linkage studies have not proved fruitful so that endothelial nitric oxide synthase[10] and 5-HT$_{2A}$ receptor[11] gene polymorphisms are not increased in migraine. Equally interesting is a possible genetic contribution[12] to cluster headache. Modern biology is only beginning to clarify this relationship.

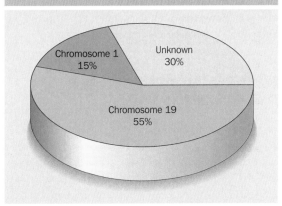

CHROMOSOMAL ALLOCATION OF GENES FOR FAMILIAL HEMIPLEGIC MIGRAINE (FHM)

Chromosome 1 15%
Unknown 30%
Chromosome 19 55%

● *Figure 5.1* *Chromosomal allocation of genes for familial hemiplegic migraine (FHM). About 55% of families can be located on chromosome 19[3] and 15% on chromosome 1[8,161] with the remaining 30% unaccounted for at the present.*

Migraine: a sum of the parts

Migraine is a syndrome that is most easily recognized when all parts are present but no less debilitating nor valid if only one element predominates. There are three essential elements to the migraine attack; the beginning, the attack and the resolution. From a biological point of view how the attack starts and how it stops are the most interesting and the least well understood, while the actual attack is the most important to the sufferer and is becoming better understood. Does the brain institute a process to terminate the attack as soon as it starts? Are the premonitory features and the aura really mechanistically similar? We shall examine some of these questions below.

Stage 1: Premonitory features of migraine — *the attack begins*

About 25% of patients report symptoms of elation, irritability, depression, hunger, thirst or drowsiness during the 24 hours preceding headache. These manifestations suggest a hypothalamic site for their origin.[13] The suprachiasmatic nucleus of the hypothalamus[14] is one of two primary oscillators which generates the circadian rhythms[15] and could be responsible for the periodicity of migraine that is such an important clinical feature. Patients frequently report that they are vaguely aware of the beginning of the attack. Despite its vagueness, the neurobiology of attack initiation is crucial to understanding migraine. The description of bilateral oligaemia in a patient with migraine without aura complaining only of visual blurring may be more relevant in understanding the complex biology of migraine than simply contribute to information about aura.[16] Since this atypical aura was associated with profound changes in brain blood flow, observations in the early parts of an attack must be a priority as better imaging strategies become more available.

Stage 2a: The attack proper — *migraine aura*

Most patients never have aura but the experience of visual disturbances (such as the scintillating scotoma; flashing lights that move across the visual field), paraesthesias or other focal neurological signs are so dramatic that so much has been said about it and so much research has been directed at the process since an early time. The migraine aura is associated with a reduction in cerebral blood flow (CBF) that moves across the cortex at a rate of 2–3 mm/min (Figure 5.2).[17] The blood flow changes begin usually in the occipital

region but generally are anterior to the occipital pole. This reduction enlarges and may involve the whole hemisphere. The spreading oligaemia does not respect vascular territories and is unlikely to be due to vasoconstriction.[18] The oligaemia may be preceded by a phase of focal hyperaemia.[19] Such a change is what would be expected if a similar phenomenon to cortical spreading depression[20-22] was involved.[23] Following the passage of the oligaemia the cerebrovascular response to hypercapnia is blunted while autoregulation is intact.[24] That is the blood vessels do not

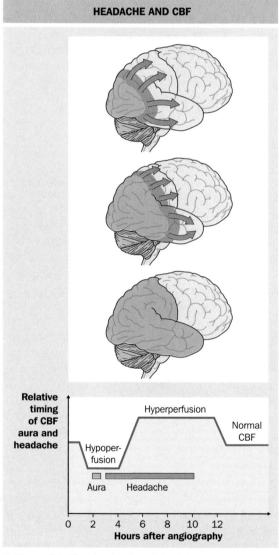

HEADACHE AND CBF

● **Figure 5.2** *Line drawing (panel A) of the spreading oligemia observed with studies of cerebral blood flow during aura after Lauritzen[25]. Panel B illustrates the variable time course and relationship of the changes in cerebral blood flow and the symptomatology of migraine.[17]*

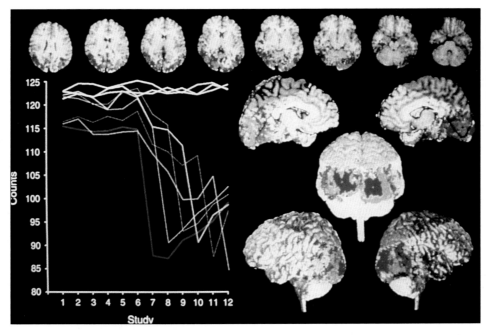

● **Figure 5.3**
Spreading oligaemia demonstrated with PET in a young female with a spontaneous attack of migraine.[16]

dilate normally in response to high CO_2 but do respond to changes in blood pressure. This pattern is also seen in spreading depression.[25] Olesen's group triggered migraine by carotid angiography, but similar changes occur in spontaneous migraine attacks measured with single-photon emission computed tomography (SPECT).[26] Some would argue that spreading oligaemia is a SPECT scan artifact due to Compton scatter; however, positron emission tomography (PET) has clearly demonstrated spreading oligaemia during

a migraine attack. Woods and colleagues[16] reported measurements of regional cerebral blood flow from the start of a spontaneous migraine attack in a 21-year-old female migraineur without aura, a normal volunteer for a PET CBF study (Figure 5.3). The patient never had a clear neurological deficit either before, during, or after the PET study. Bilateral decreases in CBF began in the occipital cortex and spread anteriorly. Since the patient had transient visual blurring but no aura, it is possible that blood flow changes occur in both migraine with and without aura. It is remarkable that spreading oligaemia can occur and be clinically silent.

Lashley[27], who suffered from migraine, calculated that the growth of his own migrainous fortification spectrum corresponded to an event moving across the cortex at a rate of 2–3 mm/min (Figure 5.4). Leao[20] found that noxious stimulation of the exposed cerebral cortex of a rabbit produced a spreading decrease in electrical activity that moved at a rate of 2–3 mm/min (spreading depression of Leao) (Figure 5.5). The rates of progression of spreading oligaemia, migrainous scotoma and spreading depression are equal, suggesting that these phenomena may be related. Magnetoencephalography measures changes in the magnetic activity of the cerebral cortex. Some signals found in migraine patients are not found in control subjects. This is felt to be consistent with changes seen with spreading depression in rabbits and provides indirect evidence that this phenomenon exists in humans.[28] Migraine with aura may be associated with a state of neuronal hyperexcitability including the excitatory amino acids: glutamate and possibly aspartate.[29] A low brain magnesium

LASHLEY'S AURA

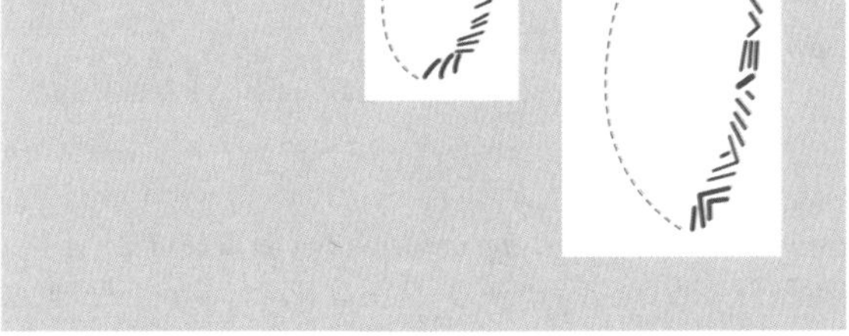

● **Figure 5.4** *Line drawings of Lashley's aura moving across his visual field.*[27]

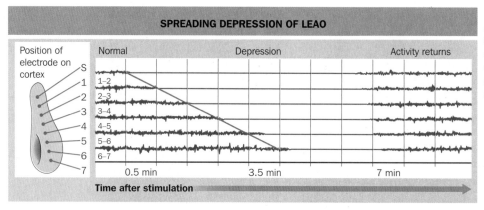

SPREADING DEPRESSION OF LEAO

Position of electrode on cortex

S 1 2 3 4 5 6 7

Normal | Depression | Activity returns

1–2
2–3
3–4
4–5
5–6
6–7

0.5 min   3.5 min   7 min

Time after stimulation

● **Figure 5.5**
Recordings from the rabbit cortex illustrating spreading depression of EEG activity.[20]

concentration (measured by 31P-NMR spectroscopy) may enhance the responsiveness of the *N*-methyl-D-aspartate (NMDA) receptor that may be involved in the genesis of both spreading depression and neuronal sensitization.[30] Headache may begin while cortical blood flow is still reduced[17] and bilateral flow changes can occur making the likelihood that the pain arises from a primary vascular abnormality untenable. Just how common the described blood flow changes are, is what we do not know. Do patients with a clouded sensorium or patients just feeling odd have similar focal changes in areas of cortex that are clinically less eloquent? Do other changes take place that do not cause tightly to coupled changes in cerebral blood flow which will only be demonstrated in studies of brain metabolism? We think these are likely although certainly untested hypotheses.

Most clinicians now believe that the migraine aura is due to neuronal dysfunction, not ischaemia, and that ischaemia rarely, if ever, occurs during the aura. The neurological changes that occur during aura parallel those that occur when the brain is directly stimulated and resemble what might be predicted if ocular dominance columns were sequentially activated. Spreading depression or its human homologue is likely to be the neurobiological basis for the migraine aura.

Stage 2b: the headache

Anatomy
The trigeminal innervation of pain-producing intracranial structures
Surrounding the large cerebral vessels, pial vessels, large venous sinuses and dura mater is a plexus of largely unmyelinated fibres that arise from the trigeminal ganglion and in the posterior fossa from the upper cervical dorsal roots.[31,32] Tracing studies have shown that fibres innervating cerebral vessels arise from within the trigeminal ganglion

from neurons that contain substance P and calcitonin gene-related peptide (CGRP).[33] Substance P and CGRP have both been shown to be released when the trigeminal ganglion is stimulated either in humans or cats.[34] The cell bodies in the trigeminal ganglion are pseudo-unipolar neurons that innervate the large cerebral arteries and dura mater and arise from the first or ophthalmic division of the trigeminal nerve. Stimulation of the cranial vessels, such as the superior sagittal sinus, is certainly painful in humans.[35,36] Human dural nerves that innervate the cranial vessels largely consist of small-diameter myelinated and unmyelinated fibres that subserve a nociceptive function.[37,38]

Physiology
Potential sources of pain in migraine
Wolff[36] believed that the aura of migraine was caused by intracerebral vasoconstriction and the headache pain was caused by reactive vasodilatation of the carotid artery. This explained the throbbing quality of the pain, its varied localizations, and its relief by ergot administration.[39] The vascular theory runs into certain difficulties since:

(1) it failed to explain the prodromal features of a migraine attack or the associated neurological features;
(2) some of the drugs used to treat migraine have no effect on blood vessels;
(3) the theory has not been supported by evidence from recent blood-flow studies; and
(4) most patients do not have aura.

Some studies have suggested that the headache of migraine could result from dilatation of the large conductance intracerebral arteries. If the carotid artery is occluded on the headache side then two-thirds of migraineurs will experience relief; however the other one-third do not respond at all.[40] Since the resistance vessels would not be affected, there would be no change in CBF, although balloon inflation of the middle cerebral artery in man produces focal headache, referred to the ophthalmic division of the trigeminal nerve.[41] The relevance of this unphysiological painful dilatation to headache is uncertain. MCA dilatation measured by transcranial Doppler during a migraine attack is not a constant finding; thus, migraine headache is not caused by MCA dilatation.

Plasma protein extravasation

Moskowitz has provided an elegant series of experiments to suggest that the pain of migraine may be a form of sterile neurogenic inflammation.[42] The trigeminal sensory C-fibres contain substance P and other neuropeptides, including CGRP and neurokinin A. Antidromic stimulation of the trigeminal nerve releases substance P, CGRP and neurokinin A from the sensory C-fibres, resulting in neurogenic inflammation. The released neuropeptides interact with the blood vessel wall, producing dilatation, plasma extravasation and sterile inflammation (Figure 5.6). Electron micrographs of the interior of these blood vessels show platelet activation. Thus platelet activation occurring during migraine may be an epiphenomenon produced by neurogenic inflammation. The sterile inflammatory process is also thought to sensitize nerve fibres to respond to previously innocuous stimuli such as

blood vessel pulsations (Figure 5.7).[43] Neurogenic inflammation results in the leakage of plasma proteins into the dura mater, which can be quantified by measuring the leakage of radiolabelled albumin (Figure 5.8). Administration of either sumatriptan or dihydroergotamine or newer 5-hydroxytryptamine (5-HT$_{1B/1D}$) agonists, such as naratriptan, rizatriptan and zolmitriptan, prevent the leakage of albumin (Figure 5.8).

Neuropeptides and headache-linking experimental and human observations

At least one-third of migraineurs have a significant extracerebral vascular component to their headache.[40] Stimulation of the trigeminal ganglion in the cat leads to an increase in cranial levels of both substance P and CGRP. Similarly, stimulation of the trigeminal ganglion in humans undergoing thermocoagulation for trigeminal neuralgia leads

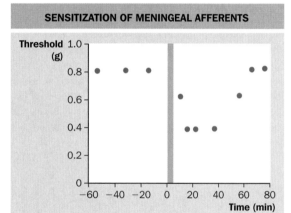

SENSITIZATION OF MENINGEAL AFFERENTS

● *Figure 5.7* *Sensitization of primary afferents to mechanical stimulation after application of an inflammatory 'soup'.*[43]

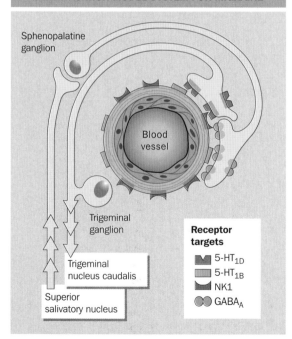

NEURALLY-INDUCED PLASMA PROTEIN EXTRAVASATION MODEL SYSTEM FOR MIGRAINE

Sphenopalatine ganglion

Blood vessel

Trigeminal ganglion

Trigeminal nucleus caudalis

Superior salivatory nucleus

Receptor targets

5-HT$_{1D}$
5-HT$_{1B}$
NK1
GABA$_A$

● *Figure 5.6* *Line drawing of the neurally-induced plasma protein extravasation model system for migraine.*[159]

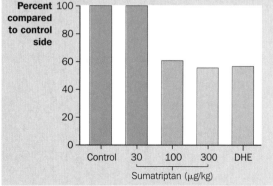

INHIBITION OF PLASMA PROTEIN EXTRAVASATION BY ANTI-MIGRAINE COMPOUNDS

● *Figure 5.8* *Bar graph comparing the leakage of plasma proteins after stimulation of the trigeminal ganglion after Buzzi.*[117]

to elevation in the cranial venous outflow of both peptides.[34] More specific stimulation of pain-producing intracranial structures, such as the superior sagittal sinus, also results in cranial venous release of CGRP and not substance P.[44] During migraine CGRP is elevated in the external jugular vein blood whereas substance P is not in both adults and in adolescents (Figure 5.9).[45,46] These data clearly demonstrate activation of trigeminovascular neurons during migraine with or without aura. Similarly, CGRP but not substance P is elevated during acute attacks of cluster headache, both spontaneous[47] and provoked[48], and during the pain of chronic paroxsymal hemicrania.[49] It is important to note in terms of understanding the pathophysiology of cluster headache that vasoactive intestinal polypeptide (VIP), a marker for cranial parasympathetic nerve activation, is also elevated in cluster headache and paroxysmal hemicrania.[47,49] Moreover, treatment with sumatriptan reduces CGRP levels in humans as their migraine subsides and in experimental animals during trigeminal ganglion stimulation.[50] Similarly, treatment with avitriptan, a potent clinically effective 5-HT$_{1B/1D}$ agonist[51,52], blocks CGRP release in experimental animals while administration of the potent blocker of neurogenic plasma protein extravasation(PPE), CP122 288, is not effective at doses specific for PPE.[53] The release of these peptides offers the prospect of a marker for migraine that can be measured in a venous blood sample and seems highly predictive of antimigraine activity in humans.

Central pain processing of trigeminovascular pain

The brainstem sites that are responsible for craniovascular pain have now begun to be mapped using fos-immunohistochemistry, a method for looking at activated cells. After meningeal irritation with blood fos expression occurs in the trigeminal nucleus caudalis[54] and after stimulation of the superior sagittal sinus fos is expressed in cat[55] and monkey[56] in the trigeminal nucleus caudalis and in the dorsal horn at the C$_1$ and C$_2$ levels (Figure 5.10). If metabolism is measured using 2-deoxyglucose similar increases are seen in the brainstem following superior sagittal sinus stimulation.[57] These data contribute to the view that the trigeminal nucleus extends beyond the traditional nucleus caudalis to the dorsal

NEUROPEPTIDE CHANGES AND MIGRAINE

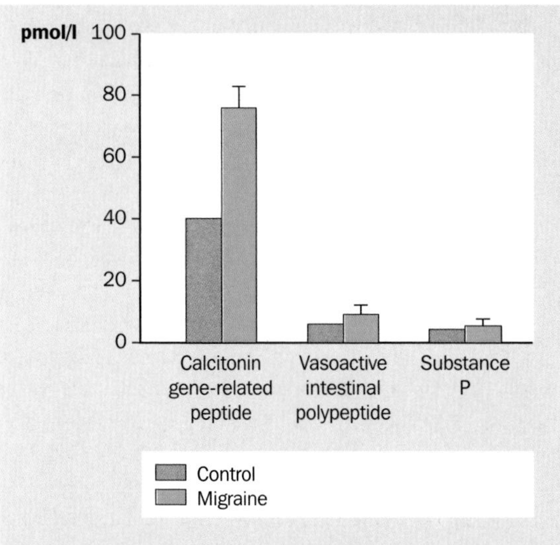

● **Figure 5.9** *Release of vasoactive peptides during migraine. Calcitonin gene-related peptide is a marker for activation of the trigeminovascular system and is elevated in primary headaches.*[160]

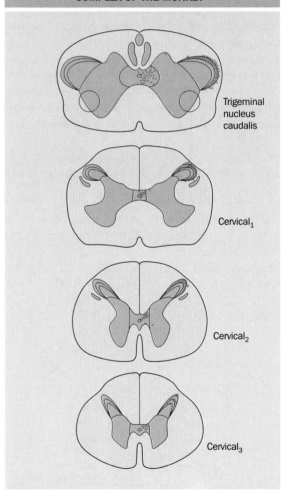

FOS ACTIVATION IN THE TRIGEMINOCERVICAL COMPLEX OF THE MONKEY

Trigeminal nucleus caudalis

Cervical$_1$

Cervical$_2$

Cervical$_3$

● **Figure 5.10** *Fos expression in the trigeminocervical complex of the monkey after stimulation of the superior sagittal sinus.*[56]

horn of the high cervical region in a functional continuum that includes a cervical extension that could be regarded as a *trigeminal nucleus cervicalis.* The entire group of cells could usefully be labelled the *trigeminocervical complex.* A substantial portion of the trigeminovascular nociceptive information comes by way of the most caudal cells in the cervical spinal cord. Indeed direct stimulation of the greater occipital nerve in the cat leads to increased metabolic activity in the entire trigeminocervical complex.[58] It is most likely then that the trigeminocervical neurons are the site for referral of head pain and that this anatomical arrangement accounts for the distribution of pain in migraine and many other forms of headache. The rather diffuse activation of neurons in the trigeminal nucleus in visceral type pain, such as that arising from intracranial vessels, is to be contrasted with what is seen when pain stimuli are applied to discrete facial structures. Neuronal activation is more restricted[59] in line with the relatively good spatial localization of more superficial pain. This provides an anatomical explanation for the referral of pain to the back of the head in migraine.

Following transmission in the caudal brainstem and high cervical spinal cord information is relayed in a group of fibres (the quintothalamic tract) to the thalamus. Processing of vascular pain in the thalamus occurs in the ventroposteromedial thalamus, medial nucleus of the posterior complex and in the intralaminar thalamus.[60] If capsaicin, the active irritant found in chilli peppers, is applied to the superior sagittal sinus trigeminal projections with a high degree of nociceptive input are processed in neurons particularly in the ventroposteromedial thalamus and in its ventral periphery.[61] In addition, cells in the medial thalamic nuclei which are likely to be involved in the affective processing of trigeminal pain are also activated by vascular stimulation.[62] The properties and further higher centre connections of these neurons are the subject of ongoing studies which will allow us to build up a more complete picture of the trigeminovascular pain pathways (Table 5.1).

● **Table 5.1** *Processing of craniovascular pain*

Order	Structures	Comments
1st	Trigeminal ganglion	Located in middle cranial fossa
2nd	Trigeminocervical complex (via quintothalamic tract)	Trigeminal nucleus caudalis and dorsal horns of C_1 and C_2 cervical spinal cord (laminae I/IIo)
3rd	Thalamus	Ventrobasal complex
		Medial nuclei
Final	Cortex	Site unknown

Stage 3: Central modulation — *starting and stopping headache*

The importance of brainstem mechanisms in the pathogenesis of migraine is underscored by the recent studies of Weiller and colleagues[63] who reported brainstem activation in spontaneous migraine attacks. Using PET to measure regional CBF (rCBF), 9 patients with right-sided migraine headache without aura were studied within hours of migraine onset. High rCBF values were found bilaterally in the cingulate, auditory association and visual association cortices and on the left side only in the inferior anterocaudal cingulate cortex. There was increased rCBF in the left brainstem anterior to the aqueduct and posterior to the corticospinal tract. Sumatriptan relieved the headache and associated symptoms and reversed the cerebral, but not the brainstem, increase in rCBF. Since the rCBF increase in the brainstem persisted despite headache resolution, it seems likely that the activation is due to factors other than, or in addition to, increased activity of the endogenous antinociceptive system. Activation of the brainstem may be inherent in the migraine process itself. The brainstem center may integrate the migraine attack. Continued activation despite symptom resolution with sumatriptan may account for headache recurrence (Figure 5.11).

Central modulation of trigeminovascular pain

In the experimental animal, stimulation of the brainstem nucleus locus coeruleus (the main central noradrenergic nucleus) reduces cerebral blood flow in a frequency-dependent manner[64] through an α_2 adrenoceptor-linked mechanism.[66,67] This reduction is maximal in the occipital cortex.[68] Cerebral blood flow is reduced up to 25% while extracerebral vasodilatation occurs in parallel.[66] In addition, activating the main serotonin-containing nucleus in the brain stem, the midbrain dorsal raphe nucleus, can increase cerebral blood flow.[69–71]

These animal studies have received considerable renewed interest with the description in humans of activation of the periaqueductal grey in the region of the dorsal raphe nucleus and in the dorsalateral pons near the locus coeruleus in PET studies during migraine without aura.[63] Moreover, these areas are active immediately after successful treatment of the headache but are not active between headache attacks. Aura can exist in isolation from pain as a 'migraine equivalent'; it is thus possible that the aura originates in the central nervous system with the vascular changes being a secondary feature (Figure 5.12). How can changes in the brainstem seen in the PET studies occur contralateral to the pain since there are no known crossed descending nociceptive control pathways from these regions?[72] These data

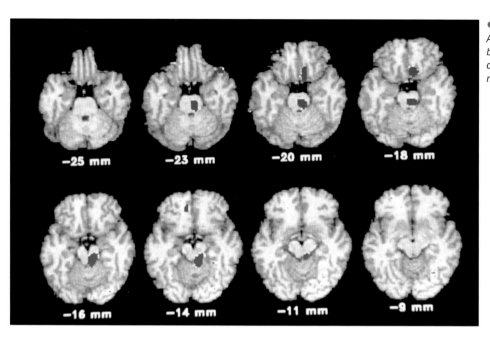

● **Figure 5.11**
Activation of the brainstem with PET during acute migraine.[63]

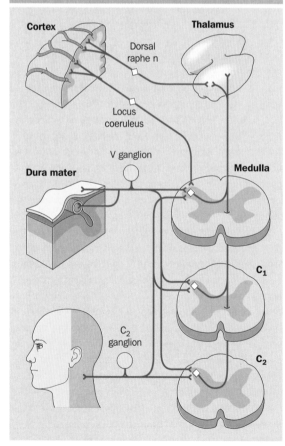

PAIN PROCESSING AND MECHANISMS AND BRAINSTEM CONTROL

● **Figure 5.12** *Diagram of the essential connections of the trigeminovascular system with the trigeminocervical complex and its control by descending pathways. Information from anterior intracranial structures, dura mater and blood vessels, projects to the superficial dorsal lamina of the trigeminal nucleus caudalis, and C_1/C_2 cervical spinal cord, the trigeminocervical complex. Projections from branches of C_2 that innervate infratentorial structures synapse on the same neurons which accounts for referred pain in primary headache syndromes. The information ascends in the quintothalamic tract synapsing in the contralateral ventrobasal and medial thalamus before projecting to cortex. Aminergic areas in the periaqueductal grey matter and dorsolateral pontine tegmentum (locus coeruleus) have effects on the incoming pain and cortical blood flow. In essence migraine is an inherited instability in this control system.*

are more easily understood in the context of ascending pain control systems. There are well described connections from both ventrobasal and medial thalamus to the ipsilateral dorsal raphe nucleus but not to the periaqueductal grey[73] and it is likely that these *ascending pathways* have been activated. Pain fibres from the trigeminal nucleus pass by way of the quintothalamic tract and decussate in the midbrain before synapsing on third order neurons in the ventrobasal thalamus and medial thalamic nuclei. This contralateral thalamic level of processing is in turn controlled or gated by ascending serotonergic fibres from the dorsal raphe nucleus and from aminergic nuclei in the pontine tegmentum, such as the locus coeruleus. This model is consistent with all known human and higher-order animal data.[74]

Aminergic modulation of trigeminovascular processing is supported by clinical observations. Placement of an electrode into the region of the periaqueductal grey matter can evoke a migraine-like headache.[75] Cells in the same region can be activated after superior sagittal sinus stimulation.[76] Contingent negative variation (CNV), an event-related slow cerebral potential, is increased in amplitude and its habituation lacking in patients with migraine without aura (Figure 5.13).[77-79] Furthermore, CNV is under aminergic control and normalizes after treatment with β-blockers.[80] The visual evoked potential is potentiated rather than habituated in migraine patients when studied between attacks.[81] These clinical observations taken together provide the human side of the argument that migraine is most likely a disorder of the central nervous system.

Migraine and the blood–brain barrier

Some very compelling data from a clinical study of aura raises the possibility that the blood–brain barrier may not be normal in migraine. This is not a new suggestion[82] although there has been little direct evidence for an altered barrier apart from a case report based on CT[83] and more recent MRI studies have been somewhat negative.[84] The era of more modern therapeutics, which has arguably started with sumatriptan, has provided more and interesting data. In a well-conducted study of patients with migraine with aura the effect of sumatriptan on the aura was examined. Sumatriptan did not shorten or lengthen the aura when compared to placebo. The most fascinating aspect of the study was that sumatriptan was not more effective than placebo for headache when it was given during the aura. Despite having good delivery and a suitable drug level with the mean length of the aura being about 20 min, headache still occurred. What is further and perhaps even more remarkable is that the developed headache responded to a further sumatriptan injection.[85] Ferrari has suggested that treatment failure is particularly associated with early use of the subcutaneous sumatriptan again suggesting that some process must take hold that facilitates the action of sumatriptan.[86] Headache severity itself may not be important as subcutaneous sumatriptan is very effective in aborting mild headache.[87] Sumatriptan may not have access to a crucial receptor site during the aura. The interaction of the drug at its receptor depends on its concentration and its access to the appropriate site. These are the elements of the equation required to terminate the migraine attack.

What is the site that sumatriptan does not have access to? The obvious is a site behind the blood–brain barrier which re-opens the very exciting possibility that the blood–brain barrier may not be normal in the headache phase of migraine. Indeed better access to sites within the central nervous system may be advantageous in drug development rather than a drawback. Results of phase II/III clinical studies with zolmitriptan[88] and eletriptan[89], two newer more lipophilic 5-HT$_{1B/1D}$ agonists, suggest that such an advantage may be of clinical benefit. A recent report of a study of zolmitriptan in treatment of aura[90] was inconclusive, attempting to analyse the outcome at 24 hours rather than when the headache would be expected after the aura. This study had several drawbacks including the use of an orally administered compound. Further studies with new agents, particularly using non-oral routes of administration, are eagerly awaited.

Perhaps a link in the overall chain of events that occurs in migraine may again be found in the brainstem particularly in the aminergic nuclei, given the recent human PET data.[63] Stimulation of the locus coeruleus, the main noradrenaline-containing cell group in the central nervous system, can alter brain blood flow and blood–brain barrier

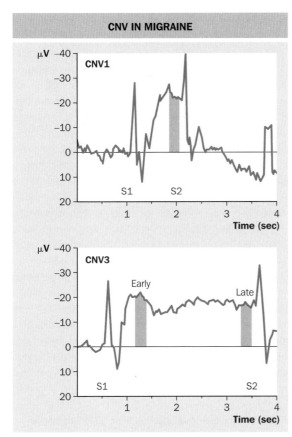

● **Figure 5.13** Contingent negative variation (CNV) recorded with a 1 second (CNV1) and 3 second (CNV3) interstimulus interval. This method has been instrumental in examining some fundamental questions concerning migraine biology.[80]

permeability.[91] Modulation of central noradrenergic systems using tricylic antidepressants can alter blood–brain barrier permeability in experimental animals.[92] Central noradrenergic innervation is essential for maintaining blood–brain barrier integrity during some pathophysiological states.[93] One differentiating feature between the central aminergic nuclei is the presence of NADPH diaphorase activity in the dorsal raphe nucleus (serotonergic) but its absence from the locus coeruleus (adrenergic).[94] NADPH-diaphorase is a marker which correlates with nitric oxide synthase activity. Given this recent interest in nitric oxide induction as a headache model, a theme can be developed from laboratory observations, through PET studies in humans and continuing into therapeutic responses in migraine suffers which implicates central aminergic dysfunction in the pathogenesis of migraine.

Observations on the pathophysiology of daily headache

The neurotrophins, a group of structurally related proteins, include nerve growth factor (NGF), brain derived nerve factor (BDNF), NT-3, NT-4 and NT-5, whose actions are mediated by specific receptors.[95] A low-affinity (so-called P75) receptor binds all the neurotrophins. High-affinity receptors are now known to be the protein tyrosine kineses, TrkA, TrkB and TrkC. NGF binds selectively to TrkA, BDNF and NT-5 to TrkB, and NT-3 to TrkC. In developing animals, NGF promotes the survival of sympathetic neurons and some sensory neurons. Evidence now links altered neurotrophin levels to the sensory disturbances (pain and hyperalgesia) associated with peripheral inflammatory states. One feature of the inflammatory response is a large upregulation of NGF production. The sensory neurons innervating the affected tissue show increased retrograde delivery of NGF and increased neuropeptide expression. Anti-NGF treatment can block hyperalgesia.[96]

Nerve growth factor may sensitize primary afferent nerve terminals, either directly through the high-affinity receptor on those terminals or indirectly following the release of mediators from other local cells.[97] Mast cells, which express the high-affinity NGF receptor, are degranulated by NGF. Mast cells occur around the cerebral blood vessels and may be involved in neurogenic inflammation[98], a model for the acute migraine attack. Increased NGF levels may also lead to a central neuronal sensitization.[99] NGF and inflammatory cytokines may change the behaviour of sensory neurons making them more sensitive to nociception. NGF increases the synthesis, transport, and neuronal content of substance P and CGRP. It also regulates two ion channels in sensory neurons: the capsaicin receptor ion channel[162] and the tetrodotoxin-resistant Na^+ channel.

Could central sensitization play a role in daily headache?

In animal models of head pain there is good evidence for Fos activation in the trigeminal nucleus caudalis.[56] In the superficial dorsal horn of the caudal most parts of the trigeminal nucleus, Fos is a marker for stimulation and may be one signal for the nervous system's adaptive responses to insult.[97,100] Fos and jun, two immediate early gene products, can alter cell proteins, receptors and other peptides, perhaps accounting for long-lasting neuronal sensitization. Sensitization of the trigeminal neurons may result in increased activation of the trigeminovascular system. Central sensitization is a well described phenomenon in animal research. It is manifested by increased spontaneous impulse discharges, increased responsiveness to noxious and non-noxious peripheral stimuli, and expanded receptive fields of nociceptive neurons. In animal models, conditioning stimuli that activate C (unmyelinated) fibres result in a marked and prolonged increase in the flexion withdrawal reflex in rats. Repetitive C-fibre stimulation at constant intensity induces the phenomenon of wind-up, which is the increase in dorsal horn nociceptive neuron responsiveness in both magnitude and duration with each subsequent stimulus above a certain frequency.[101]

Wind-up is sensitive to glutamate N-methyl-D-aspartate (NMDA) receptor antagonists. Neurons that exhibit wind-up are less sensitive to opioids than are neurons that do not exhibit this phenomenon. Wind-up is a short-lasting phenomenon and cannot explain the phenomenon of sensitization, which is of longer duration and may involve changes in neuronal plasticity.[99] Wind-up is mediated by NMDA and tachykinin receptors, is blocked by morphine pretreatment, and is accompanied by calcium entry via NMDA channels. It may be the trigger to long-lasting neuronal sensitization. The increased intracellular calcium induces translocation (from cytosolic to membrane-bound form) and activation of protein kinase C (PKC) and phosphorylation of the NMDA channel which relieves the Mg^{2+} block on the ion channel. The increased calcium may also be responsible for the induction of the genes whose products are Fos and Jun.[102] This results in increased glutamate sensitivity. This cascade can be interrupted by local anaesthesia, non-NMDA and NMDA antagonists, and gangliosides (which prevent or reduce PKC translocation and activation). Nitric oxide, a diffusible neurotransmitted gas that acts as a transmitter, is produced in response to NMDA receptor activation and may contribute to nociception.

Pain modulation in relationship to daily headache

The mammalian nervous system contains networks that modulate nociceptive transmission. In the rostroventromedial medulla are so-called 'off-cells' that inhibit and 'on-cells' that facilitate nociception. These cells are believed to modulate the activity of the trigeminal and dorsal horn neurons. Increased on-cell activity in the brainstem's pain modulation system could enhance the response to both painful and non-painful stimuli. Opiate withdrawal results in increased firing of the on-cells, decreased firing of the off-cells, and enhanced nociception.[103] A similar mechanism may occur during drug-induced headaches.[104] Some forms of chronic daily headache (see Chapter 8) may result, in part, from enhanced neuronal activity in the trigeminal nucleus caudalis as a result of enhanced on-cell or decreased off-cell activity. Other conditioned stimuli associated with pain and stress can also turn on the system and may account for some of the association between pain and stress.

Neuropharmacology of migraine treatment: what can we learn?

Serotonin and migraine

Several lines of indirect evidence suggest a relationship between serotonin and migraine. It was observed some three decades ago that urinary excretion of 5-hydroxyindoleacetic acid, the main metabolite of serotonin, is increased in association with migraine attacks[105] and that platelet 5-HT drops rapidly during the onset of the migraine attack.[106] Furthermore, 5-HT depletion can induce a migraine attack[107], while intravenous 5-HT can abort acute migraine attacks.[107,108] Headaches similar to migraine can be triggered by serotonergic drugs such as reserpine (a 5-HT releaser and depleter) and m-chlorophenylpiperazine (m-CPP) (a serotonergic agonist).[109,110] In the years following the intravenous 5-HT obser-vations, Humphrey and his colleagues clarified the 5-HT receptor responsible for selective cranial vasoconstriction[111] and this lead to the development of sumatriptan.[112] 5-HT receptors consist of at least three distinct types of molecular structures: guanine nucleotide G protein-coupled receptors, ligand-gated ion channels and transporters. There are at least seven classes of 5-HT receptors: $5-HT_1$, $5HT_2$, $5-HT_3$, $5-HT_4$, $5-HT_5$, $5-HT_6$, and $5-HT_7$ (Table 5.2).[113] In humans there are at least five $5-HT_1$ receptor subtypes: $5-HT_{1A}$, $5-HT_{1B}$, $5-HT_{1D}$, $5-HT_{1E}$, and $5-HT_{1F}$ [114] and the various *triptans* are active at a number of these sub-types (Table 5.3). At this time the $5-HT_{1B/1D}$ agonist actions seem most relevant to the action of the *triptans* but only more refined compounds will eventually clearly define the relevant receptor for the anti-migraine activity.

Pharmacology of plasma protein extravasation

The pharmacology of neurogenic plasma extravasation has recently been examined in detail in search of newer approaches to the treatment of acute attacks. Plasma

● **Table 5.2** *Classification of serotonin receptors**

5-HT receptor class	Second messenger	Antagonist	Function
1	↓Adenylate cyclase		See Table 5.3 for details
2	↑Phosphoino-sitide turnover	Methysergide Pizotifen	Contraction of smooth muscle
			Central nervous system excitation Subtypes: 2A, 2B, 2C
3	K+	Ondansetron Granisetron	Membrane depolarisation
4	↑Adenylate cyclase	GR113808	Stimulates GI contraction
5	—		Subclasses a & b
6	—		Single receptor
7	↑Adenylate cyclase	—	Subclasses a & b[157]
			Role in circadian rhythms

Modified from Hoyer and colleagues[113].

● **Table 5.3** *Classification of serotonin (5-HT) subclass 1 receptors.**

Subtype of $5-HT_1$ receptor	Agonist	Antagonist	Function
A	8-OH-DPAT† Dihydroergotamine	WAY100165†	Hypotension Behavioural (satiety)
Rat B Human B (previously known as $1_{Dβ}$)	CP-93,129† Sumatriptan Dihydroergotamine Eletriptan Naratriptan Rizatriptan Zolmitriptan	GR127935†	Central autoreceptor (rat) Craniovascular receptor
D (previously known as $1_{Dα}$)	Sumatriptan Dihydroergotamine Eletriptan Naratriptan Rizatriptan Zolmitriptan	GR127935†	Trigeminal neuronal receptor
E	Rizatriptan††	—	?
F	Sumatriptan Dihydroergotamine Naratriptan Rizatriptan Zolmitriptan LY334370**	—	?

*Modified from Hartig and colleagues[114].
**Currently in early development.
†8-OH-DPAT (8-hydroxy-2-(di-n-propylamino)tetralin), WAY100165, CP-93,129 and GR127935 are all compounds used in the laboratory for pharmacological purposes and have no current clinical indications.
††Drug agonist actions are relative and the inclusion of rizatriptan as an agonist at $5HT_{1E}$ sites is based on a published comparison with sumatriptan[158].

extravasation can be blocked by ergot alkaloids[115], indomethacin, acetylsalicylic acid[116], the serotonin (5-HT$_{1B/1D}$) agonist sumatriptan[117], GABA agonists, such as valproate and benzodiazepines[118–120], neurosteroids[121], substance P antagonists[122] and the endothelin antagonist bosentan.[123] These models do not always predict anti-migraine efficacy.[124] The lack of effect of bosentan in migraine as an unequivocal outcome from a double-blind placebo controlled study of its intravenous use[125] contrasts with data in the neurogenic inflammation model[123], but is in line with other observations.[126] Furthermore, the demonstration of a lack of clinical effect in acute migraine attacks of two orally administered substance P antagonists, RPR100893[127] and lanepitant[128], in double-blind randomized placebo-controlled trials casts some doubt upon the importance of peripherally released substance P in migraine. Furthermore, the potency of CP122 288 in neurogenically-induced PPE[129], must be viewed in the context of the fact that this compound at PPE blocking doses has no effect in acute migraine.[130] In this context CP122 288 neither blocks fos expression in the trigeminocervical complex[131] nor reduces CGRP release[132] after stimulation of the superior sagittal sinus in the cat.

Pharmacology of trigeminal neurons

Experimental pharmacological evidence indicates that many of the abortive anti-migraine drugs, such as ergots[132,133], acetylsalicylic acid[134], sumatriptan (after blood–brain barrier disruption),[135,136] zolmitriptan (311C90)[137,138], naratriptan[139], and rizatriptan[140] act at second order trigeminal neurons to reduce cell activity, suggesting trigeminocervical complex neurons in the caudal brainstem as a possible target for anti-migraine compounds. It is likely that this central action is largely mediated by the 5-HT$_{1B/1D}$ actions of the drugs since the effect of naratriptan can be antagonized by the 5-HT$_{1B/1D}$ antagonist GR127935.[139] Similarly, and perhaps bringing the 5-HT argument full circle, 5-HT when administered intravenously in experimental animals will inhibit trigeminal neuron firing an effect also blocked by GR127935.[141] Furthermore, given the results of autoradiographic studies which indicate specific binding of DHE[132] and zolmitriptan[142] in the trigeminocervical complex neurons and inhibition of firing by microiontophoretic application of zolmitriptan and ergometrine onto these neurons[143], it is highly likely that there are functional inhibitory, probably 5-HT$_{1D}$, receptors on trigeminocervical complex neurons.

Clinical observations and drug mechanisms

The clinical outcome with substance P antagonists are consistent with clinical observations of a lack of release of substance P in migraineurs during headache[45] and observations in our own model systems. Since calcitonin

gene-related peptide (CGRP) but not substance P is released in humans during migraine[45,46,50] it is likely that it is the CGRP-enriched innervation of the cerebral circulation[145,146] that plays the major role in the pain of migraine. Similarly in cluster headache[47,48] and the closely related chronic paroxysmal hemicrania[49], CGRP but not substance P is released. The latter syndromes may be lumped together under the pathophysiological rubric of trigeminal-autonomic cephalgias (TACs) and are associated with parasympathetic activation and release of vasoactive intestinal polypeptide (VIP).[147] These data suggest that the animal models of trigeminovascular activation[148] can explain the pain and some of the associated symptoms of migraine and cluster headache. To test the role of both CGRP and VIP in acute headache, specific antagonists will be required. Given that we have observed that excitatory amino acid transmission of both an NMDA and non-NMDA type takes place in the trigeminocervical complex (Storer and Goadsby, unpublished data) it is possible that a single post-synaptic solution may not be clinically helpful.

The future

The actual treatment response to the predictions made by the various migraine models will help to define the pathophysiology of the disease with more precision. There has been some effort to move away from drugs with a vascular action, which all the 5-HT$_{1B/1D}$ agonist[114] compounds possess, to more neurally active compounds, such as CP122 288[129], substance P antagonists and endothelin antagonists, although currently without success. Based on initial molecular biological studies it has been suggested that the trigeminal ganglion may preferentially contain 5-HT$_{1D}$ receptors[149] and the blood vessels 5-HT$_{1B}$ receptors.[150,151] However, both receptors may be found, to some extent, in both tissues and even in the human coronary vessels (Table 5.4), a target most clinicians would seek to avoid. While it may be possible that neurogenically-mediated sterile plasma extravasation may play a role in the expression of migraine pain it is not clear whether this is sufficient of

● **Table 5.4** Location of triptan (5-HT$_{1B/1D}$) receptors in humans

Site	5-HT$_{1B}$	5-HT$_{1D}$
Extracerebral cranial vessels	+++	±
Cerebral microvessels	–	+
Trigeminal ganglion	++	+++
Coronary vessels	+++	±

Note: + and – indicate relative strength of mRNA signal from tissues which is not quantitative nor does it indicate the relative contribution of the receptors to drug actions. Data are modified after Hamel[150,151].

itself or requires other stimulators or promotors. Certainly other receptor targets would be attractive. An exclusive 5-HT$_{1D}$ agonist which would have neuronal actions only would be attractive and such a compound has been developed[152] and could be expected to go into clinical trial. Sumatriptan and many of the other *triptans* are also 5-HT$_{1F}$ agonists which has given impetus to studying a specific 5-HT$_{1F}$ agonist in clinical trials.[153] However, the current compound may not differentiate between peripheral and central neuronal mechanisms since there are 5-HT$_{1F}$ receptors in the brainstem[154] and would only add a second mechanism of action to 5-HT$_{1B/1D}$ agonism since the clinically effective compound alniditan[155] is inactive at the 5-HT$_{1F}$ receptor.[156]

Summary

An understanding of the basic anatomy and physiology of the cranial circulation facilitates the assessment and management of patients with headache, particularly *neurovascular-type* headaches, such as migraine. Migraine should be viewed as an episodic syndrome of pain, probably involving intracranial structures, and certainly associated with other neurological disturbances. It is the syndromic nature of migraine that is its core characteristic and this attribute is conferred by the brain and the connections that process and control head pain. The aminergic nuclei, whose usual role is to gate afferent nociceptive information, modulate cerebral blood flow and blood–brain barrier permeability and control the signal-to-noise aspect of sensory inputs, are the crucial sites in migraine. Indeed they are strong candidates for the *lesion* in the classical neurological sense. When these modulatory controls are triggered or timed to dysfunction the migrainous process is driven by the brain, releasing sensory inputs to create Liveing's *nerve storm*. At once vessels pulsing normally can be felt to pulse, fluid in an otherwise satisfied stomach is perceived as nausea, normal lights, sounds or smells are perceived as pungent or unpleasant and normal movement perceived to jar and disturb the head. The trigeminovascular system provides a therapeutic target for attack treatment as it arrests the final common pathway for expression of *neurovascular* head pain, the brain, however, provides the essential key to the disorder, the key to its genesis and the key to its ultimate understanding and control.

References

1. Joutel A, Bousser MG, Biousse V, *et al*. A gene for familial hemiplegic migraine maps to chromosome 19. *Nature Genetics* 1993; 5: 40–5.

2. May A, Ophoff RA, Terwindt GM, *et al*. Familial hemiplegic migraine locus on chromosome 19p13 is involved in common forms of migraine with and without aura. *Human Genetics* 1995; 96: 604–8.

3. Ophoff RA, Terwindt GM, Vergouwe MN, *et al*. Familial hemiplegic migraine and episodic ataxia type-2 are caused by mutations in the Ca^{2+} channel gene CACNLA4. *Cell* 1996; 87: 543–52.

4. Goadsby PJ, Boyce G. Paroxysmal cerbellar ataxia. *Aust. NZ J. Med.* 1990; 20: 103.

5. Vahedi K, Joutel A, Bogaert Pv, *et al*. A gene for hereditary paroxysmal cerebellar ataxia maps to chromosome 19p. *Ann. Neurol.* 1995; 37: 289–93.

6. Ramadan NM, Halvorson H, Vande-Linde A, Levine SR, Helpern JA, Welch KMA. Low brain magnesium in migraine. *Headache* 1989; 29: 416–19.

7. Griggs RC, Nutt JG. Episodic ataxias as channelopathies. *Ann. Neurol.* 1995; 37: 285–7.

8. Ducros A, Joutel A, Vahedi K, *et al*. Familial hemiplegic migraine: mapping of the second gene and evidence for a third locus. *Cephalalgia* 1997; 17: 232.

9. Somerville BW. The role of estradiol withdrawal in the etiology of menstrual migraine. *Neurology* 1972; 22: 355–65.

10. Griffiths LR, Nyholt DR, Curtain RP, Goadsby PJ, Brimage PJ. Migraine association and linkage studies of an endothelial nitric oxide synthase (NOS3) gene polymorphism. *Neurology* 1997; 49: 614–17.

11. Nyholt DR, Curtain RP, Gaffney PT, Brimage P, Goadsby PJ, Griffiths LR. Migraine association and linkage analyses of the human 5-hydroxytryptamine (5-HT$_{2A}$) receptor gene. *Cephalgia* 1996;16: 463–7.

12. Russell MB, Andersson PG, Thomsen LL, Iselius L. Cluster headache is an autosomal dominantly inherited disorder in some families: a complex segregation analysis. *J Medical Genetics* 1995; 32: 954–6.

13. Kupfermann I. Hypothalamus and limbic system II: motivation. In: Kandel ER, Schwartz JH, eds. *Principles of Neural Science*. Amsterdam Science Publishers: Elsevier, 1985: 626–35.

14. Swaab DF, Hofman MA, Lucassen PJ, Purba JS, Raadsheer FC, Nes JAvd. Functional neuroanatomy and neuropathology of the hypothalamus. *Anat. Embryol.* 1993; 187: 317–30.

15. Moore-Ede MC. The circadian timing system in mammals: two pacemakers preside over many secondary oscillators. *Fed. Proc.* 1983; 42: 2802–8.

16. Woods RP, Iacoboni M, Mazziotta JC. Bilateral spreading cerebral hypoperfusion during spontaneous migraine headache. *N. Eng. J. Med.* 1994; 331:1689–92.

17. Olesen J, Friberg L, Skyhoj-Olsen T, *et al.* Timing and topography of cerebral blood flow, aura and headache during migraine attacks. *Ann. Neurol.* 1990; 28: 791–8.

18. Olesen J. Cerebral and extracranial circulatory disturbances in migraine: pathophysiological implications. *Cerebrovascular and Brain Metabolism Reviews* 1991; 3: 1–28.

19. Olesen J, Larsen B, Lauritzen M. Focal hyperemia followed by spreading oligemia and impaired activation of rCBF in classic migraine. *Ann. Neurol.* 1981; 9: 344–52.

20. Leao AAP. Spreading depression of activity in cerebral cortex. *J. Neurophysiol.* 1944; 7: 359–90.

21. Leao AAP. Pial circulation and spreading activity in the cerebral cortex. *J. Neurophysiol.* 1944; 7: 391–6.

22. Leao AAP. Further observations on the spreading depression of of activity in the cerebral cortex. *J. Neurophysiol.* 1947; 10: 409–14.

23. Lauritzen M. Long-lasting reduction of cortical blood flow of the rat brain after spreading depression with preserved autoregulation and impaired CO_2 response. *J. Cereb. Blood Flow Metabol.* 1984; 4: 546–54.

24. Lauritzen M, Skyhoj-Olsen T, Lassen NA, Paulson OB. Regulation of regional cerebral blood flow during and between migraine attacks. *Ann. Neurol.* 1983; 14: 569–72.

25. Lauritzen M. Pathophysiology of the migraine aura. The spreading depression theory. *Brain* 1994; 117: 199–210.

26. Andersen AR, Friberg L, Skyhoj-Olsen T, Olesen J. SPECT demonstration of delayed hyperemia following hypoperfusion in classic migraine. *Arch. Neurol.* 1988; 45: 154–9.

27. Lashley KS. Patterns of cerebral integration indicated by the scotomas of migraine. *Arch. Neurol. Psychiatry* 1941; 46: 331–9.

28. Barkley GL, Leheta BJ, Tepley N, Gaymer J, Aboukasm A, Welch KMA. Effects of dihydroergotamine on spreading depression. In: Olesen J, Saxena PR, eds. *5-Hydroxytryptamine mechanisms in primary headaches.* New York: Raven Press, 1991: 236–41.

29. Welch KMA, D'Andrea G, Tepley N, Barkeley GL, Ramadan NM. The concept of migraine as a state of central neuronal hyperexcitability. *Headache* 1990; 8(4): 817–28.

30. Welch KM, Ramadan NM. Mitochondria, magnesium and migraine. *J. Neurol. Sci.* 1995;134: 9–14.

31. Ruskell GL, Simons T. Trigeminal nerve pathways to the cerebral arteries in monkeys. *J. of Anatomy* 1987; 155: 23–37.

32. Liu-Chen LY, Mayberg MR, Moskowitz MA. Immunohistochemical evidence for a substance P-containing trigeminovascular pathway to pial arteries in cats. *Brain Res.* 1983; 268:162–6.

33. Uddman R, Edvinsson L, Ekman R, Kingman T, McCulloch J. Innervation of the feline cerebral vasculature by nerve fibers containing calcitonin gene-related peptide: trigeminal origin and co-existence with substance P. *Neurosci. Lett.* 1985; 62:131–6.

34. Goadsby PJ, Edvinsson L, Ekman R. Release of vasoactive peptides in the extracerebral circulation of man and the cat during activation of the trigeminovascular system. *Ann. Neurol.* 1988; 23: 193–6.

35. Feindel W, Penfield W, McNaughton F. The tentorial nerves and localisation of intracranial pain in man. *Neurology* 1960;10: 555–63.

36. Wolff HG. *Headache and other head pain*. New York: Oxford University Press, 1963.

37. Penfield W, McNaughton FL. Dural headache and the innervation of the dura mater. *Arch. Neurol. Psychiatry* 1940; 44: 43–75.

38. Penfield W. A contribution to the mechanism of intracranial pain. *Proc.of the Association for Research in Nervous and Mental Disease* 1934;15: 399–415.

39. Graham JR, Wolff HG. Mechanism of migraine headache and action of ergotamine tartrate. *Arch. Neurol. Psychiatry* 1938; 39: 737–63.

40. Drummond PD, Lance JW. Extracranial vascular changes and the source of pain in migraine headache. *Ann. Neurol.* 1983;13: 32–7.

41. Nichols FT, Mawad M, Mohr JP, Hilal S, Adams RJ. Focal headache during balloon inflation in the vertebral and basilar arteries. *Headache* 1993; 33: 87–9.

42. Moskowitz MA, Cutrer FM. Sumatriptan: a receptor-targeted treatment for migraine. *Ann. Rev. Med.* 1993; 44: 145–54.

43. Strassman AM, Raymond SA, Burstein R. Sensitization of meningeal sensory neurons and the origin of headaches. *Nature* 1996; 384: 560–3.

44. Zagami AS, Goadsby PJ, Edvinsson L. Stimulation of the superior sagittal sinus in the cat causes release of vasoactive peptides. *Neuropeptides* 1990;16: 69–75.

45. Goadsby PJ, Edvinsson L, Ekman R. Vasoactive peptide release in the extracerebral circulation of humans during migraine headache. *Ann. Neurol.* 1990; 28: 183–7.

46. Gallai V, Sarchielli P, Floridi A, *et al.* Vasoactive peptides levels in the plasma of young migraine patients with and without aura assessed both interictally and ictally. *Cephalalgia* 1995; 15: 384–90.

47. Goadsby PJ, Edvinsson L. Human *in vivo* evidence for trigeminovascular activation in cluster headache. *Brain* 1994; 117: 427–34.

48. Fanciullacci M, Alessandri M, Figini M, Geppetti P, Michelacci S. Increases in plasma calcitonin gene-related peptide from extracerebral circulation during nitroglycerin-induced cluster headache attack. *Pain* 1995; 60: 119–123.

49. Goadsby PJ, Edvinsson L. Neuropeptide changes in a case of chronic paroxysmal hemicrania-evidence for trigemino-parasympathetic activation. *Cephalalgia* 1996; 16: 448–50.

50. Goadsby PJ, Edvinsson L. The trigeminovascular system and migraine: studies characterising cerebrovascular and neuropeptide changes seen in man and cat. *Ann. Neurol.* 1993; 33: 48–56.

51. Couch JR, Saper J, Meloche JP. Treatment of migraine with BMS180048: response at 2 hours. *Headache* 1996; 36: 523–30.

52. Ryan RE, Elkind A, Goldstein J. Twenty-four hour effectiveness of BMS 180048 in the acute treatment of migraine headaches. *Headache* 1997; 37: 245–8.

53. Knight YE, Edvinsson L, Goadsby PJ. Blockade of release of CGRP after superior sagittal sinus stimulation in cat: a comparison of avitriptan and CP122,288. *Cephalalgia* 1997;17: 248.

54. Nozaki K, Boccalini P, Moskowitz MA. Expression of c-fos-like immunoreactivity in brainstem after meningeal irritation by blood in the subarachnoid space. *Neuroscience* 1992; 49: 669–80.

55. Kaube H, Keay K, Hoskin KL, Bandler R, Goadsby PJ. Expression of c-fos-like immunoreactivity in the trigeminal nucleus caudalis and high cervical cord following stimulation of the sagittal sinus in the cat. *Brain Res.* 1993; 629: 95–102.

56. Goadsby PJ, Hoskin KL. The distribution of trigeminovascular afferents in the non-human primate brain *macaca nemestrina*: a c-fos immunocytochemical study. *J. of Anatomy* 1997;190: 367–75.

57. Goadsby PJ, Zagami AS. Stimulation of the superior sagittal sinus increases metabolic activity and blood flow in certain regions of the brainstem and upper cervical spinal cord of the cat. *Brain* 1991;114: 1001–11.

58. Goadsby PJ, Hoskin KL, Knight YE. Stimulation of the greater occipital nerve increases metabolic activity in the trigeminal nucleus caudalis and cervical dorsal horn of the cat. *Pain* 1997: in press.

59. Strassman AM, Vos BP, Mineta Y, Naderi S, Borsook D, Burstein R. Fos-like immunoreactivity in the superficial medullary dorsal horn induced by noxious and innocuous thermal stimulation of the facial skin in the rat. *J. Neurophysiol.* 1993; 70: 1811–21.

60. Zagami AS, Lambert GA. Stimulation of cranial vessels excites nociceptive neurones in several thalamic nuclei of the cat. *Exp. Brain Res.* 1990; 81: 552–66.

61. Zagami AS, Lambert GA. Craniovascular application of capsaicin activates nociceptive thalamic neurons in the cat. *Neurosci. Lett.* 1991; 121: 187–90.

62. Zagami AS, Gordon V, Lambert GA. Medial thalamic neurones respond to electrical stimulation of cranial vessels. *J. of Clinical Neuroscience* 1996; 3: 412–13.

63. Weiller C, May A, Limmroth V, *et al.* Brain stem activation in spontaneous human migraine attacks. *Nature Medicine* 1995; 1: 658–60.

64. Goadsby PJ, Lambert GA, Lance JW. Differential effects on the internal and external carotid circulation of the monkey evoked by locus coeruleus stimulation. *Brain Res.* 1982; 249: 247–54.

65. Goadsby PJ, Lambert GA, Lance JW. The mechanism of cerebrovascular vasoconstriction in response to locus coeruleus stimulation. *Brain Res.* 1985; 326: 213–17.

66. Goadsby PJ, Lambert GA, Lance JW. Effects of locus coeruleus stimulation on carotid vascular resistance in the cat. *Brain Res.* 1983; 278: 175–83.

67. Goadsby PJ, Lambert GA, Lance JW. Stimulation of the trigeminal ganglion increases flow in the extracerebral but not the cerebral circulation of the monkey. *Brain Res.* 1986; 381: 63–7.

68. Goadsby PJ, Duckworth JW. Low frequency stimulation of the locus coeruleus reduces regional cerebral blood flow in the spinalized cat. *Brain Res.* 1989; 476: 71–7.

69. Goadsby PJ, Piper RD, Lambert GA, Lance JW. The effect of activation of the nucleus raphe dorsalis (DRN) on carotid blood flow. I The Monkey. *Am. J. Physiol.* 1985; 248: R257–62.

70. Goadsby PJ, Piper RD, Lambert GA, Lance JW. The effect of activation of the nucleus raphe dorsalis (DRN) on carotid blood flow. II The Cat. *Am. J. Physiol.* 1985; 248: R263–9.

71. Underwood MD, Bakalian MJ, Arango V, Smith RW, Mann JJ. Regulation of cortical blood flow by the dorsal raphe nucleus: topographic organization of cerebrovascular regulatory regions. *J. Cereb. Blood Flow Metabol.* 1992; 12: 664–73.

72. Basbaum AI, Fields HL. Endogenous pain control mechanisms: review and hypothesis. *Ann. Neurol.* 1978; 4: 451–62.

73. Reichling DB, Basbaum AI. Collateralization of periaqueductal gray neurons to forebrain or diencephalon and to the medullary nucleus raphe magnus in the rat. *Neuroscience* 1991; 42: 183–200.

74. Goadsby PJ, Silberstein SD. *Headache.* New York: Butterworth-Heinemann, 1997.

75. Raskin NH, Hosobuchi Y, Lamb S. Headache may arise from perturbation of brain. *Headache* 1987; 27: 416–20.

76. Keay KA, Kaube H, Hoskin KL, Bandler R, Goadsby PJ. FOS expression in the midbrain periaqueductal gray of the cat evoked by electrical stimulation of the superior sagittal sinus. *Proc. Aust. Neuro. Soc.* 1993; 4: 179.

77. Maertens de Noordhout A, Timsit-Berthier M, Timsit M, Schoenen J. Contingent negative variation and headache. *Annals Neurology* 1986; 19: 78–80.

78. Bocker KB, Timsit-Berthier M, Schoenen J, Brunia CH. Contingent negative variation in migraine. *Headache* 1990; 30: 604–9.

79. Schoenen J, Timsit-Berthier M. Contingent negative variation: methods and potential interest in headache. *Cephalalgia* 1993; 13: 28–32.

80. Maertens de Noordhout A, Timsit-Berthier M, Schoenen J. Contingent negative variation (CNV) in migraineurs before and during prophylactic treatment with beta-blockers. *Cephalalgia* 1985; 5 (suppl 3): 34–5.

81. Schoenen J, Wang W, Albert A, Delwaide PJ. Potentiation instead of habituation characterizes visual evoked potentials in migraine patients between attacks. *Eur. J. of Neurology* 1995; 2: 115–22.

82. Harper AM, MacKenzie ET, McCulloch J, Pickard JD. Migraine and the blood-brain barrier. *Lancet* 1977; 1 (8020): 1034–6.

83. Alvarez-Cermeno J, Gobernado JM, Aimeno A. Transient blood-brain barrier (BBB) damage in migraine. *Headache* 1986; 26: 437.

84. Nissila M, Parkkola R, Sonninen P, Salonen R. Intracerebral arteries and gadolinium enhancement in migraine without aura. *Cephalalgia* 1996; 16: 363.

85. Bates D, Ashford E, Dawson R, *et al.* Subcutaneous sumatriptan during the migraine aura. *Neurology* 1994; 44: 1587–92.

86. Visser WH, Vriend RHMd, Jaspers NMWH, Ferrari MD. Sumatriptan in clinical practice. *Neurology* 1996; 47: 46–51.

87. Aube M. Treatment of slow-developing migraine with subcutaneous sumatriptan. *Cephalalgia* 1995; 15 (Suppl 14): 231.

88. Visser WH, Klein KB, Cox RC, Jones D, Ferrari M. 311C90, a new central and peripherally acting 5-HT-1D receptor agonist in the acute oral treatment of migraine: a double-blind, placebo-controlled dose-range finding study. *Neurology* 1996; 46: 522–6.

89. Jackson NC. A comparison of oral eletriptan (UK-116,044) (20-80mg) and oral sumatriptan (100mg) in the acute treatment of migraine. *Cephalalgia* 1996; 16: 368–9.

90. Dowson A, Ramphul-Gokulsing S, Klein K, Cox R, Wilkinson M, Gross M. Can oral 311C90, a novel 5-HT$_{1D}$ agonist, prevent migraine headache when taken during an aura? *Cephalalgia* 1995; 15 (Suppl 14): 173.

91. Raichle ME, Hartman BK, Eichling JO, Sharpe LG. Central noradrenergic regulation of cerebral blood flow and vascular permeability. *Proc. Natl. Acad. Sci. (USA)* 1975; 72: 3726–30.

92. Preskorn SH, Hartman BK, Raichle ME, Clark HB. The effect of dibenzazepine (tricyclic antidepressants) on cerebral capillary permeability in the rat in vivo. *J. Pharmacol. Exp. Ther.* 1980; 213: 313–20.

93. Harik SI, McGunigal T. The protective influence of the locus ceruleus on the blood-brain barrier. *Ann. Neurol.* 1984;15: 568–74.

94. Johnson MD, Ma PM. Localization of NADPH diaphorase activity in monoaminergic neurons of the rat brain. *J. Comp. Neurol.* 1993; 332: 391–406.

95. Montalcini RL, Daltoso R, Dellavalle F, Skaper SD, Leon A. Update of the NGF saga. *J. Neurol. Sci.* 1995;130: 119–127.

96. Dray A, Urban L, Dickenson A. Pharmacology of chronic pain. *Trends in the Pharmacological Sciences* 1994; 15: 190–7.

97. Mungliani R, Hunt SP. Molecular biology of pain. *Brit. J. of Anaesthesia* 1995; 75: 186–92.

98. Dimitriadou V, Buzzi MG, Theoharides TC, Moskowitz MA. Ultrastructural evidence for neurogenically mediated changes in blood vessels of the rat dura mater and tongue following antidromic trigeminal stimulation. *Neuroscience* 1992; 48: 187–203.

99. Woolf CJ. Somatic pain: pathogenesis and prevention. *Brit. J. of Anaesthesia* 1995; 75: 169–76.

100. Hunt SP, Pini A, Evan G. Induction of c-fos like protein in spinal cord neurons following sensory stimulation. *Nature* 1987; 328: 1686–1704.

101. Mendell LM. Physiologic properties of unmyelinated fibre projection to the spinal cord. *Exp. Neurol.* 1966; 16: 316–332.

102. Price DD, Mao J, Mayer DJ. Central neural mechanisms of normal and abnormal pain states. In: Fields HL, Liebeskind JC, eds. *Progress in Pain Research and Management*. Washington: IASP Press, 1994: 61-84. vol 1).

103. Fields HL, Heinricher MM, Mason P. Neurotransmitters in nociceptive modulatory circuits. *Ann. Rev. of Neuroscience* 1991; 14: 219–45.

104. Scholz E, Diener H-C, Geiselhart S, Wilkinson M. Drug-induced headache: does a critical dosage exist? In: Diener H-C, ed. *Drug-induced headache*. Berlin: Springer-Verlag, 1988: 29–43.

105. Sicuteri F. Vasoneuroactive substances and their implications in vascular pain. *Research and Clinical Studies in Headache* 1967; 1: 6–45.

106. Curran DA, Hinterberger H, Lance JW. Total plasma serotonin, 5-hydroxyindoleacetic acid and p-hydroxy-m-methoxymandelic acid excretion in normal and migrainous subjects. *Brain* 1965; 88: 997–1010.

107. Anthony M, Hinterberger H, Lance JW. The possible relationship of serotonin to the migraine syndrome. In: Friedman AP, ed. *Research and Clinical Studies in Headache*. Basel: Karger, 1969: 29–59. vol 2).

108. Kimball RW, Friedman AP, Vallejo E. Effect of serotonin in migraine patients. *Neurology (Minneap.)* 1960; 10: 107–11.

109. Brewerton TD, Murphy DL, Mueller EA, Jimerson DC. Induction of migraine like headaches by the serotonin agonist m-chlorophenlypiperazine. *Clin. Pharmacol. Therap*. 1988; 43: 605–9.

110. Brewerton TD, Murphy DL, Lesem MD, Brandt HA, Jimerson DC. Headache responses following m-chloro-phenylpiperazine in bulimics and controls. *Headache* 1992; 32: 217–22.

111. Feniuk W, Humphrey PPA, Perren MJ. The selective carotid arterial vasoconstrictor action of GR43175 in anaesthetised dogs. *Br. J. Pharmacol.* 1989; 96: 83-90.

112. Humphrey PPA, Feniuk W, Marriott AS, Tanner RJN, Jackson MR, Tucker ML. Preclinical studies on the anti-migraine drug, sumatriptan. *Eur. Neurol.* 1991; 31: 282–90.

113. Hoyer D, Clarke DE, Fozard JR, *et al.* International Union of Pharmacology classification of receptors for 5-hydroxytryptamine (Serotonin). *Pharmacol. Rev.* 1994; 46: 157–203.

114. Hartig PR, Hoyer D, Humphrey PPA, Martin GR. Alignment of receptor nomenclature with the human genome: classification of 5-HT-1B and 5-HT1D receptor subtypes. *Trends in the Pharmacological Sciences* 1996; 17: 103–5.

115. Markowitz S, Saito K, Moskowitz MA. Neurogenically mediated plasma extravasation in dura mater: effect of ergot alkaloids. A possible mechanism of action in vascular headache. *Cephalalgia* 1988; 8: 83–91.

116. Buzzi MG, Sakas DE, Moskowitz MA. Indomethacin and acetylsalicylic acid block neurogenic plasma protein extravasation in rat dura mater. *Eur. J. Pharmacol.* 1989; 165: 251–8.

117. Buzzi MG, Moskowitz MA. The antimigraine drug, sumatriptan (GR43175), selectively blocks neurogenic plasma extravasation from blood vessels in dura mater. *Br. J. Pharmacol.* 1990; 99: 202–6.

118. Lee WK, Limmroth V, Ayata C, *et al.* Peripheral GABA-A receptor mediated effects of sodium valproate on dural plasma protein extravasation to substance P and trigeminal stimulation. *Br. J. Pharmacol.* 1995; 116: 1661–7.

119. Cutrer FM, Limmroth V, Ayata G, Moskowitz MA. Attenuation by valproate of c-fos immunoreactivity in trigeminal nucleus caudalis induced by intracisternal capsaicin. *Br. J. Pharmacol.* 1995; 116 :3199–204.

120. Cutrer FM, Limmroth V, Ayata G, Moskowitz MA. Valproate reduces c-Fos expression in the trigeminal nucleus caudalis (TNC) after noxious meningeal stimulation. *Cephalalgia* 1995;15 (Suppl 14): 96.

121. Limmroth V, Lee WS, Cutrer FM, Waeber C, Moskowitz MA. Progesterone and its ring-A-reduced metabolites suppress dural plasma protein extravasation by activation of peripheral GABA$_A$-receptors. *Cephalalgia* 1995; 15 (Suppl 14): 98.

122. Lee WS, Moussaoui SM, Moskowitz MA. Blockade by oral or parenteral RPR100893 (a non-peptide NK1 receptor antagonist) of neurogenic plasma protein extravsation in guinea-pig dura mater and conjunctiva. *Br. J. Pharmacol.* 1994; 112: 920–4.

123. Brandli P, Loffler B-M, Breu V, Osterwalder R, Maire J-P, Clozel M. Role of endothelin in mediating neurogenic plasma extravasation in rat dura mater. *Pain* 1995; 64: 315–22.

124. Goadsby PJ. Animal models of migraine: which one and for what? In: Rose FC, ed. *Towards Migraine 2000*. Amsterdam: Elsevier, 1996: 85–99.

125. May A, Gijsman HJ, Wallnoefer A, Jones R, Diener HC, Ferrari MD. Endothelin antagonist bosentan blocks neurogenic inflammation, but is not effective in aborting migraine attacks. *Pain* 1996; 67: 375–8.

126. Goadsby PJ, Adner M, Edvinsson L. Characterisation of endothelin ET_A receptors in the cerebral vasculature and their lack of effect upon spreading depression. *J. Cereb. Blood Flow Metabol.* 1996; 16: 698–704.

127. Diener HC. Substance-P antagonist RPR100893-201 is not effective in human migraine attacks. In: Olesen J, Tfelt-Hansen P, eds. *Proceedings of the International VIth Headache Seminar*. Copenhagen: 1996:

128. Goldstein DJ, Wang O, Saper JR, *et al.* Ineffectiveness of neurokinin-1 antagonist in acute migraine: a crossover study. *Cephalalgia* 1997; 17: 785–90.

129. Lee WS, Moskowitz MA. Conformationally restricted sumatriptan analogues, CP-122,288 and CP-122,638, exhibit enhanced potency against neurogenic inflammation in dura mater. *Brain Res.* 1993; 626: 303–5.

130. Roon K, Diener HC, Ellis P, *et al.* CP-122,288 blocks neurogenic inflammation, but is not effective in aborting migraine attacks: results of two controlled clinical studies. *Cephalalgia* 1997; 17: 245.

131. Hoskin KL, Goadsby PJ. CP122,288 has no effect on c-fos expression in the trigeminal nucleus caudalis after superior sagittal sinus stimulation. *Cephalalgia* 1997; 17:402.

132. Goadsby PJ, Gundlach AL. Localization of [³H]-dihydroergotamine binding sites in the cat central nervous system: relevance to migraine. *Ann. Neurol.* 1991; 29: 91–4.

133. Hoskin KL, Kaube H, Goadsby PJ. Central activation of the trigeminovascular pathway in the cat is inhibited by dihydroergotamine: a c-Fos and electrophysiology study. *Brain* 1996; 119: 249–56.

134. Kaube H, Hoskin KL, Goadsby PJ. Intravenous acetylsalicylic acid inhibits central trigeminal neurons in the dorsal horn of the upper cervical spinal cord in the cat. *Headache* 1993; 33: 541–50.

135. Kaube H, Hoskin KL, Goadsby PJ. Sumatriptan inhibits central trigeminal neurons only after blood-brain barrier disruption. *Cephalalgia* 1993; 13: 41.

136. Shepheard SL, Williamson DJ, Williams J, Hill RG, Hargreaves RJ. Comparison of the effects of sumatriptan and the NK1 antagonist CP-99,994 on plasma extravasation in the dura mater and c-fos mRNA expression in the trigeminal nucleus caudalis of rats. *Neuropharmacol.* 1995; 34: 255–61.

137. Goadsby PJ, Edvinsson L. Peripheral and central trigeminovascular activation in cat is blocked by the serotonin (5-HT)-1D receptor agonist 311C90. *Headache* 1994; 34: 394–9.

138. Goadsby PJ, Hoskin KL. Inhibition of trigeminal neurons by intravenous administration of the serotonin (5-HT)-1-D receptor agonist zolmitriptan (311C90): are brain stem sites a therapeutic target in migraine? *Pain* 1996; 67: 355–9.

139. Goadsby PJ, Knight YE. Naratriptan inhibits trigeminal neurons after intravenous administration through an action at the serotonin ($5-HT_{1B/1D}$) receptors. *Br. J. Pharmacol.* 1997; 122: 918–22.

140. Cumberbatch MJ, Hill RG, Hargreaves RJ. Rizatriptan has central antinociceptive effects against durally evoked responses. *Eur. J. Pharmacol.* 1997; 328: 37–40.

141. Goadsby PJ, Hoskin KL. Is the action of serotonin in migraine due in part to inhibition of neurons in the trigeminal nucleus? *Cephalalgia* 1997; 17: 400.

142. Goadsby PJ, Knight YE. Direct evidence for central sites of action of zolmitriptan (311C90): an autoradiographic study in cat. *Cephalalgia* 1997; 17: 153–8.

143. Storer RJ, Goadsby PJ. Microiontophoretic application of serotonin (5-HT)-1B/1D agonists inhibits trigeminal cell firing in the cat. *Brain* 1997;120: in press.

144. Hoskin KL, Goadsby PJ. The substance P antagonist, GR205171, does not inhibit trigeminal neurons activated by stimulation of the sagittal sinus: does NK1 blockade have a role in migraine? *Cephalalgia* 1997; 17: 347.

145. O'Connor TP, van der Kooy D. Enrichment of a vasoactive neuropeptide (calcitonin gene related peptide) in trigeminal sensory projection to the intracranial arteries. *J. Neurosci.* 1988; 8: 2468–76.

146. O'Connor TP, van der Kooy D. Pattern of intracranial and extracranial projections of trigeminal ganglion cells. *J. Neurosci.* 1986; 6: 2200–7.

147. Goadsby PJ, Lipton RB. A review of paroxysmal hemicranias, SUNCT syndrome and other short-lasting headaches with autonomic features, including new cases. *Brain* 1997;120:193–209.

148. Goadsby PJ, Zagami AS, Lambert GA. Neural processing of craniovascular pain: a synthesis of the central structures involved in migraine. *Headache* 1991; 31: 365–71.

149. Rebeck GW, Maynard KI, Hyman BT, Moskowitz MA. Selective 5-HT1D alpha serotonin receptor gene expression in trigeminal ganglion: implications for antimigraine drug development. *Proceedings of the National Academy of Science (U.S.A.)* 1994; 91: 3666–9.

150. Hamel E, Fan E, Linville D, Ting V, Villemure J-G, Chia L-S. Expression of mRNA for the serotonin 5-hydroxytryptamine-$_{1D\beta}$ receptor subtype in human bovine and cerebral arteries. *Molecular Pharmacology* 1993; 44: 242–6.

151. Bouchelet I, Cohen Z, Case B, Hamel E. Differential expression of sumatriptan-sensitive 5-hydroxytryptamine receptors in human trigeminal ganglia and cerebral blood vessels. *Molecular Pharmacology* 1996; 50: 219–23.

152. Waeber C, Cutrer FM, Yu X-J, Moskowitz MA. The selective $5-HT_{1D}$ receptor agonist U-109291 blocks dural plasma extravasation and c-fos expression in the trigeminal nucleus caudalis. *Cephalalgia* 1997; 17.

153. Phebus LA, Johnson KW, Audia JE, *et al.* Characterization of LY334370, a potent and selective $5-HT_{1F}$ receptor agonist, in the neurogenic dural inflammation model of migraine pain. *Proceedings of the Society for Neuroscience (U.S.A.)* 1996; 22:1331.

154. Waeber C, Moskowitz MA. [³H]sumatriptan labels both 5-HT1D and 5-HT-1F receptor bindings sites in the guinea pig brain: an autoradiographic study. *Naunyn-Schmiedeberg's Arch. Pharmacol.*1995; 352: 263–75.

155. Goldstein J, Dahlof CGH, Diener H-C, et al. Alniditan in the acute treatment of migraine attacks: a subcutaneous dose-finding study. *Cephalalgia* 1996; 16: 497–502.

156. Leysen JE, Gommeren W, Heylen L, et al. Alniditan, a new 5-hydroxytryptamine$_{1D}$ agonist and migraine-abortive agent: ligand-binding properties of human 5-hydroxytryptamine$_{1Da}$, human 5-hydroxytryptamine$_{1D\beta}$, and calf 5-hydroxytryptamine$_{1D}$ recetpors investigated with [^{3}H]-5-hydroxytryptamine and [^{3}H]alniditan.

Molecular Pharmacology 1996; 50: 1567–80.

157. Jasper JR, Kosaka A, To ZP, Chang DJ, Eglen RM. Cloning, expression and pharmacology of a truncated splice variant of the human 5-HT$_7$ receptor (h5-HT$_{7(b)}$). *Br. of J. of Pharmacology* 1997; 122: 126–132.

158. Beer M, Middlemiss D, Stanton J, et al. *In vitro* pharmacological profile of the novel 5-HT$_{1D}$ receptor agonist MK-462. *Cephalalgia* 1995; 15(Suppl 14): 203.

159. Cutrer FM, Limmroth V, Woeber C, Yu X, Moskowitz MA. New targets for antimigraine drug development. In:

Goadsby PJ, Silberstein SD, eds. *Headache.* Philadelphia: Butterworth-Heinemann, 1997: pp. 59–120

160. Edvinsson L, Goadsby PJ. Neuropeptides in headache. *Eur. J. of Neurology* 1997: in press.

161 Gardner K, Barmada M, Ptacek LJ, Hoffman EP. A new locus for hemiplegic maps to chromosome 1q31. *Neurology* 1997; 489: 1231–8.

162 Caterina MJ, Schumacher MA, Tominaga M, Rosen TA, Levine JD, Julius D. The capsaicin receptor: a heat-activated ion channel in the pain pathway. *Nature* 1997; 389: 816–24.

Primary headache disorders

chapter 6

Migraine: diagnosis and treatment

Introduction

Migraine is a primary episodic headache disorder characterized by various combinations of neurological, gastrointestinal and autonomic changes. In the United States, more than 17% of women and 6% of men had at least had one migraine attack in the last year.[1,2] Many famous and creative individuals have suffered from migraine (Table 6.1). Migraine diagnosis is based on the retrospective reporting of headache characteristics and associated symptoms.[3] The physical and neurological examinations, as well as laboratory studies, are usually normal and serve to exclude other, more ominous, causes of headache (see Chapters 2 and 4). Formal diagnostic criteria for migraine and other headache disorders were published by the International Headache Society (IHS) in 1988, but these remain a guide with a well-recognized group of false-negatives. The IHS system recognizes seven subtypes of migraine with two major varieties: migraine without aura (formerly common migraine) and migraine with aura (formerly classic migraine).[4,5] The IHS system provides criteria for a total of seven subtypes of migraine (Table 6.2). In this chapter, we will describe the migraine attack and its variants and their acute and preventive treatment based, in part, on the presence of any coexistent or comorbid disease.

Description of the migraine attack

Migraine has been recognized as a clinical entity for millennia. Cornelius Celsus, a Roman physician, described migraine (heterocrania) and its associated mood changes and photophobia. 'There is much torpor, heaviness of head, anxiety, and weariness. For they flee the light; the darkness soothes their disease; nor can they bear readily to look upon or hear anything disagreeable . . .' The migraine attack can be divided into four phases: the *prodrome phase*, which occurs hours or days before the headache; the *aura phase*, which immediately precedes the headache; the *headache phase* itself; and the *headache resolution* phase. Although most people experience more than one phase, no phase is obligatory for the diagnosis of migraine. A description of the four phases provides a convenient way of reviewing the protean manifestation of migraine (Figure 6.1).

● **Table 6.1** *Some famous migraineurs*

Julius Caesar	Thomas Jefferson	Ulysses S. Grant
Saint Paul	Friedrich Nietzsche	Peter Tchaikovsky
John Calvin	Immanuael Kant	Alfred Nobel
Queen Mary Tudor	Edgar Allan Poe	Leo Tolstoy
Blaise Pascal	Frédéric Chopin	Sigmund Freud
Carolus Linnaeus	Charles Darwin	Virginia Woolf
Lewis Carroll	Karl Marx	Princess Margaret

Adapted from Adler et al.[69]

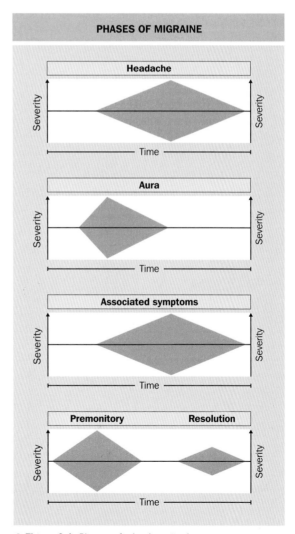

● **Figure 6.1** *Phases of migraine attack.*

Table 6.2 *IHS migraine classification*

1	Migraine
1.1	Migraine without aura
1.2	Migraine with aura
1.2.1	Migraine with typical aura
1.2.2	Migraine with prolonged aura
1.2.3	Familial hemiplegic migraine
1.2.4	Basilar migraine
1.2.5	Migraine aura without headache
1.2.6	Migraine with acute onset aura
1.3	Ophthalmoplegic migraine
1.4	Retinal migraine
1.5	Childhood periodic syndromes that may be precursors to or associated with migraine
1.5.1	Benign paroxysmal vertigo of childhood
1.5.2	Alternating hemiplegia of childhood
1.6	Complications of migraine
1.6.1	Status migrainosus
1.6.2	Migrainous infarction
1.7	Migrainous disorder not fulfilling above criteria

Table 6.3 *Prodrome (premonitory phenomena)*

Mental state	Neurological	General
Depressed	Photophobia	Stiff neck
Hyperactive	Difficulty concentrating	Food cravings
Euphoric	Phonophobia	Cold feeling
Talkative	Dysphasia	Anorexia
Irritable	Hyperosmia	Sluggish
Drowsy	Yawning	Diarrhoea or constipation
Restless		Thirst
		Urination
		Fluid retention

Table 6.4 *Characteristics of the visual aura*

Positive phenomena, negative phenomena, or both	Either may occur alone; positive phenomena often occur first and are followed by negative phenomena
Visual field	Scotoma often start centrally and migrate peripherally.
Shape	Fortification spectra often 'C'-shaped; scotoma bean shaped
Motion	Objects may rotate, oscillate, or boil
Flicker	Rate 10 cycles per second; may change during the course of the aura
Colour	Grey, red, green, gold, yellow, blue, or purple; often have no specific colour except excessively bright white
Clarity	May be blurry or fuzzy
Brightness	Often very bright.
Expansion	Build-up occurs in both fortification spectra and scotoma
Migration	Spectra may 'march' from the central area to periphery or sometimes vice versa

Prodrome (premonitory phenomena)

Premonitory phenomena occur in about 60% of migraineurs, often hours to days before headache onset. Usually patients describe a characteristic change in mood or behaviour which may include psychological, neurological, constitutional or autonomic features (Table 6.3). Some people simply report a poorly characterized feeling that a migraine attack is coming. While the prodromal features are quite variable among individuals, they are often rather consistent within an individual (Figure 6.2).

The prodrome is common. It occurs in more than half of migraineurs, with equal frequency in migraine with and without aura. The features of the prodrome, such as depression, cognitive dysfunction and episodic bouts of food cravings may be difficult to diagnose as part of the migraine complex if they occur in isolation or with a mild headache or if a careful headache history is not taken. A diary may be helpful to show the relationship of these periodic events to migraine (Table 6.3 and Figure 6.3).[6]

Aura

The migraine aura is a complex of focal neurological symptoms (positive or negative phenomena) which precedes or accompanies an attack. Most aura symptoms develop over 5–20 minutes and usually last less than 60 minutes.[5] The aura can be characterized by visual, sensory, or motor phenomena, and may also involve language or brainstem disturbances (Table 6.4).

Headache usually occurs within 60 minutes from the end of the aura but may not occur for several hours if at all.[7,8] In one prospective study headache followed the aura only 80% of the time.[7] Most patients do not feel normal during the gap between the aura and headache. Fears, somatic complaints, alterations in mood, disturbances of speech or thought, or detachment from the environment or other people may occur. The headache may begin before or simultaneously with the aura, or the aura may occur alone. Patients can have more than one type of aura, with a progression from one symptom to another. Most patients with a sensory aura also have a visual aura.[9]

Auras may occur repeatedly, as frequently as many times an hour for as long as several months. These have been termed 'migraine aura status'.[6] Scotomata may occur

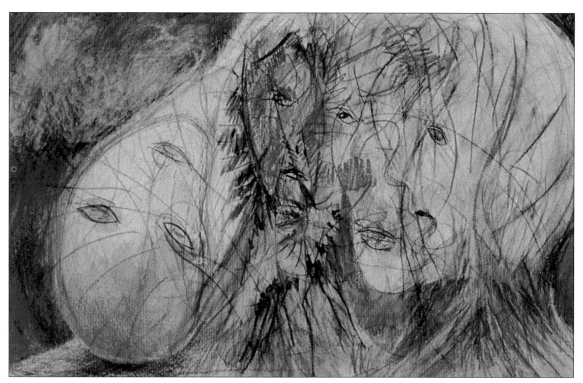

● **Figure 6.2** *'Mentally insufficient' by Angela Mark of Jamaica Plain, Massachusetts, USA. (© Sandoz Pharmaceuticals Corp.)*

EXAMPLE OF A MIGRAINE DIARY

	Date	Headache start time	Headache stop time	Severity (0-3 scale) 0=none 1=mild 2=moderate 3=severe	Associated symptoms (0-4 scale) 0=none 1=nausea 2=vomiting 3=photophobia 4=phonophobia	Disability (0-3 scale) 0=none 1=mild 2=moderate 3=severe	Medications taken to relieve headache	Any known triggers
Sunday								
Monday								
Tuesday								
Wednesday								
Thursday								
Friday								
Saturday								

● **Figure 6.3** *Example of a migraine diary.*

repeatedly, even alternating sides; closely repeating cycles of migrating sensory auras may occur for hours on end.[10] This presentation requires careful investigation before the diagnosis can be made.

Auras vary in their complexity. Elementary visual disturbances include scotomata, simple flashes (phosphenes), specks or geometric forms. They may move across the visual field, sometimes crossing the midline. Shimmering or undulations in the visual field may also occur. These 'minor visual disorders' are more likely to occur during than before the headache.[11] Because they are bilateral they are believed to arise from the occipital cortex. More complicated auras include teichopsia (Greek for 'town wall and vision') or fortification

spectrum, the most characteristic visual aura of migraine (Figure 6.4). An arc of scintillating lights, usually but not always beginning near the point of fixation, may form into a herringbone-like pattern that expands to encompass an increasing portion of a visual hemifield. It migrates across the visual field with a scintillating edge of often zigzag, flashing or occasionally coloured phenomena (Figure 6.5). Some characteristics of the aura are listed in Table 6.4. Migraine scotoma may occur simultaneously in both visual fields, but this is rare. They may even be synchronized to create an altitudinal, not a hemianoptic, pattern. The visions of Hildegard of Bingen, an 11th century mystic, have been attributed in part to her migrainous scintillating scotomas (Figure 6.6). Characteristic of the visions

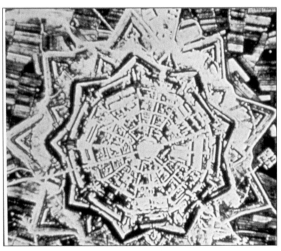

● **Figure 6.4** *Migraine with aura (aerial view of the fortified, walled city of Palmanova, Italy.)*

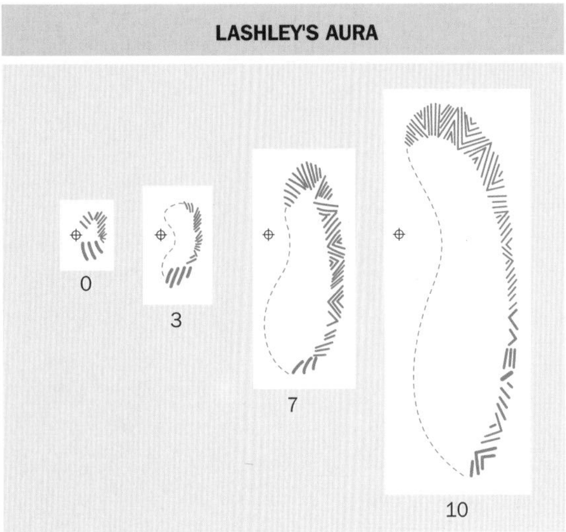

LASHLEY'S AURA

0

3

7

10

● **Figure 6.5** *Fortification spectra as depicted by Lashley.*

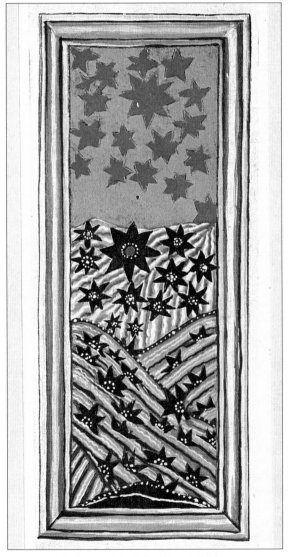

● **Figure 6.6** *'Vision of the fall of the angels' from a manuscript of Hildegard's Scivias, written in Bingen, AD 1180.*

that she and other visionary prophets, including Ezekiel, saw were working, boiling or fermenting lights.

Visual distortions and hallucinations can occur. These attacks occur more commonly in children, are usually followed by a headache, and are characterized[6] by a complex disorder of visual perception that may include metamorphopsia, micropsia, macropsia, zoom vision (opening up or closing down in the size of objects) or mosaic vision (fracture of image into facets). In addition, non-visual association cortex symptoms occur and include: complex difficulties in the perception and use of the body (apraxia and agnosia); speech and language disturbances; states of double or multiple consciousness associated with *déjà vu* or *jamais vu*; and elaborate dreamy, nightmarish, trance-like or delirious states.[6]

Paraesthesias, the second most common aura, typically are often cheiroaural, with numbness starting in the hand, migrating up the arm, and then jumping to involve the face, lips and tongue. The leg is occasionally involved.[12] As with visual auras (with positive, followed by negative, symptoms), paraesthesias may be followed by numbness and, in a few cases, loss of position sense. Paraesthesias start or become bilateral in half of patients. Sensory auras rarely occur in isolation and usually follow a visual aura (Figure 6.7).[3,4,6,12,13]

Motor symptoms can occur in up to 18% of patients, most often in association with sensory symptoms[7]; however, true weakness is rare and is always unilateral.[12] Sensory ataxia is often reported as weakness;[12] hyperkinetic movement disorders, including chorea, have been reported.[6] Aphasic auras (speech abnormalities) including aphasia have been reported in 17–20% of patients.[7,12] However, since patients are rarely examined during an aura, many of these reported cases may be dysarthria, not aphasia.[12]

Headache phase

The typical headache of migraine is unilateral, throbbing, moderate to marked in severity and aggravated by physical activity. Not all of these features are required: pain may be bilateral at onset (in 40% of cases) or start on one side and become generalized.[11] The headache of migraine can occur at any time of the day or night, but it occurs most frequently on arising in the morning.[11] The onset is usually gradual; the pain peaks and then subsides, and usually lasts between 4 and 72 hours in adults and 2 to 48 hours in children (Figure 6.8).[5]

The head pain varies greatly in intensity, although most people with migraine report pain ratings of 5 on a 0 to 10 scale.[14] It is described as throbbing in 85% of cases, although throbbing pain is often described in other types of headache.[14] The pain is commonly aggravated by physical activity or simple head movement.[5]

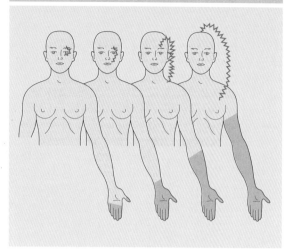

MIGRAINE AURA

● *Figure 6.7* Paraesthesias, the second most common migraine aura. (Adapted from ref.88 with permission.)

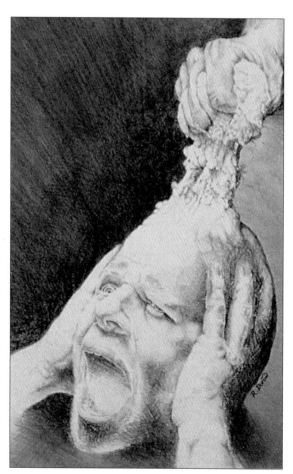

● *Figure 6.8* 'Gripping headache' by Richard Dorrow II of Athol, Massachusetts, USA. (© Sandoz Pharmaceuticals Corp.)

The pain of migraine is invariably accompanied by other features. Anorexia is common, although food craving can occur. Nausea occurs in almost 90% of patients, while vomiting occurs in about one-third of migraineurs (Figure 6.9).[15] Many patients experience sensory hyperexcitability manifested by photophobia, phonophobia, and osmophobia, and seek a dark, quiet room (Figure 6.10).[4,15] Other systemic symptoms, including blurry vision, nasal stuffiness, anorexia, hunger, tenesmus, diarrhoea, abdominal cramps, polyuria (followed by decreased urinary output after the attack), pallor (or, less commonly, redness) of the face, sensations of heat or cold, and sweating, may be noted during the headache phase. There may be localized oedema of the scalp, the face, or under the eyes, tenderness of the scalp, unusual prominence of a vein or artery in the temple, or stiffness and tenderness of the neck. Impairment of concentration is common; less often there is memory impairment. Depression, fatigue, anxiety, nervousness and irritability are common. Lightheadedness, rather than true vertigo, and a feeling of faintness may occur. The extremities tend to be cold and moist. As discussed below, the IHS selects particular associated features as cardinal manifestations for diagnosis.

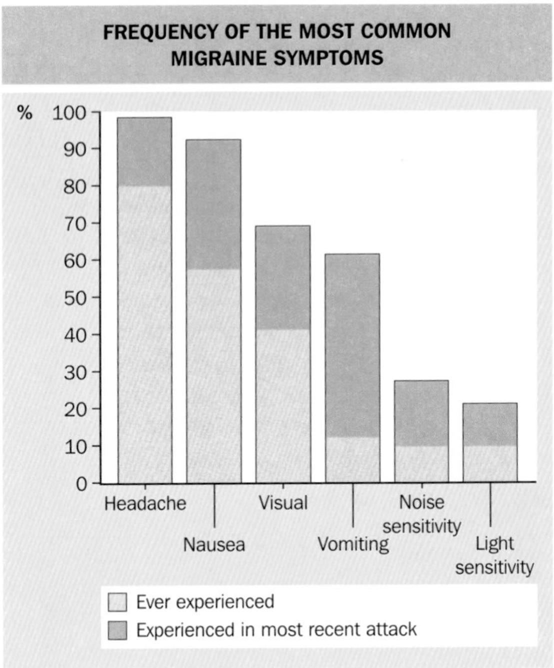

FREQUENCY OF THE MOST COMMON MIGRAINE SYMPTOMS

Ever experienced

Experienced in most recent attack

● **Figure 6.9** *Frequency of the most common migraine symptoms.(Adapted from ref.15 with permission.)*

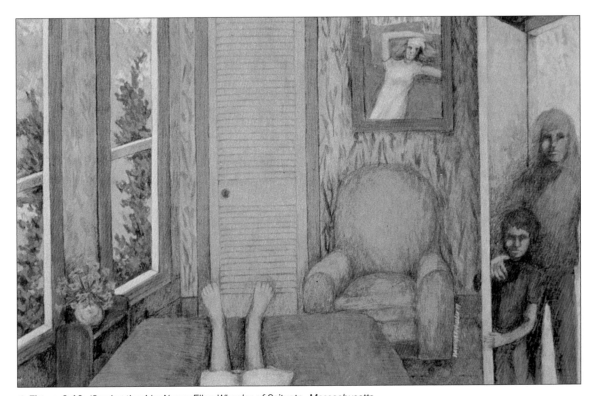

● **Figure 6.10** *'Serving time' by Nancy Ellen Wheeler of Scituate, Massachusetts, USA. (© Sandoz Pharmaceutical Corp.)*

Resolution phase

In the termination phase, the pain wanes. Following the headache, the patient may feel tired, washed out, irritable, and listless and may have impaired concentration, scalp tenderness or mood changes. Some people feel unusually refreshed or euphoric after an attack, while others note depression and malaise.

Formal diagnostic criteria

Overview of the International Headache Society (IHS)

To improve the classification of headache disorders both in clinical practice and in research, the IHS recently published diagnostic criteria for a broad range of headache disorders. These criteria, based on expert consensus, have had a major impact on clinical trials and on epidemiological research, although they have not been widely employed in clinical practice.[16]

Despite its limitations,[3] the IHS system stands as a singular advance in headache classification. Although the criteria will undoubtedly be revised as empirical evidence and clinical experience accumulate, they provide the best available diagnostic 'gold standard' for the clinician and investigator. The terms 'migraine with aura' and 'migraine without aura' were adopted to favour translations into other languages and allow unambiguous exchange of information from country to country.

Migraine without aura (common migraine) (Table 6.5)

To establish a diagnosis of IHS migraine without aura, five attacks are needed, each lasting 4 to 72 hours and having two of the following four pain characteristics: unilateral location; pulsating quality; moderate-to-severe intensity; and aggravation by routine physical activity. In addition, the attacks must have at least one of the following: nausea or vomiting or photophobia and phonophobia. Using these criteria, no single associated feature is mandatory for diagnosing migraine, although recurrent episodic attacks must be documented. A patient who has pulsatile pain aggravated by routine activity, photophobia and phonophobia meets the criteria, as does the more typical patient with unilateral throbbing pain and nausea.[5]

Migraine usually lasts several hours or all day; when it persists for more than 3 days, the term 'status migrainosus' is applied. Although migraine often begins in the morning, sometimes awakening the patient from sleep at dawn, it can begin at any time of the day or night. The frequency of attacks is extremely variable, from a few in a lifetime to several a week. The average migraineur experiences from one to three headaches a month (Figure 6.11).[1,15] Migraine is,

by definition, a recurrent phenomenon. The requirement for at least five attacks is imposed because headaches simulating migraine may be caused by organic disease ranging from brain tumors to sinusitis to glaucoma.

The IHS also requires the exclusion of secondary headache disorders in one of several ways. Thus, migraine is both a diagnosis of inclusion, as specific combinations of features are required, and a diagnosis of exclusion, as alternative causes of headache must be systematically eliminated.

● **Table 6.5** *Migraine without aura (previously used terms: common migraine, hemicrania simplex). Diagnostic criteria*

A	At least five attacks fulfilling B–D.
B	Headache lasting 4–72 hours (untreated or unsuccessfully treated).
C	Headache has at least two of the following characteristics: **1** Unilateral location. **2** Pulsating quality. **3** Moderate or severe intensity (inhibits or prohibits daily activities). **4** Aggravation by walking stairs or similar routine physical activity.
D	During headache at least one of the following: **1** Nausea and/or vomiting. **2** Photophobia and phonophobia.
E	At least one of the following: **1** History, physical and neurologic examinations do not suggest one of the disorders listed in groups 5–11. **2** History and/or physical and/or neurological examinations do suggest such disorder, but it is ruled out by appropriate investigations. **3** Such disorder is present, but migraine attacks do not occur for the first time in close temporal relation to the disorder.

MIGRAINE ATTACKS PER MONTH

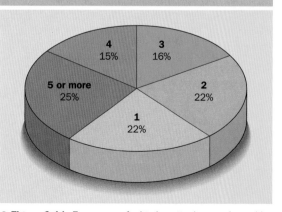

● **Figure 6.11** *Frequency of migraine attacks experienced by migraineurs per month.*

Migraine with aura (classic migraine) (Table 6.6)

A diagnosis of migraine with aura (IHS migraine classification 1.2), the new term for classic migraine, requires at least two attacks with any three of the following four features: one or more fully reversible aura symptoms; aura developing over more than 4 minutes; aura lasting less than 60 minutes; and headache following aura with a free interval of less than 60 minutes. Fewer attacks are required than for a diagnosis of migraine with aura, based on the assumption that the typical aura is highly specific for migraine. Once again, other causes of headache must be excluded.[5]

Migraine with aura is subdivided (see Table 6.2) into: migraine with typical aura (1.2.1) (homonymous visual disturbance, unilateral numbness or weakness, or aphasia); migraine with prolonged aura (1.2.2) (aura lasting more than 60 minutes); familial hemiplegic migraine (FHM) (1.2.3); basilar migraine (1.2.4); migraine aura without headache (1.2.5); and migraine with acute-onset aura (1.2.6). Other varieties of migraine include ophthalmoplegic (1.3), retinal (1.4) and childhood periodic syndromes (1.5).

The headache and associated symptoms of migraine with aura are similar to those of migraine without aura. Most migraineurs with aura also have attacks without aura. The aura usually lasts 20–30 minutes and typically precedes the headache, but occasionally it occurs only during the headache. In contrast to a transient ischaemic attack, the aura of migraine evolves gradually and consists of both positive (e.g. scintillations, tingling) and negative features (e.g. scotoma, numbness). If the aura is typical and stereotyped, the diagnosis of migraine with aura is warranted, even if the subsequent headache does not have the migrainous features described above. Virtually any symptom or sign of brain dysfunction may be a feature of the aura, but the most common auras are visual.

Focal symptoms and signs of the aura may persist beyond the headache phase. Formerly termed 'complicated migraine', the IHS classification has introduced two more specific labels. If the aura lasts for more than one hour but less than one week, the term migraine with prolonged aura is applied. If the signs persist for more than one week or a neuroimaging procedure demonstrates a stroke, a migrainous infarction has occurred. Particularly in mid or late life, the aura may not be followed by the headache; it is then considered a migraine equivalent.

Migraine variants
Basilar migraine

Basilar migraine was originally called 'basilar artery migraine'[5] or 'Bickerstaff's migraine'[17] (Table 6.7). Although it was originally believed to be mainly a disorder of adolescent girls, it affects all age groups and both sexes, with the female predominance which typifies migraine. The aura often lasts less than one hour, is usually followed by a headache and is nothing more than migraine with an aura clinically localized to the brainstem. A typical hemianoptic aura may rapidly involve both visual fields, leading at times to temporary blindness. The visual aura is usually followed by ataxia, vertigo, tinnitus, diplopia, nausea and vomiting, nystagmus, dysarthria, bilateral paraesthesia, or a change in level of consciousness and cognition. Spells of basilar migraine can present a confusing picture. This disorder should be considered in patients with paroxysmal brainstem disturbances.

● Table 6.6 *Migraine with aura (classic migraine). Diagnostic criteria*

A	At least two attacks fulfilling (B).
B	At least three of the following four characteristics:
	1 One or more fully reversible aura symptoms indicating brain dysfunction.
	2 At least one aura symptom develops gradually over more than 4 minutes or 2 or more symptoms occur in succession.
	3 No single aura symptom lasts more than 60 minutes.
	4 Headache follows aura with a free interval of less than 60 minutes (it may also begin before or simultaneously with the aura).
C	History, physical examination and, where appropriate, diagnostic tests exclude a secondary cause.

● Table 6.7 *1.2.4 Basilar migraine*. Diagnostic criteria*

Description:
Migraine with aura symptoms clearly originating from the brainstem or from both occipital lobes

A	Fulfills criteria for 1.2 (Table 6.2)
B	Two or more aura symptoms of the following types:
	Visual symptoms in both the temporal and nasal fields of both eyes
	Dysarthria
	Vertigo
	Tinnitus
	Decreased hearing
	Double vision
	Ataxia
	Bilateral paraesthesias
	Bilateral pareses
	Decreased level of consciousness

* See Table 6.2

Confusional migraine

Confusional migraine[5,18] is characterized by a typical aura, a headache (which may be insignificant), and confusion, which may precede the headache or follow it. This again is nothing more than an aura which affects the centres controlling consciousness. The confusion is characterized by inattention, distractibility, and difficulty maintaining speech and other motor activities.

Hemiplegic migraine

The IHS[5] has subdivided hemiplegic migraine into two forms, *sporadic* and *familial*, both of which typically begin in childhood and cease with adulthood. This separation may not be justified and both forms may be part of the same syndrome.[13] The age of onset of hemiplegic migraine may be earlier than that of typical migraine. The attacks are frequently precipitated by minor head injury. Changes in consciousness ranging from confusion to coma are a feature of hemiplegic migraine, especially in childhood.[13] The hemiplegia may be part of the aura and last less than one hour (migraine with typical aura) or it may last for days or weeks. Headache may precede the hemiparesis or be absent. The onset of hemiparesis may be abrupt and simulate a stroke.

The prevalence of hemiplegic migraine is uncertain and varies from 4 to 30% of cases of migraine.[11] The differential diagnosis of hemiplegic migraine includes stroke, homocystinuria, focal seizures and MELAS syndrome.[18]

Familial hemiplegic migraine (FHM)

Familial hemiplegic migraine (Table 6.8) has an autosomal dominant mode of inheritance with variable penetrance. The gene for 60% of affected families has been localized to the short arm of chromosome 19p13, and has been cloned, thus clinical and genetic heterogeneity exists. A case has been made to classify FHM as a subtype of migraine because of:

(i) the paroxysmal occurrence of headache, and the nausea, vomiting, and transient focal neuralgic symptoms, all of which are similar to migraine with aura;

(ii) the fact that individuals with migraine with and without aura coexist in one family;

(iii) the changes that occur in an affected individual over a lifetime.

For example, a person who has FHM in adolescence may develop migraine with aura as an adult and migraine without aura later in life.[19] Such a subclassification will be useful to determine the genetic and molecular basis of the problem. The gene defect for FHM has been found to be due to a mutation in a brain-specific P/Q calcium-channel subunit (Chapter 5).[24,71,72]

CADASIL

Cerebral autosomal dominant arteriopathy with subcortical infarcts and leukoencephalopathy (CADASIL) is an inherited arterial disease of the brain that has recently been mapped to chromosome 19 in two unrelated French families (Table 6.9).[20] Hutchinson et al.[21] found four family members of an Irish family with CADASIL who had a history and preceding diagnosis of FHM. The complete CADASIL syndrome consists of recurrent episodes of focal brain deficits (recurrent strokes) starting in mid-adult life, often leading to dementia, residual motor disability and pseudobulbar palsy. Even before clinical symptoms or signs have developed, MRI of at-risk individuals may be abnormal, with extensive areas of increased T2 signals in the white matter. Familial hemiplegic migraine also maps to chromosome 19, close to the gene locus for CADASIL. Familial hemiplegic migraine is usually distinguished from CADASIL by its earlier onset, benign prognosis and normal MRI findings. It is defined as migraine with aura with some hemiparesis, with at least one first-degree relative with identical attacks. Cases with associated cerebellar degeneration may be localized to chromosome 19.

Table 6.8 Familial hemiplegic migraine. Diagnostic criteria

Description:
Migraine with aura including hemiparesis and where at least one first degree relative has identical attacks.

A Fulfils criteria for 1.2*

B The aura includes some degree of hemiparesis and may be prolonged.

C At least one first-degree relative has identical attacks.

* See Table 6.2

Table 6.9 Familial hemiplegic migraine (FHM) and cerebral autosomal dominant arteriopathy with subcortical infarcts and leukoencephalopathy (CADASIL)

	FHM	CADASIL	Migraine with white matter abnormalities
Genetics	AD	AD	AD
Chromosomal locus	19*, ?	19	19 (?)
MRI	WNL	ABN	ABN
Migraine	Yes	Yes	Yes
Migraine with aura and hemiparesis	Yes	Yes	Yes
Stroke	No	Yes	No
Dementia	No	Yes	No

* When associated with cerebellar abnormalities

This suggests that a unique process, not typical of migraine, occurs in these families (Figures 6.12 and 6.13).

CADASIL can be diagnosed by the characteristic MRI abnormalities in a genetically at-risk family member with a pattern of autosomal dominant inheritance.[21] MRI shows leukoencephalopathy of varying severity on T2-weighted images and multiple deep white matter infarcts on both T1- and T2-weighted images. Four out of five members of the Irish family with the syndrome of FHM had the MRI findings of CADASIL (Figure 6.14).[21]

Chabriat et al.[22] used MRI and genetic linkage analysis to study 148 subjects belonging to seven families with CADASIL. Forty-five family members (23 men and 22 women) were clinically affected. The most frequent symptoms included recurrent subcortical ischaemic events (84%), progressive or stepwise subcortical dementia with pseudobulbar palsy (31%), migraine with aura (22%), and mood disorders with severe depressive episodes (20%). All the symptomatic subjects had prominent signal abnormalities on MRI, with hyperintense lesions on T2-weighted images in the subcortical white matter and basal ganglia (these were also present in 19 asymptomatic subjects). The mean age at onset of symptoms was 45 years (S.D. 10.6 years), with attacks of migraine with aura occurring earlier in life (38.1 years; S.D. 8.03 years) than ischaemic events (49.3 years; S.D. 10.7 years). The mean age at death was 64.5 (S.D. 10.6) years. On the basis of MRI data, the penetrance of the disease appears complete between 30 and 40 years of age.

Chabriat et al.[23] also described the medical history of one family without evidence of migrainous infarct or prolonged aura, remarkable for the high frequency of throbbing headaches in eight of the 12 examined members of the pedigree. All other affected subjects had a parent who also had migraine. The disorder is characterized by recurrent headache attacks with many features of migraine. The attacks usually lasted a few (2–48) hours, and the patients were asymptomatic between attacks. In all but one patient, headache was preceded by focal neurologic symptoms that developed gradually over 5–15 minutes and usually resolved in less than 60 minutes. Paresthaesias and unilateral or bilateral blurring of vision were the most frequent of these symptoms. According to the IHS classification, six patients satisfy the diagnostic criteria for migraine with typical aura, one for a migrainous disorder with aura, and one for migraine without aura. Some subjects occasionally had extremely unusual and severe attacks. One patient had two attacks and another patient had one in which their usual symptoms were followed by

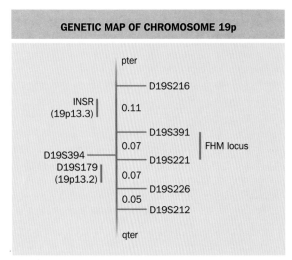

Figure 6.12 *Genetic map of chromosome 19p region based on data from the Genome Data Base: distances are given in Morgans.*[71]

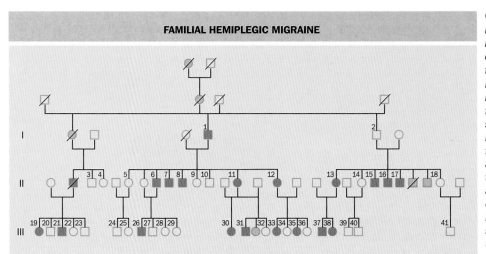

FAMILIAL HEMIPLEGIC MIGRAINE

● **Figure 6.13**
Familial hemiplegic migraine: analysis of FHM genetic family pedigree.[72] *Key: Squares, males; circles, females; affected subjects are represented by a filled symbol and by a half-filled when the symptoms are assured on the basis of familial history; hatched symbols stand for subject of unknown status.*

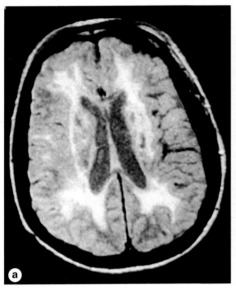 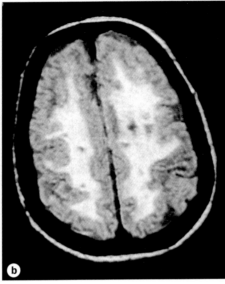

● **Figure 6.14** *MRI CADASIL. Brain MRI showing axial proton density sections at the level of the bodies of the lateral ventricles and centrum show confluent, severe, high-signal leukoencephalopathy, with discrete punctate low-signal lesions indicating cystic or necrotic lesions. (From ref. 21, with permission.)*

hyperthermia and stupor that resolved in less than 24 hours. Such a decreased level of consciousness and hyperthermia are features of 'basilar migraine'. One patient had an extremely severe attack with headache, coma, fever and aseptic meningitis that resolved within 15 days. The most unusual characteristic of this syndrome was the presence, in six of eight subjects with migraine, of striking MRI abnormalities. Numerous areas of decreased signal intensity on T1-weighted images and of increased signal intensity were found in the basal ganglia and the subcortical white matter. Some researchers have found abnormalities on T2-weighted images in up to 45% of cases of migraine, including those with complicated migraine. In control studies, abnormalities were present in 4.3–22% of controls and in 13–55% of migraine sufferers.

The main clinical presentation of CADASIL is recurrent subcortical events, either transient or (more often) permanent. However, the vascular presentation is not constant and other symptoms such as dementia or migraine with aura and depression can occur. Although these symptoms are usually associated with a history of recurrent strokes, they may be prominent or the only manifestation of the disease. Dementia is found in one-third of the overall affected family members and in 90% of subjects before death. It satisfies all the criteria for vascular dementia. It is characterized by frontal-like symptoms and memory impairment and is usually associated with gait disturbances, pyramidal signs, pseudobulbar palsy and sphincter incontinence. Attacks of migraine with aura were observed in 22% of the cases, while its prevalence in the general population is about 6%.

White matter abnormalities

White matter abnormalities (WMA) have been reported in migraine, particularly migraine with aura. Some believe this results from repeated ischaemic insults that could occur during the migrainous auras. However, they were also found in the family described by Chabriat et al.[23] without evidence of stroke. Another explanation is that migraine with aura and WMA could be the consequence of the same underlying vascular disorder that is present in mitochondrial diseases or the antiphospholipid antibody syndrome. A mutation near the CADASIL locus could thus be a new cause of migraine associated with WMA on MRI (Table 6.9).

Aura without headache (Table 6.10)

Periodic neurological dysfunction, which may be part of the migraine aura, can occur in isolation without the headache.[24] These phenomena (scintillating scotomata and recurrent sensory, motor and mental phenomena) can be part of migraine, but they are accepted as migraine only after a full investigation and prolonged follow-up. Headaches occurring in association with aura symptoms help confirm the diagnosis.[4] Aura without headache often occurs at some time in patients with migraine with aura.[4]

Levy[25] found that 32% of Cornell neurologists had a history of transient neurological loss, most commonly visual (field cuts, obscurations, scotomata), and less commonly non-visual (hemiparesis, clumsiness, paraesthesias, dysarthria). Migraine was reported in 29%, occurring in 44% of those reporting and 22% of those not reporting transient CNS dysfunction. None of the responders had developed any residual deficit

Table 6.10 *Main criteria for the diagnosis of late-life migrainous accompaniments (Fisher)*

- Scintillations (or other visual display), paraesthesias, aphasia, dysarthria and paralysis.
- Build-up of scintillations. Not seen in cerebrovascular disease.
- 'March' of paraesthesias. Not seen in cerebrovascular disease.
- Progression from one accompaniment to another, often with a delay.
- Two or more similar attacks. Helps exclude embolism.
- Headache occurs in 50% of attacks.
- Episodes last 15–25 minutes.
- Characteristic mid-life 'flurry' of attacks.
- Generally benign course.
- Normal angiography: excludes thrombosis.
- Rule out: cerebral thrombosis, embolism and dissection, epilepsy, thrombocythemia, polycythemia and thrombotic thrombocytopenia

Table 6.11 *Migrainous accompaniments*

Visual-scintillating scotoma	Hemiplegia
Ophthalmoplegia	Cyclical vomiting
Paraesthesias	Brainstem symptoms
Oculosympathetic palsy	Seizures
Aphasia	Blindness
Mydriasis	Diplopia
Dysarthria	Blurring of vision
Confusion-stupor	Deafness
Dizziness	Hemianopia
Recurrence of old stroke deficit	

many of these spells meet the IHS criteria for migraine aura without headache, others meet the diagnosis of acute-onset aura without headache, which is not recognized by the IHS.

or chronic neurological disorder at five years follow-up, suggesting that these symptoms are benign migrainous accompaniments.

Fisher[26] described late life migrainous accompaniments, which are transient neurological phenomena frequently not associated with headache. He reported on 188 patients over the age of 40 years; 60% were men and 57% had a history of recurrent headache. They had one or more attacks of episodic neurological dysfunction, which lasted from 1 minute to 72 hours with variable recurrence (one attack 27%, two to ten attacks 45%, more than ten attacks 28%). Fisher considered scintillating scotoma to be diagnostic of migraine even when it occurred in isolation, whereas other episodic neurological symptoms (paraesthesias, aphasia, and sensory and motor symptoms) needed more careful evaluation (Table 6.11).

Transient migrainous accompaniments — scintillating scotomata, numbness, aphasia, dysarthria and motor weakness — may occur for the first time after the age of 45 years and be easily confused with transient ischaemic attacks of cerebrovascular origin (Table 6.11). In all but the most classic cases, the diagnostic method is still exclusion.[27] While

Treatment

Effective migraine treatment begins with making an accurate diagnosis,[3] explaining it to the patient, and developing a treatment plan that considers the patient's diagnosis, symptoms, and any coincidental or comorbid conditions and deals with the most disturbing symptoms in the most appropriate way.[28] Comorbidity indicates an association between two disorders that is more than coincidental. Conditions that occur in migraineurs with a higher prevalence than would be expected include stroke, epilepsy, mitral valve prolapse, Raynaud's syndrome and psychological disorders, which include depression, mania, anxiety and panic (Table 6.12). Co-occurring disease presents both therapeutic opportunities and limitations. For example, if nausea and vomiting are prominent, a non-oral route of drug administration is needed. Medication must be prescribed cautiously, since a specific migraine medication may be useless or even dangerous if given for a migraine mimic or if certain comorbid conditions are present. For example, a patient with an acute symptomatic headache due to a stroke or subarachnoid haemorrhage may respond to selective 5-hydroxytryptamine-1 (or

Table 6.12 *Migraine comorbid disease*

Cardiovascular	Neurological	Gastrointestinal tract	Psychiatric	Other
Hyper- or hypotension	Epilepsy	Functional bowel disorders	Depression	Asthma
Raynaud's phenomenon	Positional vertigo		Mania	Allergies
Mitral valve prolapse			Panic disorder	
Angina/myocardial infarction			Anxiety disorder	
Stroke				

serotonin) (5-HT$_1$) agonists with a worsening of the neurological deficit, while a patient who is overusing analgesics often does not respond to preventive migraine treatment.

Patients are given a headache calendar and told to record the duration and severity of their headaches as well as their response to treatment. Relaxation, biofeedback and behavioral interventions, such as maintaining a regular schedule, getting adequate sleep and exercise, and giving up tobacco, are helpful in some patients (Table 6.13).[3] Biofeedback is a useful treatment that serves to engage patients in cognitive behavioural therapy. It is especially useful in children, pregnant women, and patients in whom stress is a trigger. Although behavioural interventions are important, drugs are the mainstay of treatment for most patients (Figure 6.15).

The pharmacological treatment of migraine may be acute (abortive) or preventive (prophylactic),[3] and patients who are experiencing frequent severe headaches often require both approaches. Acute treatment attempts to abort (reverse or stop the progression of) a headache once it has started. Preventive therapy is given, even in the absence of a headache, to reduce the frequency and severity of anticipated attacks. Symptomatic treatment is appropriate for most attacks, even in patients who are on preventive medication, and should be used two to three days a week at most. Preventive treatment is used more selectively, for example, to decrease the occurrence of frequent attacks.

Abortive headache treatment medication can be specific or non-specific (Table 6.14). Non-specific medications are used to control the pain and associated symptoms of migraine or other pain disorders, while specific medications control the headache attack but are not useful for non-headache pain disorders.

● **Table 6.13** *Behavioural modifications*

May help	Less likely to help
Regulate sleep	Avoid milk products
Regular exercise	Avoid citrus products
Regular meals	
Avoid chocolate	
Avoid tyramine-containing food	
Avoid monosodium glutamate	
Avoid alcoholic beverages	
Limit caffeine	
Limit medications	
Biofeedback or stress management	

● **Table 6.14** *Headache treatment*

Acute (symptomatic)	Specific:	for only headache
	Non-specific:	for any pain disorder or associated symptoms
Preventive (prophylactic)	Episodic:	immediately prior to triggering event
	Subacute:	for limited time
	Chronic:	continuous

Medications used for acute headache treatment include analgesics, antiemetics, anxiolytics, non-steroidal anti-inflammatory drugs (NSAID), ergots, steroids, major tranquillizers, narcotics, and, more recently, selective 5-HT$_1$ agonists (sumatriptan and zolmitriptan). Of these, the ergots (ergotamine and dihydroergotamine) and the 5-HT$_1$ agonists are considered specific migraine medications. One or more of these med-

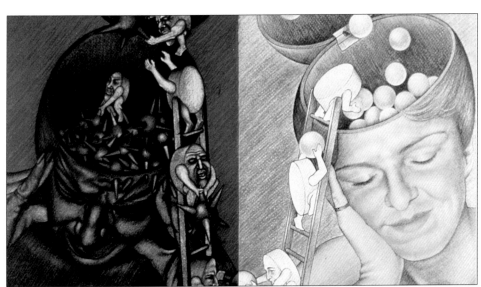

● **Figure 6.15**
'Relief' by Deborah Barrett of Everett, Massachusetts, USA. (© Sandoz Pharmaceuticals Corp.)

ications can be used for headaches of differing severities.[4] Preventive treatments include a selective group of medications from a broad range of drug classes, including notably beta-blockers, calcium-channel blockers, antidepressants, serotonin antagonists, anticonvulsants and NSAID.

Optimizing therapy requires knowledge of alternative treatments and awareness of the patient's preferences. Some patients want to minimize their attack frequency and are willing to accept significant side effects to achieve this goal. Some patients are eager to try new therapies, while others are afraid to change an established regimen even

though it may have only limited benefits. Some patients accept parenteral routes of administration readily, but others reject the idea of injections or suppositories.[3]

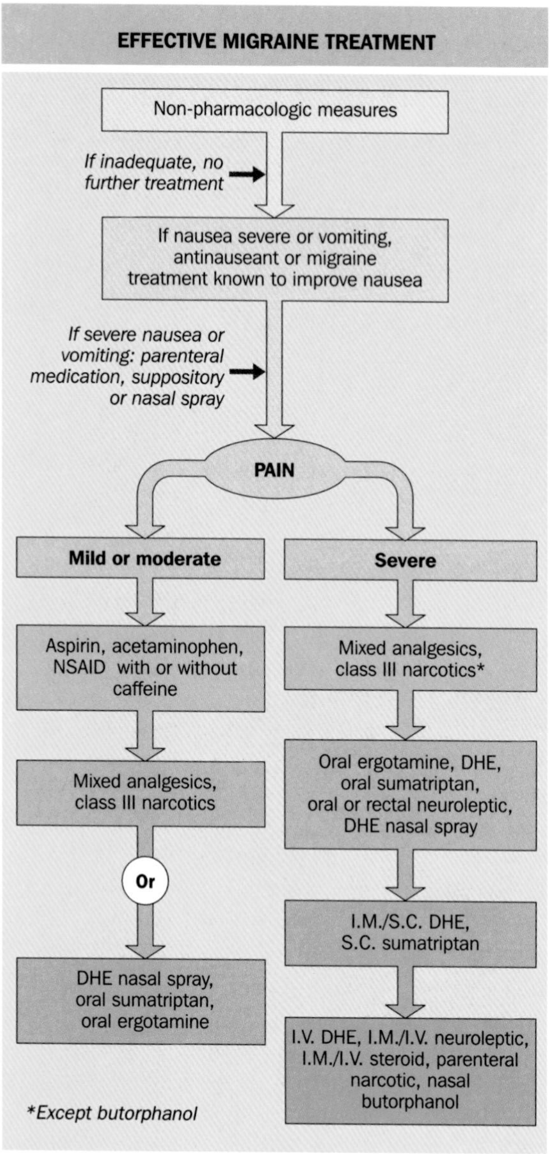

Acute treatment (Figure 6.16)
Combined treatment

Many acute treatments are available for migraine. The choice depends on the severity and frequency of the headaches, the pattern of the associated symptoms, the presence of comorbid illnesses and the patient's treatment response profile (Table 6.15). For patients with mild-to-moderate headaches, we start with oral medications, such as analgesics, NSAID, or a caffeine adjuvant compound. If this initial treatment fails, we move on to dihydroergotamine or a 5-HT$_1$ agonist (sumatriptan or zolmitriptan). If prominent nausea or vomiting is present, we prescribe an antiemetic and more readily recommend non-oral treatment. If oral medication is ineffective or cannot be used due to gastrointestinal symptoms, we recommend suppositories, nasal spray or injections, based on the patient's preferred route of administration. Suppositories include ergotamine, indomethacin and prochlorperazine. Nasal sprays include transnasal butorphanol and soon dihydroergotamine and sumatriptan. Injections include subcutaneous sumatriptan and intramuscular dihydroergotamine, among others. We often prescribe more than one acute treatment at the time of the initial visit. For example, we may advise patients to use naproxen sodium for mild-to-moderate headaches and a 5-HT$_1$ agonist for more severe headaches (Figure 6.17).[3,4]

Simple and combination analgesics, and NSAIDs

We often begin with simple analgesics for patients with mild-to-moderate headaches. Many individuals find headache relief with a simple analgesic such as aspirin or acetaminophen (paracetamol), either alone or in combination with caffeine. Butalbital is another effective analgesic adjuvant which is not generally available outside the United States. We also use the combination of acetaminophen, isomethptene (a sympathomimetic) and dichloralphenazone (a chloral hydrate derivative). For patients who are nauseated, we use antiemetics. When available, we prefer domperidone because of its lack of CNS problems; as a back-up we use metoclopramide. We often try naproxen sodium first, but we use all the NSAID, often in combination with an antiemetic. Indomethacin, available as a 50 mg rectal suppository, and intramuscular ketorolac are useful in patients with severe nausea and vomiting.[4]

Ergotamine and dihydroergotamine (Figure 6.17)

We use ergotamine and its derivative, dihydroergotamine,[29] to treat moderate-to-severe migraine if analgesics do not

EFFECTIVE MIGRAINE TREATMENT

Non-pharmacologic measures

If inadequate, no further treatment

If nausea severe or vomiting, antinauseant or migraine treatment known to improve nausea

If severe nausea or vomiting: parenteral medication, suppository or nasal spray

PAIN

| Mild or moderate | Severe |

Aspirin, acetaminophen, NSAID with or without caffeine

Mixed analgesics, class III narcotics*

Mixed analgesics, class III narcotics

Oral ergotamine, DHE, oral sumatriptan, oral or rectal neuroleptic, DHE nasal spray

Or

I.M./S.C. DHE, S.C. sumatriptan

DHE nasal spray, oral sumatriptan, oral ergotamine

I.V. DHE, I.M./I.V. neuroleptic, I.M./I.V. steroid, parenteral narcotic, nasal butorphanol

*Except butorphanol

● **Figure 6.16** *Effective migraine treatment begins with making an accurate diagnosis.*

● **Table 6.15** *Acute medications: efficacy, side effects, relative contraindications and indications*

Drug	Efficacy	Side effect	Comorbid	
			Relative contraindications	**Relative indication**
Acetaminophen (Paracetamol)	1+	1+	Liver disease	Pregnancy
Aspirin	1+	1+	Kidney disease, ulcer disease, PUD, gastritis (age <15 years)	CAD, TIA
Butalbital, caffeine and analgesics	2+	2+	Use of other sedative; history of medication overuse	
Caffeine adjuvant	2+	1+	Sensitivity to caffeine	
Isometheptene	2+	1+	Uncontrolled hypertension, CAD, PVD	
Narcotics	3+	3+	Drug or substance abuse	Pregnancy; rescue medication
NSAIDs	2+	1+	Kidney disease, PUD, gastritis	
Dihydroergotamine				
Injections	4+	2+	CAD, PVD, uncontrolled hypertension prominent nausea or vomiting	Orthostatic hypotension,
Intranasal	3+	1+		
Ergotamine				
Tablets	2+	2+	Prominent nausea or vomiting, CAD, PVD, uncontrolled hypertension	
Suppositories	3+	3+		
Sumatriptan				
SC Injection	4+	1+	CAD, PVD, uncontrolled hypertension	Prominent nausea or vomiting
Intranasal	3+	1+	CAD, PVD, uncontrolled hypertension	Prominent nausea or vomiting
Tablets	3+	1+	CAD, PVD, uncontrolled hypertension	
Zolmitriptan				
Tablets	3+	1+	CAD, PVD, uncontrolled hypertension	Prominent nausea

*Ratings are on a scale from 1+ (lowest) to 4+ (highest) based on response rates and consistency of response in double-blind placebo-controlled trials and our clinical experience.
**Abbreviations: PUD = peptic ulcer disease; PVD = peripheral vascular disease; CAD = coronary artery disease; TIA = transient ischaemic attack; NSAID = nonsteroidal anti-inflammatory drugs; SC = subcutaneous

provide satisfactory headache relief or if they produce significant side effects. Since rectal absorption is more reliable than oral, we prefer the suppository form of ergotamine. Patients who cannot tolerate ergotamine because of nausea are pretreated with an antiemetic.

ERGOTAMINE AND DIHYDROERGOTAMINE

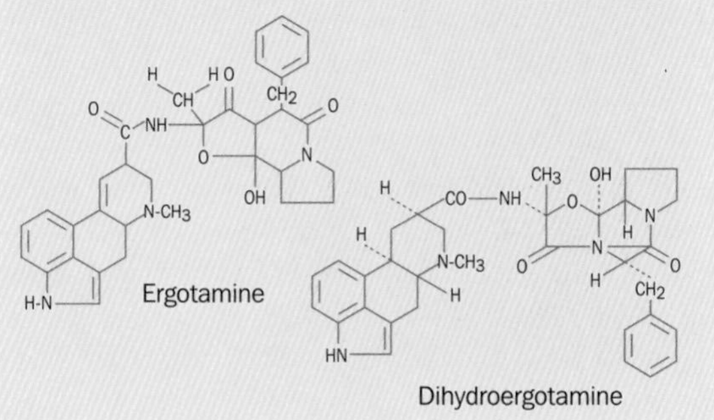

● **Figure 6.17** *Molecular structure of ergotamine and dihydroergotamine.*

Dihydroergotamine has fewer side effects than ergotamine and can be administered intranasally, intramuscularly, subcutaneously, or intravenously. Dihydroergotamine is given in doses of up to 1 mg i.m. or i.v. per treatment with a maximum of 3 mg/day, or 2mg i.n per treatment with a maximum of 4mg/day. We limit monthly use to 18 ampoules or 12 events. Dihydroergotamine is a mainstay of treatment because it is effective in most patients, it is associated with a low headache recurrence rate (<20%), and it is less likely than ergotamine to exacerbate nausea or produce rebound headache.

Avoid ergotamine and dihydroergotamine in women who are attempting to become pregnant and in patients with uncontrolled hypertension, sepsis, renal or hepatic failure, and coronary, cerebral or peripheral vascular disease. While nausea is a common side effect of ergotamine, it is less common with dihydroergotamine (unless it is given intravenously). Other side effects include dizziness, paraesthesias, abdominal cramps and chest tightness; rare idiosyncratic arterial and coronary vasospasm can occur. We recommend an electrocardiogram on all patients before their first dose of dihydroergotamine, particularly if there are any cardiac risk factors (including age >40 years).

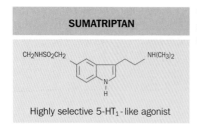

SUMATRIPTAN

Highly selective 5-HT$_1$ - like agonist

● *Figure 6.18*
Molecular structure of sumatriptan.

Selective 5-HT$_1$ agonists

Sumatriptan (Figure 6.18)

Sumatriptan, a selective 5-HT$_1$-receptor agonist, is available as an injectable (6 mg s.c.), as 25, 50 or 100 mg tablets depending upon the country and as a nasal spray (20 mg i.n.) Subcutaneous sumatriptan has a very rapid onset of action. Sumatriptan relieves headache pain, nausea, photophobia and phonophobia, and restores the patient's ability to function normally. We often prescribe sumatriptan at the initial consultation as a first line drug for severe attacks and as an escape medication for less severe attacks that do not adequately respond to simple or combination analgesics. We prefer the subcutaneous injection or the nasal spray for patients who need rapid relief or have severe nausea or vomiting. Oral sumatriptan is used for gradual onset headache when rapid pain relief is not required. Although 80% of patients get pain relief from an initial subcutaneous dose of sumatriptan, headache recurs in about 40% of patients. Recurrences are most likely in patients with long-duration headaches. Recurrences respond well to a second dose of sumatriptan or to simple and combination analgesics.[30,31]

Sumatriptan should not be used in patients with clinical or at high risk of ischaemic heart disease, Prinzmetal's angina or vertebrobasilar migraine. Common side effects include pain at the injection site, tingling, flushing, burning and warm or hot sensations. Dizziness, heaviness, neck pain and dysphoria also can occur. These side effects generally abate within 45 minutes. Sumatriptan causes non-cardiac chest pressure in approximately 4% of patients. We get an electrocardiogram on patients over the age of 40 years and with risk factors for heart disease before using sumatriptan.

We often give the first dose of sumatriptan in the office at a time the patient does not have a headache.

New 5-HT$_1$ agonists (Table 6.16)

Acute migraine treatment advanced significantly with the introduction of *sumatriptan*, the first specific 5-HT$_{1B/1D}$ agonist; however, there is still room for improvement. Approximately half of patients do not respond at two hours after administration and about three-quarters had at least some residual headache pain. Up to 40% of patients experience a headache recurrence after initial treatment. A number of new 5-HT$_{1B/1D}$ agonists, whose mechanism of action is similar to sumatriptan but whose pharmacokinetics differ, are in development. These may produce better migraine response rates, lower recurrence, or be better tolerated. Drugs that work by other mechanisms are also being studied.

Alniditan, eletriptan, naratriptan, rizatriptan and *zolmitriptan* all have affinity for the 5-HT$_{1B}$ and 5-HT$_{1D}$ receptors. All are full agonists except for eletriptan, which is a partial agonist. All can penetrate the CNS except for eletriptan, for which data is unavailable. All are being initially developed as oral tablets except for alniditan, which is being developed as an injectable (Table 6.16). All constrict the cerebral and coronary arteries and inhibit neurogenic inflammation in the Moskowitz model.

Oral *eletriptan* is rapidly absorbed (C$_{max}$ 0.5 to 1 hour), with a 50% bioavailability and a half-life of 4–5 hours.[32] Oral eletriptan (20, 40 or 80 mg) was compared to oral sumatriptan (100 mg) and placebo for abortive treatment within 6 hours of the onset of a migraine headache. Eletriptan 40 mg was at least as good as sumatriptan 100 mg at 2 hours and eletriptan 80 mg was superior to sumatriptan 100 mg. A clear improvement in headache was evident at 1 hour, with a response rate of 43% in patients receiving eletriptan 40 mg and 40% in patients on eletriptan 80 mg, compared with only 21% and 19% for those receiving sumatriptan and placebo, respectively. Treatment-related adverse events were reported by 23% of patients on placebo, 18% on eletriptan 20 mg, 25% on eletriptan 40 mg, 36% on eletriptan 80 mg and 37% on sumatriptan 100 mg.[33]

● **Table 6.16** *Selective serotonin agonists*

Action	Sumatriptan	Rizatriptan	Zolmitriptan	Naratriptan	Eletriptan
5-HT$_{1B/1D}$ affinity	✔	✔	✔	✔	✔
Agonist activity	F	F	F	F	P
Cranial vasoconstrictor	✔	✔	✔	✔	✔
Coronary vasoconstrictor	✔	✔	✔	✔	?
Inhibitor NI	✔	✔	✔	✔	✔
CNS penetration	–	✔	✔	✔	?

F = full agonist; P = partial agonist

Oral *naratriptan* has a bioavailability of 60–70% and a T_{max} of 3–5 hours. Naratriptan has been studied in a series of randomized, double-blind, placebo-controlled studies that examined a dose range from 0.1 mg to 10 mg in over 4000 patients. The drug has a well defined dose–response relationship for headache relief with a mean response of 48% at 2 hours after administration. Looking across the entire dose range the rate of recurrence was lowest for the 2.5 mg dose at 25% when compared to a recurrence rate for sumatriptan of 38% for the comparative studies done in the development programme. In a crossover study of patients enrolled with a higher than average rate of recurrence, their rate of recurrence was statistically significantly less when directly compared to sumatriptan. Tolerability for the 2.5 mg dose of naratriptan was very good in the studies in the development programme with a rate of adverse events for naratriptan at doses of 2.5 mg and below equal to that of placebo.[34,35]

Rizatriptan has high oral bioavailability. Two multicentre, double-blind, parallel-group, dose-finding studies assessed the clinical efficacy and safety of 2.5–40 mg oral rizatriptan compared with placebo and 100 mg oral sumatriptan. At 1 hour, significantly more patients on 20 and 40 mg rizatriptan reported headache response than did those on placebo. From 1 and 1.5 to 4 hours, patients treated with 5–40 mg rizatriptan showed significantly higher response rates than placebo-treated patients. Compared with 100 mg sumatriptan, the proportion of patients with headache relief at 2 hours was similar in the 10 mg and 20 mg rizatriptan groups and significantly higher in the 40 mg group.

Zolmitriptan

Zolmitriptan is the second 5-HT$_{1B/1D}$ agonist to be marketed in the UK and is now available in the USA. Zolmitriptan displays high affinity at human recombinant 5-HT$_{1B/1D}$ receptors and modest affinity for 5-HT$_{1A}$ and 5-HT$_{1F}$ receptors; it lacks significant affinity for other 5-HT receptors and a wide variety of monoamine receptors.[36,81–85] It is more lipophilic than sumatriptan.[81] It has an elimination half-life ($T_{1/2}$) of 3 hours[86], a T_{max} of 1 hour[87] and an oral bioavailability of 40%[88]. It is metabolized by MAO-A through the P450 system and has an active metabolite (N-desmethyl-zolmitriptan) that is also degraded by MAO-A. This limits the total dose to 5 mg/day in patients taking MAO inhibitors. The maximum concentration (C_{max}) of zolmitriptan (10 mg) increases with propranolol co-administration (160 mg/day)[88] but this does not limit use of the 5 mg dose. A meta-analysis of the phase II/III placebo-controlled studies of zolmitriptan demonstrated, at 2 hours, a headache response of 64% (95% CI:59–69%) with a therapeutic gain of 34% (95% CI: 27–41%) for 2.5 mg and a headache response of 66% (95% CI: 62–70%) with a corresponding therapeutic gain of 37% (30–44%) for the 5 mg dose[89]. (Therapeutic gain refers to the difference in response between active drug and placebo.) The headache-free endpoint at 2 hours for 2.5 mg was 25% (95% CI: 21–29%) with a therapeutic gain of 19% (14–24%) and for 5 mg was 34% (95% CI: 30–38%) with a therapeutic gain of 28% (23–33%). Increasing the dose increased adverse events; the therapeutic penalty rates were 17% (95% CI: 11–23%) and 29% (95% CI: 23–35%) for 2.5 mg and 5 mg respectively. Therefore, the recommended starting dose of 2.5 mg provides the best balance of benefit and side effects, although some patients may benefit from the higher 5 mg dose. At this time, no direct valid comparison trial with sumatriptan is available. One study with a high placebo response had no clear conclusion (Diener, Third European Headache Federation Meeting, Sardinia, 1996). Zolmitriptan's early onset of action will make it a useful treatment for many patients. In all studies, zolmitriptan reduced the incidence of photophobia, phonophobia and nausea compared to placebo.

Narcotics

If non-opioid medications do not provide adequate pain relief, we use codeine in combination with simple analgesics and sometimes butalbital or caffeine in the United States. We also use in restrictive circumstances, more potent narcotic analgesics such as propoxyphene, butorphanol, meperidine (pethidine), morphine, hydromorphone and oxycodone, alone and in combination with simple analgesics.[3,4] Because medication overuse and rebound headache pose a threat with narcotic use, these agents are most appropriate for patients whose severe headaches are relatively infrequent. Opiates that are mixed agonist–antagonist, such as butorphanol, have a lower drug abuse potential although it is not clear if these agents offer any protection from rebound headache. Transnasal butorphanol tartrate (1 mg followed by 1 mg 1 hour later) is an effective acute outpatient treatment which rapidly relieves the pain of migraine. It circumvents problems with oral absorption. Opiates should not be used more than 2 days a week on average (Table 6.17).

Table 6.17 *Oral doses of narcotic analgesics that achieve the same pain relief as 10 mg parenteral morphine for severe pain*

Drug		Oral dose (mg)	Oral-to-parenteral dose ratio	Parenteral dose (mg)
Morphine	Single dose	60	6:1	10
	Repeated dose	30	3:1	10
Hydromorphone		7.5	5:1	1.5
Methadone		20	2:1	10
Levorphanol		4	2:1	2
Meperidine (pethidine)		300	4:1	75
Codeine		200	1:5:1	130

In specific groups of patients, such as women with intractable menstrual migraine, we use narcotics on a more regular basis. These drugs are also especially helpful to patients who either do not respond to simple analgesics cannot take ergots or sumatriptan. Pregnant women can use codeine or meperidine (pethidine) with caution.[37] Narcotics are also useful for patients who awaken in the middle of the night with a headache. Sedation, which is sometimes an undesirable side effect, may help the patient go back to sleep and awaken headache-free in the morning.

Adjunctive treatment

Nausea and vomiting can be as disabling as the headache itself. Gastric stasis and delayed gastric emptying decrease the effectiveness of oral medication.[4] We use metoclopramide or domperidone as an antiemetic and a prokinetic, to enhance the absorption of oral medications. Promethazine and ondansetron (a selective $5\text{-}HT_3$-receptor antagonist) intravenously (0.15 mg/kg diluted in 50 ml of 5% dextrose or normal saline) or orally (8 mg tablet) can be used by patients who cannot tolerate metoclopramide because of side effects. We use the neuroleptics, chlorpromazine and prochlorperazine, intravenously, intramuscularly and by suppository, for nausea, vomiting and pain. Prochlorperazine suppositories (25 mg) are used as a primary treatment for headache and nausea and also as a rescue medication.

Preventive treatment

Preventive medication is usually given daily for months or years; however, treatment can be episodic, subacute or chronic. Episodic treatment is used when there is a known headache trigger, such as exercise or sexual activity; these patients can be instructed to pretreat prior to the exposure or activity. Patients who are undergoing a time-limited exposure to a trigger, such as ascent to a high altitude, or a reduced migraine threshold such as menstruation, can be treated subacutely by having them medicate before and during the exposure. Preventive medication can also be taken on a regular basis (chronic treatment) to decrease the frequency of migraine attacks.[4,38]

Circumstances that warrant chronic treatment include:

(i) two or more attacks a month that produce disability that lasts three or more days;

(ii) contraindication to, or ineffectiveness of, symptomatic medications;

(iii) the use of abortive medication more than twice a week, or

(iv) special circumstances, such as hemiplegic migraine or rare headache attacks producing profound disruption or risk of permanent neurologic injury.[3,33]

These rules are stricter during pregnancy, during which time severe disabling attacks accompanied by nausea, vomiting, and possibly dehydration are required for chronic treatment to be prescribed.[32]

The major medication groups for preventive migraine treatment include beta-adrenergic blockers, antidepressants, calcium channel antagonists, serotonin antagonists, anticonvulsants and NSAID. If preventive medication is indicated, the agent should be chosen from one of the major categories, based on side-effect profiles and coexistent comorbid conditions (Table 6.18).[3]

Preventive medications should be started at a low dose and increased slowly until therapeutic effects develop or until the ceiling dose for the agent in question is reached. Migraineurs frequently require a lower dose of a preventive medication than is needed for other indications. Tricyclic antidepressants such as amitriptyline are used in doses of 100–200 mg/day for depression, while 10–20 mg/day is often effective for migraine. In addition, migraineurs may be more sensitive to the side effects of medication. A starting dose of 25–50 mg/day of amitriptyline is common in patients with depression, whereas it can produce intolerable side effects in migraineurs. Divalproex or valproate is often effective at a dose of 500–750 mg/day for migraine, while higher doses may be necessary to effectively treat epilepsy and mania.[33,39] It is important to remember that some patients may respond to lower doses of preventive medications, but it may be necessary to increase the dose to tolerance before assuming the agent is ineffective.

A full therapeutic trial may take two to six months. In controlled clinical trials, efficacy is often first noted at four weeks and continues to increase for three months. It is not uncommon for a patient to be treated with a new preventive medication for one to two weeks without effect and then prematurely discontinue it, and both patient and physician believe it was not effective.

To obtain maximal benefit from preventive medication, the patient should not overuse analgesics or ergot derivatives. In addition, oral contraceptives, hormonal replacement therapy or vasodilating drugs such as nifedipine or nitroglycerine may interfere with preventive drugs.

Migraine headaches may improve with time independent of treatment; if the headaches are well controlled, a drug holiday can be undertaken following a slow taper programme. Many patients experience continued relief after discontinuing the medication or may not need the same dose. Dose reduction may provide a better risk-to-benefit ratio.

A woman of childbearing potential should be on adequate contraception before starting migraine medication. However, some women who are pregnant or who are attempting to become pregnant may still require preventive medications.

● **Table 6.18** *Choices of preventive treatment in migraine: influence of comorbid conditions*

Drug	Efficacy*	Side effects*	Comorbid condition**	
			Relative contraindication	Relative indication
Beta-blockers	4+	2+	Asthma, depression, CHF, Raynaud's disease, diabetes	Hypertension, angina
Antiserotonin				
Pizotifen	3+	2+	Obesity	
Methysergide	4+	4+	Angina, PVD	Orthostatic hypotension
Calcium-channel blockers				
Verapamil	2+	1+	Constipation, hypotension	Migraine with aura, hypertension, angina, asthma
Flunarizine	4+	2+	Parkinson's disease	Hypertension, familial hemiplegic migraine
Antidepressants				
Tricyclic	4+	2+	Mania, urinary retention, heart block	Other pain disorders, depression, anxiety disorders, insomnia
SSRI	2+	1+	Mania	Depression, OCD
MAOI	4+	4+	Unreliable patient	Refractory depression
Anticonvulsants				
Divalproex/valproate	4+	2+	Liver disease, bleeding disorders	Mania, epilepsy, anxiety disorders
NSAID				
Naproxen	2+	2+	Ulcer disease, gastritis	Arthritis, other pain disorders

*Ratings are on a scale from 1+ (lowest) to 4+ (highest).
** Abbreviations: CHF = congestive heart failure; OCD = obsessive compulsive disorder; PVD = peripheral vascular disease; MAOI = monoamine oxidase inhibitor; SSRI = serotonin specific re-uptake inhibitor; NSAID = non-steroidal anti-inflammatory drug

If this is absolutely necessary, inform the patient and her significant other of any potential risks and pick the medication with the least adverse effects on the fetus.

Medication

Beta-blockers

Since the relative efficacy of the different beta-blockers (propranolol, metoprolol, timolol, nadolol and atenolol) has not been clearly established, choose a beta-blocker based on beta-selectivity, convenience of drug formulation, side effects and the patient's individual reaction.[3,4] We prefer nadolol and atenolol because of their long half-life and favourable side-effect profile, although propranolol remains a very useful drug. Since beta-blockers can produce behavioural side effects, such as drowsiness, fatigue, lethargy, sleep disorders, nightmares, depression, memory disturbance and hallucinations, we avoid them in patients with depression or low energy. Decreased exercise tolerance limits their use by athletes. Less common side effects include impotence, orthostatic hypotension, significant bradycardia and aggravation of intrinsic muscle disease. We find beta-blockers especially useful in patients with comorbid angina or hypertension. They are relatively contraindicated in patients with congestive heart failure, asthma, Raynaud's disease and insulin-dependent diabetes.

Antidepressants

We use both tricyclic antidepressants and selective serotonin reuptake inhibitors (SSRI). The tricyclic antidepressants we use most commonly are nortriptyline and doxepin, and dothiepin outside the United States, although only amitriptyline has demonstrated benefits in placebo-controlled, double-blind studies.[3,4] We often use tricyclic antidepressants for the patient with a sleep disturbance. We frequently use SSRI such as fluoxetine, paroxetine and sertraline, based on their favourable side-effect profiles, not their established efficacy. Fluoxetine is of proven value in chronic daily headache.[40] We believe that venlafaxine, the first specific serotonin and norepinephrine reuptake inhibitor, may be effective, but no studies have been performed.

Side effects of tricyclic antidepressants are common. Most involve antimuscarinic effects, such as dry mouth and sedation. The drugs also cause increased appetite and weight gain; cardiac toxicity and orthostatic hypotension occur occasionally. Sexual dysfunction is not uncommon with SSRI and can be treated with amantadine.[41] Antidepressants are especially useful in patients with comorbid depression and anxiety disorders.

Calcium-channel blockers

Of the calcium-channel blockers available in the USA, verapamil is the most effective.[3,4] It is especially useful in patients with comorbid hypertension or with contraindications to beta-blockers such as asthma and Raynaud's disease. We use verapamil in patients with migraine with prolonged aura or migrainous infarction. Because the drug has an especially favourable side-effect profile, we use it preferentially on patients unlikely to tolerate cognitive side effects. Constipation is verapamil's most common side effect. Flunarizine is the most effective drug of this class, but is not available everywhere. The symptoms of parkinsonism, produced by its antidopaminergic activity, limits its use.

Anticonvulsant medications

The most effective anticonvulsant is valproic acid in the USA; we use it in the form of divalproex.[33,34] Divalproex and valproate are very effective preventive medications for migraine, as has been demonstrated by four placebo-controlled studies. It is effective in many patients at a low dose of 500–750 mg/day. In patients who do not respond to lower doses, we push the dose of divalproex to a trough level of 120 mg/ml.

Side effects include sedation, hair loss, tremor and changes in cognitive performance. Nausea, vomiting and indigestion can occur but these are self-limited side effects. Hepatotoxicity is the most serious side effect, but irreversible hepatic dysfunction is extremely rare in adults. Baseline liver-function studies should be obtained, but routine follow-up studies are probably not routinely needed in adults on monotherapy. Follow-up is necessary to adjust the dose and monitor side effects.

Divalproex is especially useful when migraine occurs in patients with comorbid epilepsy, anxiety disorders or manic-depressive illness. It can be safely administered to patients with depression, Raynaud's disease, asthma and diabetes, circumventing the contraindications to beta-blockers.

Serotonin antagonists

Methysergide is an effective migraine prophylactic drug. Side effects include transient muscle aching, claudication, abdominal distress, nausea, weight gain and hallucinations. Frightening hallucinations after the first dose are not uncommon. The major complication of methysergide is the rare (1/2500) development of retroperitoneal, pulmonary or endocardial fibrosis, the unreasonable fear of which prevents its more widespread use. To prevent this complication, a medication-free interval of four weeks following each six-month course of continuous treatment is recommended. We find methysergide to be a very effective drug with minimal side effects, but we reserve its use because of the need for a drug holiday.[4]

Pizotifen

Pizotifen is a benzocycloheptathiophene derivative structurally similar to cyproheptadine and the tricyclic antidepressants. It has a long elimination half life (about 23 hours) and can be given as a single evening dose. Pizotifen is 5-HT$_2$ and histamine-1 antagonist with the side effects of drowsiness and increased appetite with associated weight gain. Pizotifen has proven effective in controlled trials[74] and placebo-controlled trials[75–77]. In an open trial it was less effective than methysergide[78] but more effective than placebo. In another placebo-controlled trial it was as effective as naproxen sodium and both were more effective than placebo. Pizotifen (2–3 mg) daily was as effective as flunarazine 10 mg daily. Pizotifen is often used in adolescent migraineurs at doses of 0.5–1.5 mg daily. Adults, in contrast, may require up to 3 mg daily. Pizotifen has no interaction with specific antimigraine compounds, such as ergotamine or the triptans.

Setting treatment priorities

The goals of treatment are to relieve or prevent the pain and associated symptoms of migraine and to optimize the patient's ability to function normally. The medications used to treat migraine can be divided into two major categories:

(i) alternatives of high efficacy, which include beta-blockers, tricyclic antidepressants, pizotifen, divalproex, and alternatives of lower efficacy, which include SSRI, calcium-channel antagonists and NSAID, and

(ii) second-line choices of high efficacy, which include methysergide and monoamine oxidase inhibitors (MAOI), and second-line choices of unproven or low efficacy, which include cyproheptadine, gabapentin and lamotrigan (Table 6.19).

● **Table 6.19** *Preventive drugs*

Alternatives	High efficacy:	Beta-blockers, tricyclic antidepressants, divalproex, pizotifen
	Low efficacy:	Verapamil, NSAID, SSRI
Second-line choices	High efficacy:	Methysergide*
		Flunarizine
		MAOI*
	Unproven efficacy:	Cyproheptadine
		Gabapentin
		Lamotrigan

Significant adverse effects

● Table 6.20 *Drug combinations*

Suggested	Antidepressants	Beta-blocker
		Calcium-channel blocker
		Divalproex
		Methysergide
	Methysergide	Calcium-channel blocker
	SSRI	Tricyclic antidepressants
Caution	Beta-blocker	Calcium-channel blocker
		Methysergide
	MAOI	Amitriptyline or nortriptyline
Contraindications	MAOI	SSRI
		Most tricyclic antidepressants (except amitriptyline or nortriptyline)
		Carbamazepine

Choose a drug from one of the high-efficacy alternatives based on the patient's profile and the presence or absence of coexisting or comorbid disease (Table 6.12). Use the drug with the best risk-to-benefit ratio for the individual patient and take advantage of the side-effect profile of the drug. An underweight patient would be a candidate for one of the medications that commonly produce weight gain, such as a tricyclic antidepressant; in contrast, one would avoid these drugs in the overweight patient. Sedating tertiary tricyclic antidepressants would be useful at bedtime for patients with insomnia. The older patient with cardiac disease may not be able to use tricyclic antidepressants or calcium-channel or beta-blockers but could easily use divalproex. In the athletic patient, beta-blockers should be avoided. Medication that can impair cognitive functioning should be avoided in patients who are dependent on their wits.

Comorbid and coexistent diseases have important implications for treatment. The presence of a second illness provides therapeutic opportunities but also imposes certain therapeutic limitations. In some instances, two or more conditions may be treated with a single drug. When migraine and hypertension and/or angina occur together, beta-blockers or calcium-channel blockers may be effective for all conditions.[3,4] For the patient with migraine and depression, tricyclic antidepressants or SSRI may be especially useful.[42] For the patient with migraine and epilepsy[34] or migraine and manic depressive illness,[34] divalproex sodium is the drug of choice. The pregnant migraineur who has a comorbid condition that needs treatment should be given a medication that is effective for both conditions and has the lowest potential for adverse effects on the fetus. In individuals with more than one disease, certain categories of treatment may be relatively contraindicated. For example, beta-blockers should be used with caution in the depressed migraineur,

while tricyclic antidepressants, neuroleptics or sumatriptan may lower the seizure threshold and should be used with caution in the epileptic migraineur.

Drug combinations are commonly used for patients with refractory headache disorders. Some combinations, such as antidepressants and beta-blockers, are suggested; others, such as beta-blockers and calcium-channel blockers, should be used with caution; and some, such as MAOI and SSRI, are contraindicated because of potentially lethal interactions (Table 6.20). Many clinicians find that the combination of an antidepressant (such as a tricyclic antidepressant or SSRI) and a beta-blocker, act synergistically. Lance has advocated combining methysergide with a vasodilator such as a calcium-channel blocker to decrease side effects. Divalproex, used in combination with antidepressants, is a logical choice to treat refractory migraine that is complicated by depression or bipolar disease. Some clinicians cautiously use the combination of phenelzine and amitriptyline in refractory headache patients.

Use of abortive medication in patients on preventive treatment

Preventive medication is considered to be effective if it decreases the frequency of attacks more than 50%. Thus patients treated with preventive medication may continue to have attacks of episodic migraine and tension-type headache. Menstrual migraine attacks often persist to a greater extent than non-menstrual attacks. Preventive medication may also decrease the intensity and duration of the attacks, and in some cases may make abortive medications more effective. The use of preventive and abortive medication in concert presents a new set of complexities. First, the amount of acute medication must be limited to prevent the development of drug-induced daily rebound headache and loss of efficacy of the preventive medication. This is one of the causes of secondary failure of preventive medication. Secondly, certain abortive medications should be used with

● Table 6.21 *Cautions in acute medication use*

Agent	Caution	Contraindicated
Methysergide	Ergotamine, dihydroergotamine, 5-HT_1 agonists	
Monoamine oxidase inhibitors	Oral sumatriptan	Meperidine
		Sympathomimetics (Midrid)
Non-steroidal anti-inflammatory drugs	Other NSAID or aspirin-containing compounds	
Divalproex	Overuse of short-acting barbiturates	

caution in the presence of certain preventive medications (see Table 6.21). Ergotamine, dihydroergotamine, and sumatriptan could potentially have enhanced vasospastic properties in the presence of methysergide. However, many authorities have found that the ergots are more effective in patients treated with methysergide. Monoamine oxidase inhibitors increase the half-life and the area under the curve of oral sumatriptan. Therefore, the dose of oral sumatriptan should be reduced and used cautiously, if at all, in patients taking MAOI. Meperidine and sympathomimetics are a potentially lethal addition to MAOI and may result in serotonin syndrome or hypertensive crisis.

Status migrainosus

Status migrainosus is a condition characterized by severe, persistent headache often associated with intractable nausea and vomiting. Prior to instituting treatment serious organic causes of headache must be excluded.[43] We start treatment by rehydrating the patient with intravenous fluids and using one of the treatment options in Table 6.22. If the headache persists and is associated with intractable nausea and vomiting (migraine status), hospital admission may be required. Some indications for admission are listed in Table 6.23. Various treatment options have been explored for treating this type of headache.

Intravenous chlorpromazine and prochlorperazine are effective in controlling intractable headache.[3,4,44,45] Chlorpromazine was found to be more effective than the combination of meperidine and dimenhydrinate and prochlorperazine was more effective than placebo in treating emergency department patients.[46] Although neuroleptics are locally irritating when given intravenously, they are more effective than when given intramuscularly or by suppository. We have found that haloperidol (5 mg) and thiothixene (5 mg) given intramuscularly are effective as adjunct or primary treatment for the severe migraine headache.[47] Intravenous haloperidol and intravenous droperidol have recently been used successfully.

Intravenous prochlorperazine 5 mg followed by intravenous DHE is a safe and effective means of terminating a migraine attack.[40] The combination of intravenous metoclopramide and intravenous DHE is more effective in treating an acute migraine attack than is intramuscular meperidine.[3,4] Prochlorperazine (10 mg, 2 ml) and dihydroergotamine (1 mg, 1 ml) can be mixed in a syringe and 2 cc of the mixture can be injected intravenously. If the headache is not relieved in 15–30 minutes the remainder of the dose can be injected. At times the addition of 5–10 mg of i.v. diazepam will help terminate the headache attack.

Repetitive intravenous dihydroergotamine

Patients who have truly intractable headaches should be admitted to the hospital and treated with repetitive intravenous dihydroergotamine.[6] The patient should be pretreated with metoclopramide 10 mg i.v. and then given dihydroergotamine 0.5 mg (Figure 6.19). If the patient has no nausea and the headache persists, another 0.5 mg dihydroergotamine is given. If the patient's headache is gone, 0.5 mg dihydroergotamine is continued every eight hours. If nausea develops, the dose of dihydroergotamine is decreased and the metoclopramide increased. Both drugs are continued as needed, the dihydroergotamine every eight hours until the patient is headache-free, at which time it is tapered and discontinued.

● **Table 6.23** *Indications for admission to hospital*

Emergency or urgent admission*

* Migraine variants such as hemiplegic migraine.
* Suspected CNS infection.
* Acute vascular disorder.
* Drug toxicity.
* Status migrainosus.
* Failed outpatient treatment of severe headache.

Non-emergent admission

* Headache causing interruption and compromise of the ability to carry out activities of daily living.
* Chronic daily refractory headache or cluster headache that does not respond to aggressive outpatient treatment.
* Headache complicated by significant depression or psychiatric disturbance.
* Headache accompanied by significant medical or surgical problem.
* Headache treatment requiring polypharmacy with potentially dangerous drug interactions or requiring close observation during initiation (monoamine oxidase inhibitors).
* Headache complicated by drug overuse that could not be safely or effectively treated overnight.

* Diagnosis itself warrants admission

● **Table 6.22** *Treatment of status migrainosus*

* Start i.v.
* Pretreat with prochlorperazine 5–10 mg i.v. or metoclopramide 10 mg i.v.
* Treat with dihydroergotamine 0.5–1 mg i.v.
* If headache persists after 1 hr give additional 0.5 mg dihydroergotamine i.v.
* Additions: dexamethasone 4 mg i.v.; diazepam 5–10 mg i.v.
* Alternatives:
    ketorolac 30–60 mg i.m.
    narcotics
    chlorpromazine 0.1 mg/kg

INTRAVENOUS DIHYDROERGOTAMINE (DHE)

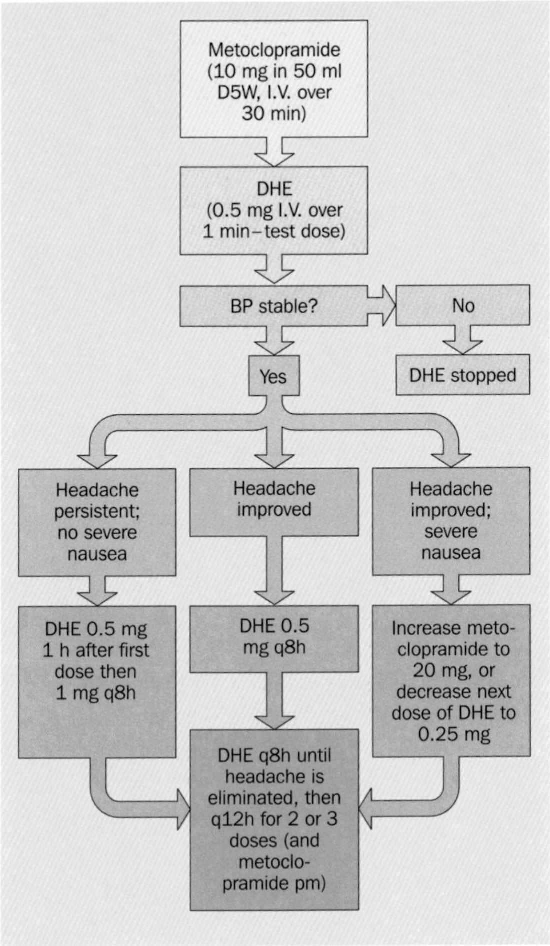

● **Figure 6.19** *Treatment protocol of repetitive intravenous dihydroergotamine (DHE).*

Repetitive intravenous dihydroergotamine was effective in eliminating chronic intractable headache in 89% of patients within 48 hours in one series. Intravenous diazepam was only partially effective in eliminating such headaches (13% within 3–6 days). We found that repetitive intravenous dihydroergotamine was effective in eliminating prolonged migraine, cluster headache, and chronic daily headaches with or without rebound.

By breaking the headache cycle and making the patient's headaches more manageable, intravenous dihydroergotamine seems to have a prolonged effect on the patient's well-being. Whether this is a result of dihydroergotamine, the active metabolite 8-hydroxydihydroergotamine, the cessation of overused drugs, or the removal of the patient from a stressful environment is uncertain, but the patients frequently do well after hospital discharge.[42]

Some clinicians advocate the use of parenteral corticosteroids, either alone or in combination with other symptomatic medications, to treat the severe resistant headache. Controlled studies have shown corticosteroids to be effective in the treatment of headache associated with altitude sickness.[3,4] Dexamethasone 4 mg i.v. following pretreatment with intravenous metoclopramide may be effective in the treatment of acute migraine headache.[3,4] The addition of dexamethasone to a narcotic regimen seems to provide additional relief.[3,4] Clinical experiences also support the view that steroids, such as a rapidly-tapering short course of prednisone (starting with 80–100 mg/day) or dexamethasone (Decadron, starting with 8–20 mg/day), will assist in terminating an otherwise refractory migraine headache.[42] Inpatients can be treated with high-dose intravenous corticosteroids, alone or in conjunction with neuroleptics or dihydroergotamine, to help terminate a headache cycle.

Menstrual migraine

Migraine can occur before, during, or after menstruation, or at the time of ovulation.[48] When migraine occurs before menstruation (premenstrual migraine, PMS) it may have other features of premenstrual syndrome (LLPDD) (Table 6.24). Migraine that occurs during menstruation is often associated with dysmenorrhoea and is frequently refractory to treatment. It is important to differentiate between the two conditions, because medications that may be useful in treating headache related to dysmenorrhoea may not help headache associated with PMS.[43] Based on clinical experience, the frequency of menstrual migraine has been reported to be as high as 60–70%. Based on retrospective analysis, prevalence ranges from 26–60% in headache clinic patients. The prevalence is lower in non-headache clinic patients. The relative frequency of menstrual migraine depends on the means of ascertainment.[49]

Most women have increased headache attacks at the time of menses (Figure 6.20). Women preselected on the basis of PMS have more headaches prior to the onset of menses, but most women have more headaches just before or with menstruation. Some women have migraine (usually without aura)

● **Table 6.24** *Premenstrual syndrome*

Depression	Backache
Anxiety	Breast tenderness
Crying spells	Swelling
Difficulty in thinking	Nausea
Lethargy	

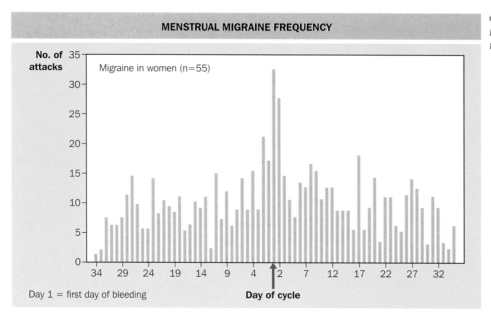

Figure 6.20
Menstrual migraine frequency.[89]

only with menses. Menstrual migraine can be defined by looking at attacks triggered by menstruation on a regular basis (Table 6.25). Attacks occurring only with menstruation, even if infrequent, would be called 'true menstrual migraine'. Attacks occurring both at menstruation and at other times of the month could be called 'menstrually triggered migraine'. A frequency indicator (e.g. frequent >70%, common 35–70% and infrequent <35%) would look at the tightness of this association. The quality of these attacks, their response to treatment, and the hormonal changes in such patients could then be analysed based on this association. Migraine attacks occurring –2 to –7 days before the onset of menses would be called 'premenstrual'; those occurring from –1 to +4 days, 'menstrual'. This cut-off is arbitrary and needs to be further examined.[43]

Menstrual migraine occurs at the time of the greatest fluctuation in oestrogen levels (Figure 6.21). Attempts to find consistent differences in ovarian hormone levels between women with menstrual migraine and controls have not yielded consistent results. Some authors have reported higher oestrogen and progestin levels; others have not;[43] most find that testosterone, follicle-stimulating hormone, and luteinizing levels are similar to controls. In Beckham's study, headache activity correlated with high progesterone during the luteal phase. Since progesterone is the marker for the luteal phase, it tells us nothing as to any causal association between luteal headaches and progesterone.[43]

Somerville[50] reported that menstrual migraine headache occurs during or after the simultaneous fall of oestrogens and progesterone. Oestrogens given premenstrually delay the onset of migraine but not menstruation.[43] In contrast, progesterone administration delays menstruation but does

not prevent migraine.[43] Somerville concluded that oestrogen withdrawal may trigger migraine attacks in susceptible women (Figure 6.22).

Oestrogen-withdrawal migraine requires several days of exposure to high levels of oestrogen. When Somerville used an erratic delivery system of long-acting oestrogen implants to suppress migraine, his patients developed irregular bleeding and headaches associated with fluctuating oestrogen levels.

The initial treatment of women who have migraine throughout their menstrual cycle should include general measures such as reassurance, identification and elimination of triggers, use of abortive and prophylactic medications, psychological modalities and sleep hygiene.[43]

Table 6.25 Menstrual migraine definition

Premenstrual migraine	Menstrual migraine
Attacks occur –7 to –2 days*	Attacks occur –1 to +4 days*

* Day 0 onset of menses

Table 6.26 Treatment of menstrual migraine

- Non-steroidal anti-inflammatory drugs (NSAID)
- Ergotamine and its derivatives
- Perimenstrual use of standard prophylactic drugs
- Short course of corticosteroids or major tranquillizers
- Hormonal therapy
    Oestrogens (with or without androgens or progestogen)
    Synthetic androgens (danazol)
    Anti-oestrogen (tamoxifen)
    Dopamine agonists (bromocriptine)

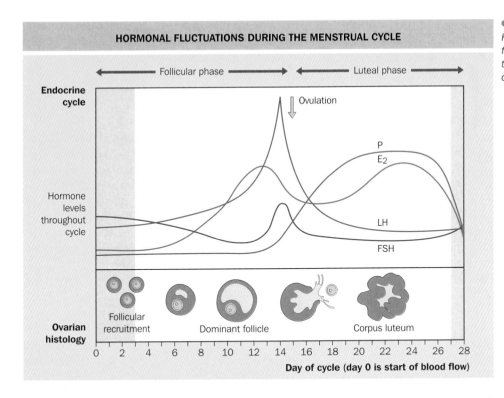

Figure 6.21
Hormonal fluctuations during the menstrual cycle.

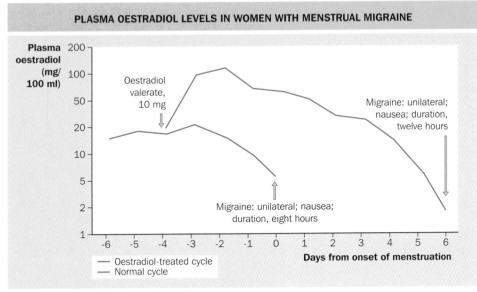

Figure 6.22
Plasma oestradiol levels in women with menstrual migraine (adapted from ref. 50).

These measures may eliminate all headaches except those associated with the menses.[43] Menstrually-related migraine typically occurs at the same time of month or in association with symptoms that herald its occurrence, allowing the timed use of medications.[43] Treatment of coexistent PMS may help control premenstrual headache (Table 6.26).

Women who have migraine exclusively with their menses can be treated by the perimenstrual use of prophylactic med-ication (antidepressants, beta-blockers, calcium-channel blockers or methysergide).[43] Women already using prophy-lactic medication for non-menstrual migraine can increase the dose of medication prior to their menses.

NMR spectroscopy has shown magnesium deficiency in the cerebral cortex of migraineurs.[51] Ionized serum mag-nesium is low in some women who selectively respond to bolus intravenous magnesium.[52] A placebo-controlled double-blind study of 24 women with PMS and migraine has shown that oral magnesium (360 mg magnesium pyrolidone carboxylic acid) decreases the severity of the PMS symptoms and the duration and intensity of menstrual migraine occurring prior to the onset of menstruation.[43] Perhaps responders belong to the subset of women with low serum ionized magnesium.[43]

An attack of menstrual migraine may be controlled by the use of NSAID, ergotamine, dihydroergotamine and sumatriptan.

Prostaglandin production may be enhanced in menstrual migraine. The effectiveness of the NSAID[43] may be a result of blocking prostaglandin synthesis by inhibiting the enzyme cyclooxygenase. The meclofenamates, in addition, are prostaglandin receptor antagonists. One NSAID, ketoprofen, inhibits the formation of leukotrienes by inhibiting 5-lipooxygenase. Non-steroidal anti-inflammatory drugs in adequate doses can be used abortively or prophylactically one to two days before the expected onset of headache and continued for the duration of vulnerability. If the first NSAID is ineffective, other classes of NSAID should be tried (Figure 6.23).[43]

Ergotamine and dihydroergotamine can be used prophylactically at the time of menses without significant risk of developing ergot dependence. Ergotamine tartrate, at bedtime or twice a day, is an effective prophylactic agent.

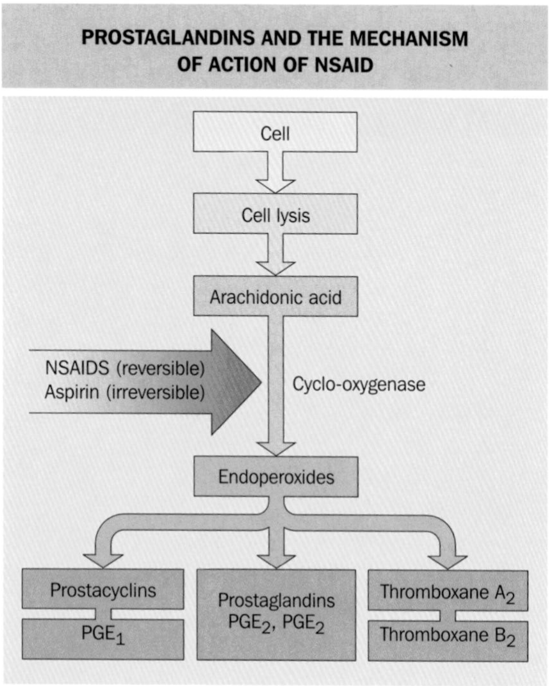

Ergotamine in combination with belladonna and phenobarbital (Bellergal) may be useful in treating other PMS (LLPDD) symptoms in addition to headache.[43]

Subcutaneous sumatriptan is as effective for menstrually associated migraine[53] as for non-menstrually related migraine and, in addition, controls the nausea and vomiting associated with attacks.

If severe menstrual migraine cannot be controlled with NSAID, ergots, dihydroergotamine, or sumatriptan, then analgesics in combination with narcotics, high-dose corticosteroids, major tranquillizers (chlorpromazine, haloperidol, thiothixene) or a course of intravenous dihydroergotamine can be tried. If these fail, a trial of hormonal therapy may be indicated.[43]

Successful hormonal therapy of menstrual migraine has been reported with oestrogens,[54] oestrogen antagonists, prolactin-release inhibitors and oestrogens in combination with progesterone or testosterone. Progesterone is not effective in the treatment of headache or other symptoms of PMS despite many favourable anecdotal reports.[43]

The decrease in oestrogen levels during the late luteal phase of the menstrual cycle is a trigger for migraine.[45] Oestrogen replacement prior to menstruation has been used to prevent migraine. In two double-blind crossover studies, percutaneous oestradiol gel perimenstrually significantly reduced headache.[43] Magos, in both an open study and a double-blind study, found oestradiol implants (available investigationally in the USA) and cyclic progesterones to be effective in menstrual migraine.[55] The oestradiol cutaneous patch provides a relatively stable plasma-oestrogen level over the time of application.[56] Levels are less stable with higher dose patches. Serum oestrogen levels rise within four hours of applying the transdermal patch and are proportional to the dose (patch TTS 25, serum level of 23 pg/ml; TTS 50, 39 ng/ml and TTS 100 74 pg/ml).[57]

The TTS 25 patch used from four days before to four days after menstruation was not as effective as the TTS 100 patch.[58] Serum oestradiol level between 60 and 80 pg/ml may be needed during the crucial week to prevent menstrual migraine.[43] TTS 50 patches (TTS = 39 pg/ml), were not significantly different from placebo in a placebo-controlled double-blind trial[59] and in another placebo-controlled trial, except for patients who had abnormal CNV and normal ES2.[60]

Combinations of oestrogens and progestogens or progestogens alone in the form of oral contraceptives (discussed below) may be a reasonable approach for some patients with intractable menstrual migraine, particularly if associated with severe dysmenorrhoea.[43]

Danazol, an androgen derivative, may be effective in the prophylaxis of menstrual migraine at a dose of 200–600 mg/day, starting before the expected onset of the headache and continuing through the menses.[43]

PROSTAGLANDINS AND THE MECHANISM OF ACTION OF NSAID

Cell

↓

Cell lysis

↓

Arachidonic acid

NSAIDS (reversible)
Aspirin (irreversible) → Cyclo-oxygenase

↓

Endoperoxides

Prostacyclins — PGE_1

Prostaglandins PGE_2, PGE_2

Thromboxane A_2 — Thromboxane B_2

● *Figure 6.23* Prostaglandins and the mechanism of action of NSAID.

Tamoxifen, an anti-oestrogen, may be effective in resistant menstrual migraine. A dose of 5–15 mg/day for days 7–14 of the luteal cycle has provided significant relief of menstrual headache without side effects.[43]

Bromocriptine,[43] a dopamine D_2-receptor agonist, is an inhibitor of prolactin release. A dose of 2.5–5 mg/day during the luteal phase of the menstrual cycle may decrease the premenstrual symptoms of breast engorgement, irritability and headache. In an open trial,[61] 24 women with severe, disabling menstrual migraine (occurring within three days of menstruation) were treated with bromocriptine 2.5 mg three times daily. Seventy-five per cent of the women had at least a 25% reduction in headache compared to baseline. Overall headache frequency decreased 72%. None of the patients had >10% increase in headache; three could not tolerate bromocriptine, and three did not benefit.

Hysterectomy and oophorectomy have not been shown to be effective in unselected cases in the treatment of migraine and we do not recommend this approach. However, medical ovariectomy using gonadotrophin-releasing hormone (GnRH) analogues to suppress ovulation are effective in refractory PMS. Since GnRH analogues induce menopause, treatment is usually limited to six months unless replacement oestrogens are used.[43]

Premenstrual migraine sufferers who have had a hysterectomy without an oophorectomy continue to have cyclic mental and physical symptoms during the late luteal phase of the menstrual cycle, demonstrating that neither the presence of the uterus nor the occurrence of menstruation is necessary for the maintenance of PMS.[43]

Some physicians are again advocating the use of hysterectomy and oophorectomy in women with severe intractable PMS or menstrual migraine who respond to medical ovariectomy.[62,63] There are no long-term follow-up or controlled studies to suggest the effectiveness of this radical procedure.

The effects of ovariectomy and hysterectomy on PMS and headache are contaminated by the postoperative use of daily oestrogen. No study is placebo-controlled, and women with PMS are very sensitive to placebo. The use of continuous oestrogen alone could account for the positive results.[64]

Migraine in the menopause

The menopause presents a particular set of problems in women in whom oestrogen replacement is indicated but leads to a worsening of migraine symptoms.

Although migraine prevalence decreases with advancing age, migraine can regress or worsen at menopause. Neri et al.[65] investigated 556 consecutive postmenopausal women

● **Table 6.27** Treatment of oestrogen replacement headache

- Reduce oestrogen dose
- Change oestrogen type from conjugated oestrogen to pure oestradiol to synthetic oestrogen to pure oestrone
- Convert from interrupted to continuous dosing
- Convert from oral to parenteral dosing
- Add androgens

attending an outpatient clinic and found that headache was present in 13.7%. Most (82%) had headache prior to the onset of menopause. Many (62%) had migraine without aura; the remainder had tension-type headache. None had migraine with aura or cluster headache. Women with prior migraine in general (two-thirds) improved with physiological menopause. In contrast, surgical menopause usually (two-thirds) resulted in a worsening of migraine. Other studies have shown that hysterectomy or oophorectomy is not an effective treatment for migraine at any age[66] despite recent suggestions to the contrary.[57,58] Oestrogen replacement therapy can exacerbate migraine or, alone or with testosterone, relieve it.[43] This has been confirmed in one, but not another, double-blind study. The use of drugs for treatment of migraine in menopausal women who do not need replacement oestrogens should be guided by their cardiac and renal status. Refractory cases may be treated with hormonal replacement.[43,53]

Headache management can be difficult in women who require oestrogen replacement therapy for menopausal symptoms but develop headaches as a result of the therapy. Several empirical strategies may be utilized (Table 6.27). Reducing the dose of oestrogen or changing the type of oestrogen from a conjugated oestrogen to pure oestradiol, to synthetic ethinyl oestradiol, or to a pure oestrone may significantly reduce headache. Changing from interrupted to continuous administration may be very effective if the headaches are associated with oestrogen withdrawal. Parenteral oestrogens, with or without adjunct hormones, can be effective. The oestradiol cutaneous patch, which provides a physiological ratio of oestradiol to oestrone and a steady-state concentration of oestrogen, has been associated anecdotally with fewer headache side effects; however, this has not been proven in any controlled study.

Migraine associated with oral contraceptive use

Hormonal contraceptive steroids are available as oral preparations, subcutaneous implants, depo-injections and vaginal preparations (in some countries).[67] The oral contraceptives

● **Table 6.28** *Oral contraceptives*

Progestin	Dose (mg)	Oestrogen	Dose (mg)
Monophasic			
Desogestrel	0.15	Ethinyloestradiol	30, 35
Ethynodiol diacetate	1.0	Ethinyloestradiol	35, 50
Levonorgestrel	0.15	Ethinyloestradiol	30
Norethindrone	0.4, 0.5, 1.0	Ethinyloestradiol	30, 35, 50
Norethindrone acetate	1.0, 1.5	Ethinyloestradiol	20, 30, 50
Norgestimateol	0.25	Mestranol	50
Norgestrel	0.5	Ethinyloestradiol	50
Multiphasic			
Norethindrone	0.5 (7), 1.0 (14)	Ethinyloestradiol	35
Norethindrone	0.5 (7), 0.75 (7), 1.0 (7)	Ethinyloestradiol	35
Norgestamate	0.180 (7), 0.215 (7), 0.290 (7)	Ethinyloestradiol	30

● **Table 6.29** *Oral contraceptives and stroke risk*

Factor		Odds ratio
Oestrogen dose (mg)	>50	8–10
	50	2–4
	30–40	1.5– 2.5
Progestogen alone		1
Smoking		1.5–1.6

After Lidegaard 70.

most commonly used in the USA contain combinations of synthetic oestrogen (ethinyl oestradiol or mestranol) and synthetic progestin (derivatives of 9-norprogesterone) taken 21 days each month. Another method of contraception is a progestin alone, which inhibits the luteinizing hormone surge.[43] In an attempt to minimize the associated androgenic side effects, the type of synthetic progestin has been changed. The newest (desogestrol, gestodene, norgestimate) are less androgenic and have less effect on carbohydrate and lipid metabolism than prior progestins.[68] The new formulation of oral contraceptives, containing 35 mg of ethinyl oestradiol and one of the new progestins, are comparable in efficacy to each other and to established agents (Table 6.28).

There is persistent controversy concerning oral contraceptives and the risk of stroke in migraineurs. During the last two decades, at least 15 retrospective studies have looked at the influence of oral contraceptives on the risk of cerebral thromboembolic events. Most (11/15) were conducted during a period when high-dose oestrogen pills were widely used. These data suggest that oral contraceptives containing more than 50 mg, 50 mg, and 30–40 mg of oestrogen are associated with odds ratios for cerebral thromboembolic attacks of about 8–10, 2–4 and 1.5–2.5 respectively, whereas those containing only a progestin are not associated with any increased risk (Table 6.29).[70]

The older combined oral contraceptives can induce, change or alleviate headache. Oral contraceptives can trigger the first migraine attack, most often in women with a family history of migraine. Existing migraine may exacerbate and headaches may occur on the days off the oral contraceptive. The headache pattern may become more severe and frequent and may be associated with neurological symptoms. In most women, however, the headache pattern does not change, and some women may have a distinct improvement in their headaches.[43]

New onset of migraine usually occurs in the early cycles of oral contraceptive use, but it can occur after prolonged oral contraceptive usage. Stopping the oral contraceptives may not bring immediate headache relief; there may be a delay of 6–12 months, or no improvement.

Studies from neurological or migraine clinics show increased incidence and severity of migraine in users of the older oral contraceptives. While headaches frequently occur on the days off the oral contraceptive, many women have relief with oral contraceptives. Studies from contraceptive clinics and general practitioners are more favourable towards oral contraceptives. Four double-blind placebo-controlled studies showed no difference in headache incidence between oral contraceptive and placebo. Both groups had a decreasing incidence of headache with continued observation. Some uncontrolled studies show an increase in headache frequency in women on oral contraceptives.

A new oral contraceptive containing 35 mg of the new, third-generation progestin, norgestimate (Ortho-Cyclen), was associated with a low incidence of headaches over three cycle intervals.

Contraception with progestins alone is a hormonal alternative to the use of the combined oral contraceptive. Progestins have no effect on blood clotting or platelet aggregation and are the contraceptive of choice for hypertensive women.

Norplant, a system of subdermal implants that release a steady dose of levonorgestrel (a progestin), is an effective contraceptive that lasts five years. The primary side effects are irregular menstrual bleeding and headaches. Headache, which was the primary reason cited for removal other than menstrual disturbance, occurs in about 5–20% of patients.

Recently Depo-Provera (medroxyprogesterone acetate suspension), a long-acting parenteral progestin, has been approved as a contraceptive agent. The exact frequency of headache with this drug is uncertain.

Oral contraceptives may generate new headaches or aggravate or ameliorate pre-existing headaches. This variability is also noted with pregnancy and menopause and may be a consequence of a variation in intrinsic oestrogen neuronal response. Women with intractable menstrual migraine or a history of headache relief with oral contraceptives may be candidates for a trial of oral contraceptives. They must be followed for headache aggravation or the development of neurological symptoms. Progestins can be used for contraception when oestrogens have caused increased headaches or are contraindicated.

References

1. Stewart WF, Lipton RB, Celentano DD, Reed ML. Prevalence of migraine in the United States. *JAMA* 1992; 267: 64–9.
2. Lipton RB, Stewart WF. Migraine in the United States: epidemiology and healthcare utilization. *Neurology* 1993; 43(3): 6–10.
3. Silberstein SD, Lipton RB. Overview of diagnosis and treatment of migraine. *Neurology* 1994; 44(7): 6–16.
4. Silberstein SD, Saper J. Migraine: diagnosis and treatment. In: Dalessio D, Silberstein SD (eds). *Wolff's Headache and Other Head Pain*. 6th Edition. New York: Oxford University Press, 1993: 96–170.
5. Headache Classification Committee of the International Headache Society. Classification and diagnostic criteria for headache disorders, cranial neuralgia, and facial pain. *Cephalalgia* 1988; 8(Suppl. 7):1–96.
6. Silberstein SD, Young WB. Migraine aura and prodrome. *Semin Neurol* 1995; 45: 175–82.
7. Jensen K, Tfelt-Hansen P, Lauritzen M, Olesen J. Classic migraine, a prospective recording of symptoms. *Acta Neurol Scand* 1986; 73: 359–62.
8. Blau JN. Classical migraine: symptoms between visual aura and headache onset. *Lancet* 1992; 340: 355–6.
9. Olesen J. Some clinical features of the acute migraine attack. An analysis of 750 patients. *Headache* 1978; 18: 268–71.
10. Sacks O. *Migraine: Understanding a Common Disorder*. Berkeley: University of California Press, 1985.
11. Selby G, Lance JW. Observations on 500 cases of migraine and allied vascular headache. *J Neurol Neurosurg Psychiatry* 1960; 23: 23–32.
12. Manzoni G, Farina S, Lanfranchi M, Solari A. Classic migraine: clinical findings in 164 patients. *Eur Neurol* 1985; 24: 163–9.
13. Bradshaw P, Parsons M. Hemiplegic migraine, a clinical study. *Q J Med* 1965; 133: 65–85.
14. Stewart WF, Schecter A, Lipton RB. Migraine heterogeneity: disability, pain intensity, attach frequency, and duration. *Neurology* 1994; 44(4): S24–39.
15. Silberstein SD. Migraine symptoms: results of a survey of self-reported migraineurs. *Headache* 1995; 35: 387–96.
16. Lipton RB, Silberstein SD, Stewart WF. An update on migraine epidemiology. *Headache* 1994; 34: 319–28.

17. Bickerstaff ER. Migraine variants and complications. In: Blau JN (ed). *Migraine: Clinical and Research Aspects*. Baltimore: John Hopkins University Press, 1987: 55–75.
18. Hosking G. Special forms: variants of migraine in childhood. In: Hockaday JM (ed.). *Migraine in Childhood*. Boston: Butterworths, 1988: 35–53.
19. Ophoff RA, van Eijk R, Sandkuijl LA *et al*. Genetic heterogeneity of familial hemiplegic migraine. *Genomics* 1994; 22: 21–6.
20. Tournier-Lasserve E, Joutel A, Melki J *et al*. Cerebral autosomal arteriopathy with subcortical infarcts and leukoencephalopathy maps to chomosome 19q12. *Nature Genet* 1993; 3: 256–9.
21. Hutchinson M, O'Riordan J, Javed M *et al*. Familial hemiplegic migraine and autosomal dominant arteriopathy with leukoencephalopathy. *Ann Neurol* 1995; 38: 817–24.
22. Chabriat H, Vahedi K, Iba-Zizen MT *et al*. Clinical spectrum of CADASIL: a study of seven families. *Lancet* 1995; 346: 934–9.
23. Chabriat H, Tournier-Lasserve E, Vahedi K *et al*. Autosomal dominant migraine with MRI white-matter abnormalities mapping to the CADASIL locus. *Neurology* 1995; 45: 1086–91.
24. Whitty CWM. Migraine without headache. *Lancet* 1967; ii: 283–5.
25. Levy DE. Transient CNS deficits: a common, benign syndrome in young adults. *Neurology* 1988; 38: 831–6.
26. Fisher CM. Late-life migraine accompaniments as a cause of unexplained transient ischemic attacks. *Can J Neurol Sci* 1980; 7: 9–17.
27. Fisher CM. Late-life migraine accompaniments: further experience. *Stroke* 1986; 17: 1033–42.
28. Lipton RB, Silberstein SD. Why study the comorbidity of migraine? *Neurology* 1994; 44(17): 4–5.
29. Silberstein SD, Young WB (for the Working Panel of the Headache and Facial Pain Section of the American Academy of Neurology). Safety and efficacy of ergotamine tartrate and dihydroergotamine in the treatment of migraine and status migrainosus. *Neurology* 1995; 45: 577–84.
30. Johnson S, Johnson FN. Sumatriptan. *Reviews in Contemporary Pharmacotherapy* 1994: 5.

31. Edmeads J. Advances in migraine therapy: focus on oral sumatriptan. *Neurology* 1995; 45(8 Suppl. 7): 53–4.
32. Färkkilä M (for the Eletriptan Steering Committee). A dose-finding study of eletriptan (UK-116,044) (5–30 mg) for the acute treatment of migraine. *Cephalalgia* 1996; 16: 387.
33. Jackson NC. A comparison of oral eletriptan (UK-116,044) (20–80 mg) and oral sumatriptan (100 mg) in the acute treatment of migraine (for the Eletriptan Steering Committee). *Cephalalgia* 1996; 16: 368.
34. Kempsford RD, Baille P, Fuseau E. Oral naratriptan tablets (2.5 mg–10 mg) exhibit dose-proportional pharmacokinetics (abstract). *Neurology* 1997; In press.
35. Klassen A, Webster C, Laurenza A, Austin R, Asgharnejad M. Naratriptan tablets are effective and well-tolerated in the acute treatment of migraine: results of a double-blind, placebo-controlled, parallel-group trial (abstract). *Neurology* 1997; In press.
36. Visser WH, Klein KB, Cox RC, Jones D, Ferrari MD. 311C90: a new central and peripherally acting 5-HT$_{1D}$-receptor agonist in the acute oral treatment of migraine: a double-blind, placebo-controlled, dose-range finding study. *Neurology* 1996; 46: 522–6.
37. Silberstein SD. Migraine and pregnancy. *Neurol Clin* 1997; 15: 209–31.
38. Silberstein SD. Preventive headache treatment. *Cephalalgia* 1997; 17: 67–72.
39. Silberstein SD. Divalproex sodium in headache: a literature review and clinical guidelines. *Headache* 1996; 36: 547–55.
40. Saper JR, Silberstein SD, Lake AE, Winters ME. Double-blind trial of fluoxetine: chronic daily headache and migraine. *Headache* 1994; 34: 497–502.
41. Stein DJ, Hollander E. Sexual dysfunction associated with the drug treatment of psychiatric disorders: incidence and treatment. *CNS Drugs* 1994; 2(1): 78–86.
42. Silberstein SD, Lipton RB, Breslau N. Migraine: association with personality characteristics and psychopathology. *Cephalalgia* 1995; 15: 337–69.
43. Silberstein SD. Status migrainosus. In: Gilman S, Goldstein GW, Waxman SG (eds.). *Neurobase*. La Jolla: Arbor, 1995.
44. Bell R, Montoya D, Snualb A, Lee MA. A comparative trial of three agents in the treatment of acute migraine headache. *Ann Emerg Med* 1990; 19: 1079–82.

45. Callaham M, Raskin N. A controlled study of dihydroergotamine in the treatment of acute migraine headache. *Headache* 1986; 26: 168–71.

46. Jones J, Sklar D, Dougherty J, White W. Randomized double-blind trial of intravenous prochlorperazine for the treatment of acute headache. *JAMA* 1989; 261: 1174–85.

47. Silberstein SD, Schulman EA, Hopkins MM. Repetitive intravenous DHE in the treatment of refractory headache. *Headache* 1990; 30: 334–9.

48. Silberstein SD, Merriam G. Sex hormones and headache. In: Goadsby P, Silberstein SD (eds). *Blue Books of Practical Neurology: Headache*. Boston: Butterworth Heinemann, 1997: 143–76.

49. Johannes CB. *Hormonal factors in relationship to migraine headache attacks in young women*. A dissertation submitted to The Johns Hopkins University in conformity with the requirements for the degree of Doctor of Philosophy. Baltimore: Maryland, 1989.

50. Somerville BW. The role of estradiol withdrawal in the etiology of menstrual migraine. *Neurology* 1972; 22: 355–65.

51. Ramadan NM, Halvorson H, Vande-Linde A et al. Low brain magnesium in migraine. *Headache* 1989; 29: 416–19.

52. Mauskop A, Altura BT, Cracco RQ, Altura BM. Intravenous magnesium sulfate relieves acute migraine in patients with low serum ionized magnesium levels (abstr). *Neurology* 1995; 45(4): A379.

53. Solbach MP, Waymer RS. Treatment of menstruation-associated migraine headache with subcutaneous sumatriptan. *Obstet Gynecol* 1993; 82: 769–72.

54. DeLignieres B, Vincens M, Mauvais-Jarvis P et al. Prevention of menstrual migraine by percutaneous oestradiol. *BMJ* 1986; 293: 1540.

55. Magos AL, Brincat M, Studd JWW. Treatment of the premenstrual syndrome by subcutaneous oestradiaol implants and cyclical oral norethisterone: a placebo-controlled study. *BMJ* 1986; 292:1629–33.

56. Stumpf PG. Pharmacokinetics of estrogen. *Obstet Gynecol* 1990; 75(Suppl.): 9S–17S.

57. Schwartz J, Freeman R, Frishman W. Clinical pharmacology of estrogens: cardiovascular actions and cardioprotective benefits of replacement therapy in postmenopausal women. *J Clin Pharmacol* 1995; 35: 1–16.

58. Pradalier A, Vincent D, Beaulieu PH, Baudesson G, Launay JM. Correlation between oestradiol plasma level and therapeutic effect on menstrual migraine. In: Rose FC (ed.). *New advances in headache research*. 4th edition. Smith-Gordon: London. 1994: 129–32.

59. Pfaffenrath V. Efficacy and safety of percutaneous estradiol vs. placebo in menstrual migraine (abstr). *Cephalalgia* 1993.

60. Smits MG, VanDerMeer YG, Pfeil JP et al. Perimenstrual migraine: effect of estraderm TTS and the value of contingent negative variation and exterocceptive temporalis muscle suppression test. *Headache* 1993; 34: 103–6.

61. Herzog AG. Continuous bromocriptine therapy in menstrual migraine (abstr). *Neurology* 1995; 45(4): A465.

62. Casson P, Hahn PM, Van Vugt DA, Reid RL. Lasting response to ovariectomy in severe intractable premenstrual syndrome. *Obstet Gynecol* 1990; 162: 99–105.

63. Casper RF, Hearn MT. The effect of hysterectomy and bilateral oophorectomy in women with severe premenstrual syndrome. *Am J Obstet Gynecol* 1990; 162: 105–9.

64. Watson NR, Savvas M, Studd JWW, Barnett T, Baber RJ. Treatment of severe premenstrual syndrome with oestradiol patches and cyclical oral norethisterone. *Lancet* 1989; 2: 730–2.

65. Neri I, Granella F, Nappi R et al. Characteristics of headache at menopause: a clinico-epidemiologic study. *Maturitas* 1993; 17: 31–7.

66. Alvarez WC. Can one cure migraine in women by inducing menopause? Report on forty-two cases. *Mayo Clin Proc* 1940; 15: 380–2.

67. Baird DT, Glasier AF. Hormonal contraception. *N Engl J Med* 1993; 328: 1543–9.

68. Speroff L, DeCherney A and the Advisory Board for the New Progestins. Evaluation of a new generation of oral contraceptives. *Obstet Gynecol* 1993; 81: 1034–47.

69. Adler CS, Adler SM, Friedman AP. A historical perspective on psychiatric thinking about headache. In: Adler CS, Adler SM, Packard RC (eds.). *Psychiatric aspects of headache*. Baltimore: Williams and Wilkins, 1987: 3–21.

70. Lidegaard O. Oral contraception and risk of a cerebral thromboembolic attack: results of a case-control study. *BMJ* 1993; 306: 956–63.

71. May A, Ophoff RA, Terwindt GM et al. Familial hemiplegic migraine locus on 19p13 is involved in the common forms of migraine with and without aura. *Hum Genet* 1995; 96: 604–8.

72. Joutel A, Bousser MG, Biousse V et al. A gene for familial hemiplegic migraine maps to chromosome 19. *Nature Genetics* 1993; 5: 40–5.

73. Hutchinson M, O'Riordan J, Javed M et al.. Familial hemiplegic migraine and autosomal dominant arteriopathy with leukoencephalopathy (CADASIL). *Ann Neurol* 1995; 38: 817–24.

74. Speight TM, Avery GS. Pizotifen (BC-105): a review of its pharmacological properties and its therapeutic efficacy in vascular headaches. *Am J Med Sci* 1972; 240: 327–31.

75. Arthur GP, Hornabrook RW. The treatment of migraine with BC-105 (Pizotifen), a double-blind trial. *N Z Med J* 1971;73: 5–9.

76. Lawrence ER, Hossain M, Littlestone W. Sanomigran for migraine prophylaxis: controlled multicenter trial in general practice. *Headache* 1977; 17: 109–12.

77. Capildeo R, Rose FC. Single-dose Pizotifen, 1.5 mg nocte: a new approach in the prophylaxis of migraine. *Headache* 1982; 22: 272–5.

78. Curran DA, Lance JW. Clinical trial of methysergide and other preparations in the management of migraine. *J Neurol Neurosurg Psychiatry* 1964; 27: 463–9.

79. Hill AP, Hyde RM, Robertson AD, Woollard PM, Glen RC, Martin GR. Oral delivery of 5-HT$_{1D}$ receptor agonists: towards the discovery of 311C90, a novel antimigraine agent. *Headache* 1995; 34: 308.

80. Martin GR, Robertson AD, MacLennan SJ et al. Receptor specificity and trigeminovascular inhibitory actions of a novel HT 1B/1D receptor partial agonist, 311C90 (zolmitriptan). *Br J Pharmacol* 1997; 121: 157–64.

81. Goadsby PJ, Edvinsson L. Peripheral and central trigeminovascular activation in cat is blocked by the serotonin HT$_{1D}$ receptor agonist 311C90. *Headache* 1994; 34: 394–9.

82. Goadsby PJ, Hoskin KL. Inhibition of trigeminal neurons by intravenous administration of the serotonin HT$_{1D}$ receptor agonist zolmitriptan (311C90): are brain stem sites a therapeutic target in migraine. *Pain* 1996; 67: 355–9.

83. Goadsby PJ, Knight YE. Direct evidence for central sites of action of zolmitriptan (311C90): an autoradiographic study in cat. *Cephalalgia* 1997; 17: 153–8.

84. Seaber E, On N, Phillips S, Churchus R, Posner J, Rolan P. The tolerability and pharmacokinetics of the novel antimigraine compound 311C90 in healthy male volunteers. *Br J Clin Pharmacol* 1996; 41(2): 141–7.

85. Thomsen LL, Dixon R, Lassen LH et al. 311C90 (zolmitriptan), a novel centrally and peripheral acting oral 5-hydroxytryptamine-1D agonist: a comparison of its absorption during a migraine attack and in a migraine-free period. *Cephalalgia* 1996;16(4): 270–5.

86. Palmer KJ, Spencer CM. Zolmitriptan. *CNS Drugs* 1997; 7: 468–78.

87. Goadsby PJ. 311C90, a novel HT$_{1B/1D}$ agonist: the assessment of efficacy and tolerability in the acute treatment of migraine. *Neurology* 1997; 43(3): A86.

88. Spierings ELH (ed.) Symptomatology and pathogenesis In:<u>Management of Migraine.</u> Newton: Butterworth-Heinemann,pp7–19

89. MacGregor EA <u>et al.</u> Migraine and menstruation. <u>Celphalalgia</u> 1990; 10: 305.

chapter 7

Tension-type headache: diagnosis and treatment

Introduction

In the past, 'tension headache' was a poorly-defined term that was inappropriately associated with psychopathology and unscientifically attributed to muscle contraction. In 1988, the International Headache Society (IHS)[1] revised the headache classification system and designated the term 'tension-type headache' (TTH) to describe what was previously called 'tension headache', 'muscle contraction headache' or 'psychogenic headache'. Previously, 'tension or muscle contraction headache' was defined as: 'ache or sensation of tightness, pressure or constriction, widely varied in intensity, frequency and duration, long-lasting, commonly occipital and associated with sustained contraction of skeletal muscles, usually as a part of the individual's reaction during life stress'.[2]

This vague, ambiguous description is not operational. It not only includes clinical features, triggers and a proposed mechanism (contraction of skeletal muscles), but suggests that the headache has a psychological basis, a prejudiced and unproven allegation.[3,4] The new IHS definition[1] attempts to define this type of headache more precisely and to distinguish between patients with episodic tension-type headache (ETTH) and those with chronic tension-type headache (CTTH). 'CTTH' is used by the IHS[1] instead of 'chronic daily headache' (CDH) which they state was the previously used term. CDH and CTTH are not identical and the substitution has created confusion.[3] TTH of both the episodic and chronic type are now subclassified into those associated with or unassociated with disorder of the pericranial muscles. These subclassifications are based on the presence or absence of tenderness or increased electromyographic (EMG) activity. TTH is no longer presumed to be caused by chronic muscle contraction, but it may be associated with muscle tenderness and increased EMG activity. We will review the new IHS classification of TTH and discuss the pathogenesis and treatment of TTH as well as its relationship to migraine. CDH will be considered in Chapter 8.

Episodic tension-type headache

Definition and clinical characteristics
ETTH is defined[1] as recurrent episodes of headache meeting the IHS diagnostic criteria in Table 7.1. TTH is the most common headache type, with a lifetime prevalence (in Denmark) of 69% in men and 88% in women and a one-year

● **Table 7.1** *Tension-type headache (IHS)*

2.1	**Episodic tension-type headache**
Diagnostic criteria:	
A	At least 10 previous headache episodes fulfilling criteria (B–D) listed below. Number of days with such headache <180/year (<15/month).
B	Headache lasting from 30 minutes to 7 days.
C	At least two of the following pain characteristics: 1 Pressing/tightening (non-pulsating) quality. 2 Mild or moderate intensity (may inhibit, but does not prohibit activities). 3 Bilateral location. 4 No aggravation by walking stairs or similar routine physical activity.
D	Both of the following: 1 No nausea or vomiting (anorexia may occur). 2 Photophobia and phonophobia are absent, or one but not the other is present.
2.1.1	**Episodic tension-type headache associated with disorder of pericranial muscles**
Diagnostic criteria:	
A	Fulfills criteria for 2.1.
B	At least one of the following: 1 Increased tenderness of pericranial muscles. 2 Increased EMG level of pericranial muscles.
2.1.2	**Episodic tension-type headache unassociated with disorder of pericranial muscles**
Diagnostic criteria:	
A	Fulfills criteria for 2.1.
B	No increased tenderness or EMG activity of pericranial muscles.
2.2	**Chronic tension-type headache**
Diagnostic criteria:	
A	Average headache frequency >15 days/month (180 days/year) for >6 months fulfilling criteria (B–D).
B	At least two of the following pain characteristics: 1 Pressing/tightening quality. 2 Mild or moderate severity (may inhibit but does not prohibit activities). 3 Bilateral location. 4 No aggravation by walking stairs or similar routine physical activity.
C	Both of the following: 1 No vomiting. 2 No more than one of the following: nausea, photophobia or phonophobia.
2.2.1	**Chronic tension-type headache associated with disorder of pericranial muscles**
2.2.2	**Chronic tension-type headache unassociated with disorder of pericranial muscles**

prevalence of 63% in men and 86% in women.[5] In Israel, the prevalence of non-migrainous headaches in Jewish immigrants was 65% in men and 66% in women.[6] Most TTH studies present a number of methodological problems, including selection bias, inconsistent definitions and failure to control for drug use and headache duration. In comparison to epidemiological studies, clinic-based studies include patients with more severe headaches, patients with concomitant migraine and patients with CDH evolving from migraine (Figure 7.1).[3]

TTH varies in frequency as well as in severity from rare, brief episodes to frequent, often continuous, disabling headaches. In Denmark, 59% of the population had one day or less each month of TTH and 3% had more than 15 days a month.[15] In the United States, 0.5% of the population have daily severe headache.[7] The one-year prevalence of frequent (>1 month) TTH is 20–30%. TTH is more prevalent in women than in men; the prevalence declines with age in both sexes. TTH prevalence does not differ significantly with socioeconomic background.[8,9] Among Danish TTH sufferers, only 16% had ever consulted a doctor because of their headache.[8]

DIAGNOSIS OF EPISODIC TENSION-TYPE HEADACHE

Headache pain accompanied by two of the following symptoms:

- Pressing/tightening (nonpulsating) quality
- Bilateral location
- Not aggravated by routine physical activity

Headache pain accompanied by both of the following symptoms:

- No nausea or vomiting
- Photophobia and phonophobia absent or only one present

Fewer than 15 days per month with headache

No evidence of organic disease

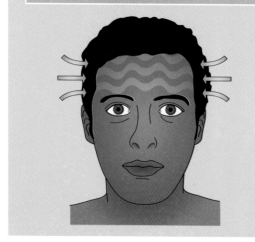

● **Figure 7.1** Diagnosis of episodic tension-type headache.

The lifetime prevalence of headache in the general population is over 90%.[5] Despite this, Friedman[10] found a positive family history of headache in only 40% of TTH patients and 70% of migraineurs. This discrepancy may be explained by the fact that many of Friedman's patients had CDH, not ETTH, and only a family history of severe headache may have been recalled. Ziegler et al.[11] reported a family history of episodic headache in 64% of all headache sufferers, with no increase in migraineurs. Bakal and Kaganov[12] reported similar findings. Friedman found that headache onset was usually between 20 and 40 years of age and was more common in women than in men. This is not consistent with the observation that many children have ETTH.[13] Most of Friedman's patients had CDH and only 15% had headache occurring less than once a week. Thus his conclusions were biased towards the more severely affected patient.

TTH has no prodrome or aura. The pain is a dull, achy, non-pulsatile feeling of tightness, pressure or constriction (vice-like or hatband-like), and is usually mild-to-moderate in severity, in contrast to the moderate-to-severe pain of migraine. Pain intensity increases with headache attack frequency.[14] Most patients have bilateral pain but the location varies considerably within and between patients, and can involve the frontal, temporal, occipital or parietal regions, alone or in combination, commonly changing locations during the attack.[15] Occipital location is less common than frontal or temporal location. Some patients have neck or jaw discomfort or have frank problems with their temporomandibular joint.[16] The presence of reciprocal clicking of the temporomandibular joint or pain with maximum jaw opening and pain upon palpation are said to be sensitive clinical signs of oromandibular dysfunction.[17] Unilateral headache occurs in 10–20% of patients.[9,14] Whether these patients had CDH secondary to transformed migraine, hemicrania continua or true ETTH is not clear. Scalp tenderness is more frequent and more severe in migraine or TTH patients during a headache than in non-headache controls, is greatest at the site of the headache, and may persist for several days after the headache subsides.[13] TTH does not usually interfere with daily activities[18] and physical activity normally has no influence on headache intensity.[19]

Some patients may have tender spots and sharply localized nodules in the pericranial or cervical muscles that can be detected by manual palpation of pericranial and neck muscles. In general, ETTH sufferers, whether or not they are having a headache, have more muscle tenderness than do headache-free controls.[20] Most patients have no associated symptoms but some may report slight photophobia or phonophobia or nausea.[15] Lack of sleep is a common precipitating factor, with TTH occurring in 39% of healthy volunteers after sleep deprivation.[21] TTH subjects have more problems sleeping than do migraineurs or non-headache controls.[22,23]

TTH is subdivided by the IHS up to the fourth digit code to indicate possible causative factors. This empiric subdivision is mainly useful for research purposes. For example, coexistence of oromandibular dysfunction and headache is frequent but could be due to chance. The prevalence of oromandibular dysfunction does not differ between subjects with frequent TTH, migraineurs and headache-free persons possibly contributing.[24] Psychological and psychiatric causative factors, defined according to the DSM-IV criteria, could be the result, rather than the cause, of recurrent pain.

A primary headache disorder requires exclusion of other organic disorders. TTH is the most frequent but the least distinct of the primary headache disorders; its clinical diagnosis is based chiefly on the absence of symptoms that characterize migraine (unilaterality, pulsatility, aggravation by physical activity, associated symptoms, etc.). There is no diagnostic test for TTH. Patients with secondary organic headache types often have symptoms that mimic TTH.[25] Pericranial tenderness can also be found in other primary as well as asymptomatic headaches, e.g. in intracerebral lesions, such as tumour or haemorrhage. Be alert for atypical symptoms or any abnormalities on neurological examination.

The prognosis and clinical course of TTH is variable. Subjects with frequent ETTH may be at increased risk of developing CTTH over a period of many years.[17] Whether subjects with more severe TTH are at increased risk for developing migraine or whether migraineurs are more likely to develop more severe and frequent TTH is still controversial.

Episodic tension-type headache and migraine

Migraine and ETTH have traditionally been considered distinct entities. The IHS continues this separation, and patients can be classified as having both migraine and TTH. However, some clinicians and epidemiologists believe that migraine and TTH are related entities that differ more in severity than kind.[26–31] Factor analysis of headache clinic patients[32] and epidemiological studies have unsuccessfully attempted to find clinical features that would distinguish TTH from migraine. Both migraine and TTH may be 'benign recurring headaches which occur in the headache-prone'. The majority of migraineurs (62%) also have TTH and 25% of TTH patients also have migraine. A migraine headache may begin as a TTH that develops migrainous features when it increases in severity.[30]

Iversen *et al.*[14] examined the clinical characteristics of migraine and ETTH in relation to the old *ad hoc* and the new IHS diagnostic criteria. Eighty-one patients diagnosed as having migraine, TTH or both, according to previous criteria,[1] were re-analysed using the new IHS diagnostic criteria. Use of the new IHS criteria did not radically change the headache diagnosis.

Sixty-three percent of patients with only ETTH, 17% of patients with only migraine and 41% of patients with both dis-

orders had pericranial and neck muscle tenderness. ETTH was usually mild to moderate in severity and changed location in half the attacks. Almost 20% of the ETTH were unilateral in location and 10% were pulsating and throbbing. ETTH was more variable and often shorter in duration than migraine.

Routine physical activity typically aggravates pain in migraine but not in TTH. However, physical activity exacerbates TTH in patients who also have migraine. Photophobia, phonophobia and nausea are less frequent in patients with only TTH than in patients who also had migraine. Iversen[14] has speculated that patients with both migraine and TTH may differ from patients with pure TTH.

What we call 'TTH' may be two distinct disorders. The first disorder may be attacks of mild migraine. The second may be a pure TTH that is not associated with other features of migraine (sensitivity to movement, nausea or photophobia) or with attacks of severe migraine. What we call 'migraine' may be the upper end in a normal distribution of painful episodic headaches.[3] Whether TTH is a milder form of migraine or is a distinct entity is still not certain.

Chronic tension-type headache

CTTH (Table 7.1) requires head pain for 15 days a month for at least six months; many patients have daily headache. Although the pain criteria are identical to ETTH, the IHS allows nausea but not vomiting, or either photophobia or phonophobia occurring alone, while the presence of nausea is consistent with the IHS diagnosis of CTTH but not ETTH. This makes no sense.[1]

In their pure episodic forms, migraine and TTH are easily distinguished, but as migraine headache frequency increases, the clinical distinctions become blurred. As the process progresses, the headaches increase in frequency but decrease in severity, and associated migrainous features decline in prominence. The headaches, which occur on a daily or near-daily basis, often come to resemble TTH, with bilateral pressure pain and little nausea, photophobia or phonophobia. Superimposed on these background headaches may be occasional full-blown migraine attacks.[33] The nomenclature for this headache disorder is controversial. Within the IHS system, the daily headache disorder is classified as 'CTTH' while the superimposed headache is classified as 'migraine'. The terms 'mixed headache' or 'combined headache' are used by some clinicians, again suggesting that this picture represents two distinct disorders. Many clinicians prefer the terms CDH evolving from migraine or transformed migraine to convey the idea that this is one headache syndrome characterized by two headache types.[34–36] This will be discussed in Chapter 8.

Mechanisms of tension-type headache

TTH was believed to arise from the sustained contraction of pericranial muscles ('muscle contraction headache'), perhaps as a consequence of emotion or tension or a reaction to head pain. Tonic muscle contraction could then lead to tissue ischaemia and a 'vascular' headache.[37] However, there may be as much if not more muscle contraction in patients with migraine as in patients with TTH.[11,25,38,39] No correlation exists between muscle contraction, tenderness and the presence of headache.[40] Biofeedback using EMG is as effective in TTH as in migraine.[41] There is no evidence of muscle ischaemia in TTH. Temporal muscle blood flow is normal in CTTH at rest and during teeth clenching[42] and amyl nitrite (a vasodilator) worsens TTH.[43,44]

Although conclusions are based on clinic-based studies with a bias towards transformed migraine or 'mixed' headache in the TTH group, a variety of evidence suggests that migraine and TTH have a similar pathogenesis: both are associated with muscle tenderness; both are associated with abnormal EMG; both are associated with abnormal exteroceptive suppression (ES2); both may be associated with abnormal platelet serotonin; and both are associated, when severe and chronic, with decreased cerebrospinal fluid β-endorphin.

During an attack, most migraineurs and TTH patients have more muscle tenderness than do non-headache controls.[45] While the total amount of muscle tenderness correlates to headache intensity, there is no pattern to the tenderness or correlation to the headache site. In addition, some non-headache controls have tender spots.[46] Thus migraine and TTH cannot be differentiated solely on the basis of muscle tenderness.

Pericranial EMG levels may be within the normal range in the majority of patients with TTH when recordings are performed at rest and in one muscle. The proportion of abnormal findings increases with multiple recording sites and under stressful conditions.[47] There is no correlation between pericranial tenderness and EMG levels, and patients with abnormal EMG levels or increased tenderness do not differ clinically from those without such an abnormality.[48] Patients with ETTH, CTTH and migraine may have increased EMG activity in some muscles when multiple muscles are sampled under different conditions.[46,49] No increase in neck-muscle EMG activity was found during continuous monitoring by ambulatory EMG during a headache attack.[50]

Muscle tenderness and EMG activity were evaluated in subjects with ETTH, comparing them to headache-free controls during a headache-free state. No significant association was found between increased EMG activity and the presence of tenderness.

Exteroceptive suppression (ES) is the inhibition of voluntary EMG activity of the temporalis muscle induced by trigeminal nerve stimulation.[51] There are two successive ES (ES1 and ES2) silent periods (Figure 7.2). ES2, a multisynaptic reflex subject to limbic and other modulation, is absent in 40% of patients with CTTH and reduced in duration in 87%. ES1, an oligosynaptic reflex, is normal. ETTH patients may have a perimenstrual reduction in ES2.[52,53] ES2 may be absent in more headache-prone patients.[54] Some studies[55] found a reduction of ES2 in migraine without aura, additional evidence for a continuum between migraine and chronic TTH.[49] ES2 reduction is not specific for TM as it occurs in other neurological disorders, such as dystonia and Parkinson's disease.

Schoenen et al.[46] measured the ES2, pain threshold, EMG activity, anxiety scores, and response to biofeedback in 32 women with CTTH, and found an abnormal EMG in 62.5% of the patients if three different muscles and three states were tested. The EMG was abnormal in only 40% if only one muscle and one state were tested. A decreased pain threshold was found in half the patients tested in one of three muscles but in only 34% if only one muscle was tested. ES2 duration was reduced in 87% of patients.

Reduced Achilles tendon pain thresholds were found in half of CTTH patients when compared to headache-free controls.[45] Biofeedback moderately but significantly increased the pain threshold, perhaps by normalizing limbic input to the brainstem pain modulating system. Increased EMG activity or decreased pain thresholds were found in 72% of the patients,[45] consistent with a diagnosis of CTTH 'associated with disorder of pericranial muscles', but these findings were not present in the remaining 28% of patients, consistent with a diagnosis of CTTH

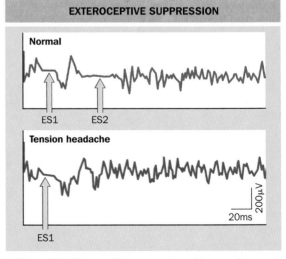

● **Figure 7.2** Exteroceptive suppression of temporalis muscle. Note absence of ES2 tension-type headache.[51]

'unassociated with such disorder'. Headache severity, anxiety, ES2 and response to biofeedback did not differ between these two groups, suggesting that their separation may be artificial or a consequence of the headache.

Göbel et al.[56] found no difference on average between the pain sensitivity or baseline EMG activity between migraineurs, ETTH patients and controls in the headache-free state. However, the surface EMG of the pericranial muscles determined before, during, and following experimental pain induction differed. Migraineurs had lower induced EMG activity than controls.

In general, patients with TTH showed significantly higher induced EMG scores during suprathreshold pain stimulation. Although, on average, there was no difference in pericranial pain sensitivity, two groups were apparent:

(i) TTH patients with low pain sensitivity who exhibited high EMG scores before and after stimulus application but low scores during stimulus application, and
(ii) TTH patients with high pain sensitivity who showed low EMG scores before and after stimulus application but elevated EMG scores during experimental headache. These groups may correspond to the two classes of TTH: those associated with a disorder of the pericranial muscles and those unassociated with this problem.

Göbel et al.[57] found that aspirin caused a highly significant increase in ES2 duration in all subjects, with or without headache, suggesting that aspirin's analgesic effect may in part be mediated by the antinociceptive brainstem reflex. The overstimulation of the pathway could lead to its exhaustion and could in part explain drug-induced headache.

Contingent negative variation, an event-related potential, and EEG and evoked potentials are normal in TTH.

Fibromyalgia, myofascial pain syndrome, tension myalgia and tension-type headache

Fibromyalgia is a chronic disorder of widespread pain and musculoskeletal tenderness throughout the body[58] that mainly affects women (90%). Associated symptoms include sleep disturbance (75%), morning stiffness (77%), fatigue (81%), paraesthesias, headache (52.8%) and anxiety (47.8%) or depression (31.5%). Because it is associated with a decreased pain threshold, pain from other disorders may be exacerbated.[59]

The myofascial pain syndrome[60] is distinguished from fibromyalgia by being a focal self-limited disorder associated with trigger points. Both fibromyalgia and TTH may have motor dysfunction (loss of the reciprocal innervation of muscles during voluntary activity),[55] tender spots, relief

with trigger point injection, and, when chronic, associated anxiety and depression. There may also be decreased pain threshold and involvement of the pain control systems, suggesting that TTH may overlap with localized fibromyalgia of the pericranial structures.

Biochemical changes in tension-type headache

Platelets, the major source of serotonin in the blood and plasma, account for 98% of the circulating blood level. Platelet serotonin content in patients with CTTH is significantly lower than in normal controls.[61] In addition, patients with CTTH inconsistently have mean levels of circulating plasma serotonin that are on the same order as the levels that migrainous patients have during a headache.[62] Some patients with ETTH have higher plasma serotonin levels[63] while others have lower plasma serotonin levels[64] during a headache. Patients with severe headache show abnormalities of cerebrospinal β-endorphin and release of luteinizing hormone induced by naloxone.[65]

Platelet gamma-aminobutyric acid (GABA) levels in patients with CTTH (43.1 ± 11.8 pmol/10^{12} platelets) are significantly higher than in migraineurs (30.9 ± 11.7) and healthy controls (34.7 ± 8.1). The platelet, a model of monamine neurons, may have elevated GABA levels to counter the state of neuronal hyperexcitability seen during an attack of migraine and continually during chronic TTH.[66] Elevated levels of GABA are found in the CSF of patients during migraine attacks.[67] Valproic acid, which among other actions is a GABA-mimetic agent, is effective in the treatment of migraine, CDH, and cluster headache, suggesting that the increased GABA levels are a reaction to, not a cause of, head pain.

Relationship to depression

Many have attempted to portray TTH as a primary psychological disorder.[68] This conclusion, based on studies of patients with CDH frequently complicated by medication overuse, says nothing about ETTH. Merikangas et al.,[69] following a cohort of ETTH patients from Zurich, have found no evidence of associated anxiety or depression, in contrast to the frequent association of anxiety and depression with migraine and the psychological distress in patients with CDH.

Some believe that CTTH can mask depression or other serious emotional disorders. A persistent, vague headache for which no organic cause can be determined (as is true for migraine) is frequently blamed on underlying psychic distress. Martin et al.,[68] in a study that did not have adequate controls and did not take medication overuse into account, found repressed hostility, sexuality issues and unresolved dependency needs in patients with chronic TTH. The psychological problems these patients have could be the result, not the cause, of their chronic pain.

The relationship between headache and depression is complicated. 'Depression headache' has been described in detail.[70,71] In one series, 84% of depressed patients complained of headache. The source of this population is not clear, nor is it clear whether the headache preceded the depression, followed the depression, or was a comorbid condition. Patients with depression headache frequently have transformed migraine[72] (see Chapter 8).

Depression may be a result, not a cause, of chronic pain. Additionally, depression, anxiety and chronic headache may be comorbid conditions with a common biologic basis, as is true for the conditions of migraine, depression and anxiety. Prior to the onset of either migraine or CTTH, patients show an increase in perceived stressful life events, whereas headache-free controls do not. This may be a result of an idiosyncratic, biologically-determined overreaction to significant life events in these patients.[73] Serotonin has been implicated in the genesis of migraine, depression and anxiety disorders, and may be the biological basis for their comorbidity.[4,74]

Probable mechanisms

TTH is postulated to be a clinical manifestation of abnormal neuronal sensitivity and pain facilitation, not abnormal muscle contraction: pain sensitivity is increased; tenderness is increased in some pericranial muscles; EMG is increased in some pericranial muscles, under some conditions independent of headache; and tenderness and increased EMG activity vary independently. Thus headache is not directly related to muscle contraction and focal tenderness. ES2 is frequently abnormal, suggesting abnormal modulation of the interneurons that connect the trigeminal nerve to the motor neurons. This abnormality may be a consequence of abnormal modulation from the basal ganglia, the limbic system, or the serotonergic neurons from the nucleus raphe dorsalis.

The nucleus caudalis of the trigeminal complex, the major relay nucleus for head and face pain, receives nociceptive input from cephalic blood vessels and pericranial muscles and dual supraspinal input, both inhibitory and facilitory.[75] Recent evidence suggests the presence of central pain facilitory neurons (on-cells) in the ventromedial medulla.[76] In addition, the trigeminal nucleus caudalis can be sensitized as a result of intense neuronal activation (Figure 7.3).

In both migraine and CTTH there may be hypersensitivity of neurons in the trigeminal nucleus caudalis neurons as a result of supraspinal facilitation. The vascular nociceptor may be hypersensitive in migraine; in CTTH associated with a disorder of the pericranial muscles, the myofascial nociceptor may be hypersensitive. In CTTH not associated with a disorder of the pericranial muscles, there may be less myofascial nociceptor hypersensitivity and a general increase in nociception. CTTH may be the result of an interaction between

HEADACHE PAIN PATHWAYS

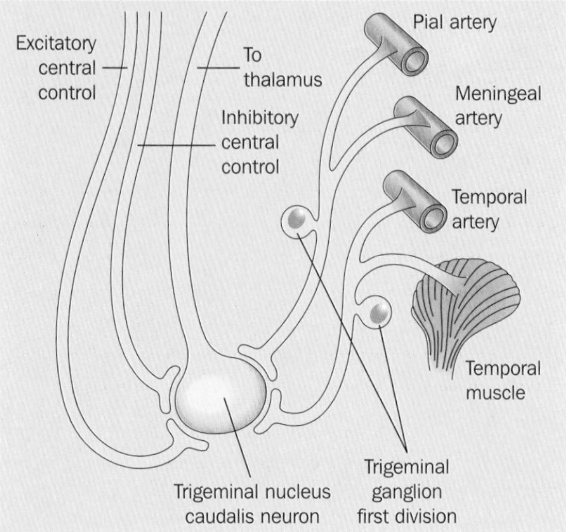

● *Figure 7.3 Headache pain pathways: vascular supraspinal myogenic model. Trigeminal nucleus caudalis has excitatory and inhibitory central control. It receives input from both arteries and muscle.[43]*

endogenous nociceptive brainstem activity and peripheral input (Figure 7.2). Acute ETTH occurs in otherwise perfectly normal individuals. It can be brought on by physical or psychological stress or by non-physiological working positions. Increased nociception from strained muscles trigger the attack in an individual with altered pain modulation. Emotional mechanisms may also reduce endogenous antinociception. Long-term potentiation of nociceptive neurons and decreased activity in the antinociceptive system could cause CTTH. Sensitization of the trigeminal nucleus caudalis neurons can result in normal non-painful stimuli becoming painful, producing trigger spots, an overlap in the symptoms of migraine and TTH, and activation of the trigeminal vascular system.

The pain from intense stimulation or injury usually diminishes as healing progresses and disappears when healing is complete. However, another type of pain occurs when the peripheral or central nervous system malfunctions. Three spatiotemporal characteristics of pain can be seen during both normal and pathophysiological pain:[77]

(i) as pain intensity increases, the area in which the pain is experienced often enlarges (radiation),
(ii) the pain often outlasts the evoking stimulus, and
(iii) repeated nociceptive stimulation may slowly increase the perceived intensity of pain, even without an increase in the peripheral input (sensitization).

Jensen and Olesen[78] used 30 minutes of sustained teeth-clenching (10% of maximal EMG signal) to trigger TTH in 58 patients with frequent, but not daily, CTTH or ETTH and 58 matched controls. Within 24 hours, 69% of patients (more than would be expected) and 17% of controls developed TTH. Shortly after clenching, EMG amplitude was significantly increased in the trapezius but not in the temporal muscle, and tenderness (which was increased at baseline in the headache patients) further increased only in the patients who subsequently developed headache. Mechanical pain thresholds remained unchanged in the group that developed headache but increased in the group that did not develop headache. Pain tolerance decreased in the patients who developed headache, was unchanged in the remaining patients and increased in controls, suggesting that headache patients do not effectively activate their antinociceptive system. This study clearly shows that peripheral mechanisms alone cannot explain TTH, but they could act as a trigger for a central process. Tenderness, not muscle contraction, correlates to headache development. Tenderness may have a central cause or result from muscle contraction causing activation and chemical sensitization on myofascial mechanoreceptors and/or their afferent fibres.

The therapeutic approaches should consider the relative importance of peripheral and central mechanisms, since they may vary, producing complex interactions.

Treatment of tension-type headache

The approach to the treatment of episodic headache, whether tension-type or migraine, is similar, and consists of psychophysiological therapy, physical therapy and pharmacotherapy.

Psychophysiological therapy involves reassurance, counselling, stress management, relaxation therapy, and biofeedback. (The use of traditional acupuncture is controversial and was not more effective than placebo in one study.)[79] Physical therapy consists of: modality treatments (heat, cold packs, ultrasound and electrical stimulation); improvement of posture through stretching, exercise and traction; trigger point injections or occipital nerve blocks; and a programme of regular exercise, stretching, balanced meals and adequate sleep.[80]

Pharmacotherapy

Acute (abortive) therapy, to stop or reduce the severity of the individual attack, consists of the structured use of simple analgesics alone or in combination with caffeine, anxiolytics or codeine and non-steroidal anti-inflammatory drugs (NSAID). Because of the potential of drug-induced headache, use of these drugs must be limited (Table 7.2). Optimizing therapy requires knowledge of alternative treatments and awareness of the patient's preferences. Many acute treatments are available. The choice depends on the severity and frequency of the headaches, the associated symptoms, the presence of coexistent illness and the patient's treatment profile. Oral medications, such as analgesics, NSAID or a caffeine adjuvant compound are useful for patients with mild-to-moderate headaches not complicated by nausea. We begin with simple analgesics for patients with mild-to-moderate headaches. Many individuals find headache relief with OTC analgesics such as naproxen sodium, ibuprofen, aspirin or acetaminophen (paracetamol), alone or in combination with caffeine. When we use prescription drugs we add butalbital or use the combination of acetaminophen, isometheptene and dichloralphenazone. This combination may be more effective than simple analgesics or NSAID, but great care must be used when prescribing butalbital-containing components since the addiction potential is so high. Avoid overuse of all analgesics because of the risk of dependency, abuse and development of CDH.

Simple analgesics and NSAID are effective in TTH as demonstrated by the headache attack model for acute pain.

● **Table 7.2** *Acute medications for tension-type headache**

Drug		Efficacy	Side effects
Analgesics	Aspirin	2+	2
	Acetaminophen**	2+	1
Non-steroidal anti-inflammatory drugs	Indomethacin	3	2
	Ibuprofen	2+	2
	Naproxen	3+	2
	Fenoprofen	2	2
	Ketoprofen	2	2
	Ketorolac	3	3
Combination	Aspirin and/or acetaminophen plus caffeine	3+	2
	Aspirin or acetaminophen plus butalbital with caffeine	3+	3
Muscle relaxants	Orphenadrine	0 (?)	3
	Carisoprodol	0 (?)	3
	Methocarbamal	0 (?)	3
	Diazepam	0 (?)	3
	Cyclobenzaprine	0 (?)	3
	Chlorphenesin	0 (?)	3
	Chloroxazone	0 (?)	3

* Rated on a 1–3 scale.
** Paracetamol.

Ibuprofen and naproxen are significantly more effective than placebo and may be more effective than aspirin or acetaminophen.[81] Improvement in headache occurs within 15–30 minutes. Other NSAID such as ketoprofen, ketorolac or indomethacin are also effective, but are less well studied. Based on the lower prevalence of gastrointestinal side effects,[82] some prefer ibuprofen and naproxen sodium. Aspirin is more effective than placebo and comparable to acetaminophen, which has fewer gastrointestinal side effects.

The NSAID have anti-inflammatory, analgesic, and antipyretic properties and are quickly absorbed when taken orally, with a time to peak plasma concentration (T_{max}) of <2 hours.[83] Naproxen has a plasma half-life of 14 hours, which accounts for the fact that it can provide pain relief that lasts 12 hours.

The major side effects with these medications are gastrointestinal symptoms (bleeding, nausea, vomiting, constipation, ulcers, epigastric pain and diarrhoea). Dermatological (rash, pruritus) and central nervous system side effects (headache, lethargy, confusion) are less common, and even rarer are oedema, leukopenia, thrombocytopenia and liver-function abnormalities. Contraindications include hypersensitivity to aspirin or any NSAID, peptic ulcers, treatment with anticoagulants, bleeding tendency, and severe renal, cardiac or liver impairment within the last three months.

There is no evidence that muscle relaxants, such as the mephenesin-like compounds, baclofen, diazepam, tizanidine, cyclobenzaprine or dantrolene sodium, are effective in the treatment of TTH.

Prophylactic treatment is designed to reduce the frequency and severity of headache attacks and should be considered if the frequency (more than two per week), duration (>3–4 hours) and severity might lead to the overuse of abortive medication or significant disability. We prefer to begin treatment with the tricyclic antidepressants or serotonin-specific reuptake inhibitors (SSRI), but any of the 'migraine' preventive drugs can be used empirically. If preventive medication is indicated, the agent should be chosen from one of the major categories, based on side effect profiles and coexistent comorbid conditions (Chapter 6).

The tricyclic antidepressants are drugs the most commonly used for TTH, despite few controlled studies. One major problem with the trials that show statistical differences between placebo and tricyclic antidepressants is the clinical relevancy of the observed effect. Amitriptyline is the most frequently used tricyclic antidepressant. Other antidepressants, such as doxepin, nortriptyline or protriptyline can be used. The SSRI can be used based on empiric evidence. They have fewer side effects than the tricyclic antidepressants and are often preferred by the patient. In one controlled trial, fluoxetine was more effective than placebo.[84]

These drugs should be started at a low dose and increased slowly until therapeutic effects develop or until the ceiling dose for the agent in question is reached. Tricyclic antidepressants such as amitriptyline are often used in doses of 100–200 mg/day for depression, while 10–20 mg/day is often effective for TTH. (A starting dose of 25–50 mg/day of amitriptyline is common in patients with depression, whereas it can produce intolerable side effects in migraineurs.) With fluoxetine, for example, we begin with 10 mg and slowly increase the dose. While some patients respond to lower doses of preventive medications, it may be necessary to increase the dose to tolerance before assuming the agent is ineffective. A full therapeutic trial may take two to six months. Patients may be treated with a new preventive medication for one to two weeks without effect and then prematurely discontinue it, and both patient and physician believe it was not effective. To obtain maximal benefit from preventive medication, the patient should not overuse analgesics. Headaches may improve with time independent of treatment; if the headaches are well controlled, a drug holiday can be undertaken following a slow taper programme. Many patients experience continued relief after discontinuing the medication or may not need the same dose. Dose reduction may provide a better risk-to-benefit ratio. The other medications used to treat migraine and depression have been used to treat episodic and chronic TTH (see Chapter 6).

Non-pharmacological treatments

Although behavioural treatment of TTH may produce improvement more slowly than pharmacological treatment, improvement is often maintained for long periods without contact with the therapist. Relaxation and biofeedback are useful in the management of TTH. Relaxation training, EMG biofeedback training, or a combination thereof can produce a 50% reduction in headache activity. This is a significantly greater decrease than has been observed in untreated patients or patients with false or non-contingent biofeedback.[85] Some patients who fail to respond to relaxation training may benefit from subsequent EMG biofeedback training.

Cognitive behavioural interventions, such as stress management programmes, may effectively reduce TTH activity when used alone, but these modalities may be more useful in conjunction with biofeedback or relaxation therapies, particularly in patients with a high level of daily stress.

Limited contact treatment utilizing three or four monthly clinical sessions supplemented by home use of audiotapes and written materials is a cost-effective alternative in many patients. Excessive analgesic or ergotamine use limits the therapeutic benefits. Patients with continuous headache are less responsive to relaxation or biofeedback therapies, and patients with significant psychiatric comorbidity may do poorly with behavioural treatment that does not address the comorbid problem.[86]

Physical therapy techniques include positioning, ergonomic instruction, massage, transcutaneous electrical nerve stimulation, heat or cold application, and manipulations. While none of these techniques has been proven to be effective in the long term, some such as massage may be useful for acute episodes of TTH.

Oromandibular treatment may be helpful in some TTH patients. Unfortunately, most studies claiming efficacy of treatment such as occlusal splints, therapeutic exercises for masticatory muscles, or occlusal adjustment are uncontrolled. Many headache-free subjects have signs and symptoms of oromandibular dysfunction,[23] therefore caution should be taken not to advocate irreversible dental treatments in TTH. Patients rarely benefit from oromandibular treatment.

References

1. Headache Classification Committee of the International Headache Society. Classification and diagnostic criteria for headache disorders, cranial neuralgias and facial pain. *Cephalalgia* 1988; 8(Suppl. 7): 196.
2. Ad Hoc Committee on Classification of Headache. Classification of headache. *Arch Neurol* 1962; 6:13–16.
3. Silberstein SD. Chronic daily headache and tension-type headache. *Neurology* 1993; 43: 1644–9.
4. Silberstein SD. Advances in understanding the pathophysiology of headache. *Neurology* 1992; 42(Suppl. 2): 610.
5. Rassmussen BK, Jensen R, Schroll M, Olesen J. Epidemiology of headache in a general population — a prevalence study. *J Clin Epidemiol* 1991; 44: 1147–57.
6. Abramson JH, Hopp C, Epstein LM. Migraine and nonmigrainous headaches. A community survey in Jerusalem. *J Epidemiol Community Health* 1980; 34: 188–193.
7. Newman LC, Lipton RB, Solomon S et al. Daily headache in a population sample: results from the American Migraine Study. *Headache* 1994; 34(1): 295.
8. Waters WE. Migraine: intelligence, social class and familial prevalence. *BMJ* 1971; 2: 77–81.
9. Rasmussen BK. Migraine and tension-type headache in a general population: psychosocial factors. *Int J Epidemiol* 1992; 21: 1138–43.
10. Friedman AP, Von Storch TJC, Merritt HH. Migraine and tension headaches. A clinical study: 2000 cases. *Neurology* 1964; 4: 773.
11. Ziegler DK, Hassanein R, Hassanein K. Headache syndromes suggested by factor analysis of symptom variables in a headache prone population. *J Chron Dis* 1972; 25: 353–63.
12. Bakal DA, Kaganov JA. Symptom characteristics of chronic and non-chronic headache sufferers. *Headache* 1979; 19: 285–9.
13. Silberstein SD. Twenty questions about headaches in children and adolescents. *Headache* 1990; 30: 716–24.

14. Drummond PD. Scalp tenderness and sensitivity to pain in migraine and tension headache. *Headache* 1987; 27: 45–50.
15. Iversen HK, Langemark M, Andersson PG, Hansen PE, Olesen J. Clinical characteristics of migraine and episodic tension-type headache in relation to old and new diagnostic criteria. *Headache* 1990; 30: 514–19.
16. Olesen J. Clinical characterization of tension headache. In: Olesen J, Edvinsson L (eds.). *Basic Mechanisms of Headache*. Amsterdam: Elsevier, 1988: 914.
17. Schiffman E, Haley D, Baker C, Lindgren B. Diagnostic criteria for screening headache patients for temporomandibular disorders. *Headache* 1995; 35: 121–4.
18. Langemark M, Olesen J, Poulsen DL, Bech P. Clinical characterization of patients with chronic tension headache. *Headache* 1988; 28: 590–6.
19. Rasmussen BK, Jensen R, Olesen J. A population-based analysis of the diagnostic criteria of the International Headache Society. *Cephalalgia* 1991; 11: 129–34.
20. Hatch JP, Moore PJ, Cyr-Provost M et al. The use of electromyography and muscle palpation in the diagnosis of tension-type headache with and without pericranial muscle involvement. *Pain* 1992; 49: 175–8.
21. Blau JN. Sleep deprivation headache. *Cephalalgia* 1990; 10: 157–60.
22. Rasmussen BK. Migraine and tension-type headache in a general population: precipitating factors, female hormones, sleep patterns and relation to lifestyle. *Pain* 1993; 53: 65–72.
23. Paiva T, Batista A, Martins P, Martins A. The relationship between headaches and sleep disturbances. *Headache* 1995; 35: 590–6.
24. Jensen R, Rasmussen BK, Pedersen B et al. Oromandibular disorders in a general population. *J Craniomandib Disorders Facial Oral Pain* 1993; 7: 175–82.
25. Forsyth PA, Posner JB. Intracranial neoplasms. In: Olesen J, Tfelt-Hansen P, Welch KMA (eds). *The Headaches*. New York: Raven Press, 1993: 705.
26. Bakal DA. *The psychobiology of chronic headache*. New York: Springer, 1982.

27. Waters WE. *Series in clinical epidemiology: headache*. Littleton MA: PSG, 1988.
28. Featherstone HJ. Migraine and muscle contraction headaches: a continuum. *Headache* 1985; 25:194–8.
29. Raskin NH. *Headache. 2nd edition*. New York: Churchill-Livingstone, 1988.
30. Saper JR. Changing perspectives of chronic headache. *Clin J Pain* 1986; 2: 19–28.
31. Marcus DA. Migraine and tension-type headaches: the questionable validity of current classification systems. *Clin J Pain* 1992; 8: 28–36.
32. Ziegler DK, Hassanein RS. Specific headache phenomena: their frequency and coincidence. *Headache* 1990; 30: 152–6.
33. Post RM, Silberstein SD. Shared mechanisms in affective illness, epilepsy, and migraine. *Neurology* 1994; 44(7): S37–47.
34. Saper J. Daily chronic headache. *Neurol Clin* 1990; 8: 891–901.
35. Mathew NT. Drug-induced headache. *Neurol Clin* 1990; 8: 903–912.
36. Mathew NT. Chronic daily headache: clinical features and natural history. In: Nappi G, Bono G, Sandrini G, Martignoni E, Micieli G (eds). *Headache and Depression*. New York: Raven Press, 1991: 49–58.
37. Wolff HG. Muscles of the head and neck as sources of headache and other pain. In: *Headache and other Head Pain*. 2nd edition. New York: Oxford University Press, 1963: 582–616.
38. Lichstein KL, Fischer SM, Eakin TL, Amberson JI, Bertorini T, Hoon PW. Psychophysiological parameters of migraine and muscle-contraction headaches. *Headache* 1991; 31: 27–34.
39. Sutton EP, Belar CD. Tension headache patients versus controls: a study of EMG parameters. *Headache* 1982; 22: 133–6.
40. Arena JG, Hannah SL, Bruno GM, Smith JD, Meador KJ. Effect of movement and position of muscle activity in tension headache sufferers during and between headaches. *J Psychosom Res* 1991; 35: 187–95.

41. Ziegler DK. The headache syndrome: how many entities? *Arch Neurol* 1985; 42: 273–277.

42. Langemark M, Jensen K, Olesen J. Temporal muscle blood flow in chronic tension-type headache. *Arch Neurol* 1990; 47: 654–8.

43. Silberstein SD, Lipton R, Solomon S, Mathew H. Classification of daily and near daily headaches: proposed revisions to the IHS classification. *Headache* 1994; 34: 17.

44. Martin PR, Mathews AM. Tension headaches: psychophysiological investigation and treatment. *J Psychosom Res* 1978; 22: 389–99.

45. Olesen J. Clinical and pathophysiological observations in migraine and tension-type headache explained by integration of vascular, supraspinal and myofascial inputs. *Pain* 1991; 46: 125–32.

46. Langemark M, Olesen J. Pericranial tenderness in tension headache: a blind, controlled study. *Cephalalgia* 1987; 7: 249–55.

47. Schoenen J, Bottin D, Hardy F, Gerard P. Cephalic and extracephalic pressure pain thresholds in chronic tension-type headache. *Pain* 1991; 47: 145–9.

48. Schoenen J, Gerard P, De Pasqua V, Sianard-Gainko J. Multiple clinical and paraclinical analyses of chronic tension-type headache associated or unassociated with disorder of pericranial muscles. *Cephalalgia* 1991; 11: 135–9.

49. Pritchard DW. EMG cranial muscle levels in headache sufferers before and during headache. *Headache* 1989; 29: 103–8.

50. Hatch JP, Prihoda TJ, Moore PJ et al. A naturalistic study of the relationships among electromyographic activity, psychological stress, and pain in ambulatory tension-type headache patients and headache-free controls. *Psychosom Med* 1991; 53: 576–84.

51. Schoenen J, Jamart B, Gerard P et al. Exteroceptive suppression of temporalis muscle activity in chronic headache. *Neurology* 1987; 37: 1834–6.

52. Schoenen J, Bottin D, Sulon J et al. Exteroceptive silent period of temporalis muscle in menstrual headaches. *Cephalalgia* 1991; 11: 87–91.

53. Wallasch TM, Reinecke M, Langohr HD. EMB analysis of the late exteroceptive suppression period of temporal muscle activity in episodic and chronic tension-type headaches. *Cephalalgia* 1991; 11: 109–12.

54. Paulus W, Raubüchl O, Straube A, Schoenen J. Exteroceptive suppresion of temporalis muscle activity in various types of headache. *Headache* 1992; 32: 41–44.

55. Makashima K, Takahashi K. Exteroceptive suppression of the masseter, temporalis and trapezius muscles produced by mental nerve stimulation in patients with chronic headaches. *Cephalalgia* 1991; 11: 23–8.

56. Göbel H, Weigle L, Kropp P, Soyka D. Pain sensitivity and pain reactivity of pericranial muscles in migraine and tension-type headache. *Cephalalgia* 1992; 12: 142–51.

57. Göbel H, Ernst M, Jeschke J, Keil R, Weigle L. Acetylsalicylic acid activates antinociceptive brain-stem reflex acitivty in headache patients and in healthy subjects. *Pain* 1992; 48: 187–95.

58. Wolfe F, Smythe HA, Yanus MB et al. The American College of Rheumatology 1990 criteria for the classification of fibromyalgia: report of the multicenter criteria committee. *Arthritis Rheum* 1990; 33: 160–72.

59. Wolfe F. Two muscle pain syndromes: fibromyalgia and the myofascial pain syndrome. *Pain Management* 1990; 3: 153–64.

60. Travell J, Simons DG. Myofascial pain and dysfunction: the trigger point manual. Baltimore: Williams & Wilkins, 1983.

61. Rolf LH, Wiele G, Bruno GG. 5-Hydroxytryptamine in platelets of patients with muscle contraction headache. *Headache* 1981; 21: 10–11.

62. Anthony M, Lance JW. Plasma serotonin in patients with chronic tension headaches. *J Neurol Neurosurg Psychiatry* 1989; 52: 182–4.

63. Castillo J, Martinez F, Leira R et al. Plasma monoamines in tension-type headache. *Headache* 1994 ;34: 531–5.

64. Kitano A, Shimomura T, Takeshima T et al. Increased 11-dehydrothromboxane B_2 in migraine: platelet hyperfunction in patients with migraine during headache-free period. *Headache* 1994; 34: 515–18.

65. Silberstein SD, Meriam GR. Estrogens, progestins, and headache. *Neurology* 1991; 41: 786–93.

66. Kowa H, Shimomura T, Takahashi K. Platelet gamma-aminobutyric acid levels in migraine and tension-type headache. *Headache* 1992; 32: 229–32.

67. Welch KMA, Chabi E, Bartosh K, Achar VS, Meyer JS. Cerebrospinal fluid gamma aminobutyric acid levels in migraine. *BMJ* 1975; 3: 516–17.

68. Martin MJ, Rome HP, Swenson WM. Muscle contraction headache. A psychiatric review. *Res Clin Stud Headache* 1967; 1: 184.

69. Merikangas KR, Angst J. Migraine and psychopathology: epidemiologic and genetic aspects. *Clin Neuropharm* 1992; 15(Suppl. 1): 275A.

70. Diamond S. Muscle contraction headache. In: Dalessio DJ (ed.). *Wolff's Headache and other Head Pain.* (5th edition). New York: Oxford University Press, 1987: 172–89.

71. Diamond S. Depressive headaches. *Headache* 1964; 4: 255–9.

72. Diamond S. Depression and headache. *Headache* 1983; 23: 122–6.

73. De Benedittis G, Lorenzetti A, Pieri A. The role of stressful life events in the onset of chronic primary headache. *Pain* 1990; 40: 65–75.

74. Peatfield RC. Pain, headache, and depression: a discussion. In: Sandler M, Collins GM (eds). *Migraine: a Spectrum of Ideas.* New York: Oxford University Press, 1990.

75. Basbaum AI, Fields HL. Endogenous pain control mechanisms: review and hypothesis. *Ann Neurol* 1978; 4: 451–62.

76. Fields HL, Heinricher M. Brainstem modulation of nociceptor-driven withdrawal reflexes. *Ann NY Acad Sci* 1989; 563: 34–44.

77. Scholz E, Diener H-C, Geiselhart S. Drug-induced headache — does a critical dosage exist? In: Diener H-C, Wilkinson M (eds). *Drug-Induced Headache.* Berlin, Heidelberg: Springer-Verlag, 1988: 29–43.

78. Jensen R, Olesen J. Initiating mechanisms of experimentally induced tension-type headache. *Cephalalgia* 1996; 16: 175–82.

79. Tavola T, Gala C, Conte G, Invernizzi G. Traditional Chinese acupuncture in tension type headache: a controlled study. *Pain* 1992; 48: 325–9.

80. Silberstein SD, Lipton RB. Overview of diagnosis and treatment of migraine. *Neurology* 1994; 44(Suppl. 7): S6–16.

81. Nebe J, Heier M, Diener HC. Low-dose ibuprofen in self-medication of mild to moderate headache: a comparison with acetylsalicylic acid and placebo. *Cephalalgia* 1995; 15: 531–5.

82. Ryan RE. Motrin — a new agent for symptomatic treatment of muscle contraction headache. *Headache* 1977; 16: 280–3.

83. Tfelt-Hansen P, Johnson ES. Nonsteroidal anti-inflammatory drugs in the treatment of the acute migraine attack. In: Olesen J, Tfelt-Hansen P, Weldch KMA (eds). *The Headaches.* New York: Raven Press, 1993: 305–13.

84. Saper JR, Silberstein SD, Lake AE, Winters ME. Double-blind trial of fluoxetine: chronic daily headache and migraine. *Headache* 1994; 34: 497–502.

85. Holroyd KA, Penzien DB. Client variables and behavioral treatment of recurrent tension headaches: a meta-analytic review. *J Behav Med* 1986; 9: 515–36.

86. Holroyd KA. Tension-type headache, cluster headache, and miscellaneous headaches: psychological and behavioural techniques. In: Olesen J, Tfelt-Hansen P, Welch KMA (eds). *The Headaches.* New York: Raven Press, 1993: 515–20.

chapter 8

Chronic daily headache: diagnosis and treatment

Introduction

The classification of very frequent primary headache disorders and the appropriate use of the term 'chronic daily headache' (CDH) is still controversial. Some authors use CDH to refer to 'transformed migraine', a distinct clinical syndrome described below. Others use the term for any headache disorder that occurs on a daily or near daily basis, regardless of aetiology. The International Headache Society (IHS) has not yet fully addressed the classification of very frequent primary headache disorders. In this chapter, we use the term 'CDH' to refer to the broad group of headache disorders that occur more frequently than 15 days a month and will discuss those that have an average duration of 4 hours or longer.

When a patient presents with frequent headaches that are not related to a structural or systemic illness, the physician faces a substantial diagnostic and therapeutic challenge. While only 0.5% of the population have severe headaches on a daily basis,[1] and only 3% meet IHS criteria for chronic tension-type headache (CTTH),[2] these groups account for the majority of consultations in headache subspecialty practices.[3] Often these patients are overusing medication, and this may play a role in initiating or sustaining the pattern of frequent headaches. Anxiety, depression and other psychological disturbances may accompany CDH and require treatment.[3]

Patients with CDH are difficult to classify, biologically versus phenomenologically, using the IHS system as it is currently framed.[4-7] When they can be classified, many individuals with CDH are placed in the CTTH group or have two diagnoses. If there are superimposed attacks of severe headache, a second IHS diagnosis of migraine is often assigned. Several lines of evidence (outlined below) suggest that patients with CDH evolving from migraine have the biology of the migraineur. Therefore, it seems inappropriate to classify their headaches as a form of tension-type headache (TTH). An approach to classifying CDH is presented in Table 8.1. We classify CDH into primary or secondary varieties and subclassify primary CDH on the basis of average daily headache duration (>4 or <4 hours). Transformed migraine and new daily persistent headache (NDPH) are primary CDH disorders not included in the current IHS classification.

Causes of shorter duration daily head pain include: chronic cluster headache, chronic paroxysmal hemicrania, hypnic headache and idiopathic stabbing headache; and the cranial neuralgias, which usually differ from CDH. Both the short- and long-duration primary and secondary CDH disorders can be associated with analgesic or ergotamine overuse.

Cervicogenic headache[8] is a unilateral pain disorder that does not switch sides,[9] occurs mainly in women, and may be associated with ipsilateral blurred vision, tinnitus, lacrimation, tingling, difficulty swallowing, photophobia, arm pain, and, when more severe, nausea and anorexia. 'Neck triggers' and reduced cervical range of motion are characteristic. Cervicogenic headache may be difficult to distinguish from migraine and TTH, especially if the patient is overusing symptomatic medication.[10] It is uncertain whether cervicogenic headache is an independent entity or migraine or TTH with a cervical trigger.

Headache is a common accompaniment of cervical disc lesions.[11,12] High cervical bony defects or root damage such as caused by Paget's disease, which involves the bones of the base of the skull and the upper cervical spine, are associated with headache. Since most of the population over the age of 40 years has radiological changes of cervical spondylosis, but few have symptoms, it is important not to attribute headache to the mere presence of X-ray abnormalities. However, 40% of patients with spondylosis or symptomatic cervical disc disease such as radiculopathy or myelopathy have headache as a major complaint.[46,47]

● **Table 8.1** Chronic daily headache

Primary variety

Headache duration >4 hours
    Transformed migraine
    Chronic tension-type headache (CTTH)
    New daily persistent headache (NDPH)
    Hemicrania continua

Headache duration <4 hours
    Cluster headache
    Chronic paroxysmal hemicrania
    Hypnic headache
    Idiopathic stabbing headache

Secondary variety
Post-traumatic headache (PTH)
Cervical spine disorders
Headache associated with vascular disorders: arteriovenous malformation; arteritis, including giant cell arteritis; dissection; subdural haematoma
Headache associated with nonvascular intracranial disorders (intracranial hypertension, infection (Epstein–Barr virus, HIV), neoplasm)
Other (temporomandibular joint disorder; sinus infection)

● **Table 8.2** Headache classification for chronic daily headache (CDH)

Daily or near daily headache lasting >4 hours/day for >15 days/month
1.8 Transformed migraine
1.8.1 with medication overuse
1.8.2 without medication overuse
2.2 Chronic tension-type headache (CTTH)
2.2.1 with medication overuse
2.2.2 without medication overuse
4.7 New daily persistent headache (NDPH)
4.7.1 with medication overuse
4.7.2 without medication overuse
4.8 Hemicrania continua (HC)
4.8.1 with medication overuse
4.8.2 without medication overuse
Adapted from Silberstein et al.[3]

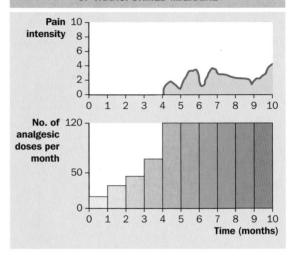

● **Figure 8.1** Temporal profile of transformed migraine provided by a 30-year-old woman who has a ten year history of headache. For many years she had bouts of episodic migraine without aura but with some nausea lasting 6–8 hours which she treated with a caffeine/analgesic mixture. About one year ago her headaches became more frequent and she started to increase her use of analgesics. After four months she experienced daily, bilateral headaches which were mild to moderate in intensity and associated with periodic migraine exacerbations.

Even in the absence of uniform terminology, a systematic approach to these difficult patients is needed. Once secondary headache has been excluded, frequent headache sufferers can be divided into two groups, based on headache duration. When headache duration is <4 hours, the differential diagnosis includes cluster headache, chronic paroxysmal hemicrania, idiopathic stabbing headache, hypnic headache, and other miscellaneous headache disorders. When the headache duration is >4 hours, the major primary disorders to consider are transformed migraine, hemicrania continua, CTTH and NDPH (Table 8.1).[3]

Several authors have examined the relative frequency of some of these conditions in clinic patients who have CDH. Most had CDH evolving from migraine, some began de novo, and a few had CDH that had evolved from episodic tension-type headache (ETTH). Many, if not most, patients had CDH associated with medication overuse.[13]

In this chapter, we discuss the classification and treatment of CDH, highlighting the four categories above. At present, the IHS provides criteria for only one of these disorders. We propose revisions to the IHS system and offer criteria for transformed migraine, hemicrania continua, CTTH and NDPH (Table 8.2).[3]

Transformed migraine

Patients with transformed migraine often have a past history of episodic migraine typically beginning in their teens or twenties.[14] In subspecialty clinics most are women, 90% of whom have a history of migraine without aura. The headaches grow more frequent over months to years and the associated symptoms of photophobia, phonophobia and nausea become less severe and less frequent than during typical migraine (Figure 8.1).[15,16] Patients often develop a pattern of daily or nearly daily headaches that phenomenologically resemble CTTH. That is, the pain is often mild to moderate and not associated with photophobia, phonophobia or gastrointestinal features. Other features of migraine, including unilaterality, gastrointestinal symptoms, and aggravation by menstruation and other trigger factors, may persist. Attacks of full-blown migraine superimposed on a background of less severe headaches occur in many patients.

About 80% of patients with transformed migraine overuse symptomatic medication.[15-19] Headaches often increase in frequency during a period of increasing medication use (Figure 8.1). Stopping the overused medication frequently results in distinct headache improvement, although improvement often develops over days to weeks (Figure 8.2). Many patients have significant long-term improvement after detoxification.

Eighty percent of patients with transformed migraine have depression.[15,19] The depression often lifts when the pattern of medication overuse and daily headache is interrupted. Although transformed migraine is widely recognized as a clinical entity, widely accepted formal diagnostic criteria are lack-

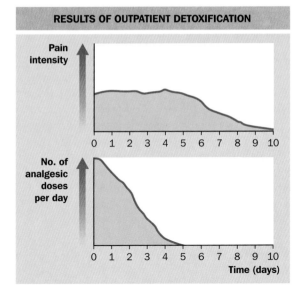

RESULTS OF OUTPATIENT DETOXIFICATION

● **Figure 8.2** *Results of outpatient detoxification. An improvement in CDH occurred within days of stopping the overuse of analgesics. Breakthrough headaches were treated with intramuscular dihydroergotamine administration.*

● **Table 8.3** *Proposed '1995' criteria for transformed migraine.*

1.8 Transformed migraine	
A	Daily or almost daily (>15 days/month) head pain for >1 month
B	Average headache duration of >4 hours/day (if untreated)
C	At least one of the following: • History of episodic migraine meeting any IHS criteria 1.1 to 1.6 • History of increasing headache frequency with decreasing severity of migrainous features over at least 3 months • Headache at some time meets IHS criteria for migraine 1.1 to 1.6 other than duration
D	Does not meet criteria for new daily persistent headache (4.7) or hemicrania continua (4.8)
E	At least one of the following: • There is no suggestion of one of the disorders listed in groups 5–11 • Such a disorder is suggested, but it is ruled out by appropriate investigations • Such disorder is present, but first migraine attacks do not occur in close temporal relation to the disorder

Adapted from Silberstein et al.[3]

ing. We proposed and then revised criteria for transformed migraine (Table 8.3). We believed that transformed migraine is a form of migraine and that the diagnosis of transformed migraine depended upon a past history of IHS migraine with a process of transformation leading to CDH. The period of transformation was characterized by increasing headache frequency and decreasing prominence of associated migrainous features.

Our criteria provide three alternative diagnostic links to migraine:

(i) a prior history of IHS migraine,
(ii) a clear period of escalating headache frequency with decreasing severity of migrainous features (which were both required in the 1994 criteria), or
(iii) current superimposed attacks of headaches that meet all the IHS criteria for migraine except duration.

To avoid undue diagnostic overlap we proposed hierarchical rules. If a patient meets the criteria for two disorders, the rules establish which diagnosis should be used. Thus the diagnosis of transformed migraine precludes a diagnosis of either episodic migraine (IHS 1.11.7) or CTTH.

Although migraine transformation most often develops in the setting of medication overuse, transformation may occur without overuse.[17,20] Using the IHS criteria, a firm diagnosis of 'headache induced by substance use or exposure' requires that the headaches remit after the overused medication is discontinued. In Figure 8.2 we illustrate a patient with daily headache which remitted when medication overuse was eliminated, but whose episodic migraine continued. In such a patient the diagnosis changes from episodic migraine to transformed migraine with medication overuse back to episodic migraine. This criterion is difficult to apply reliably and diagnosis is impossible until the overused medication is discontinued. As an alternative, we provide definitions for medication overuse based on a review of published reports and clinical experience (see below).[3]

Other forms of chronic daily headache

Chronic tension-type headache (Table 8.4)
Daily headaches may also develop in patients with a history of ETTH. These headaches are more often diffuse or bilateral and frequently involve the posterior aspect of the head and neck. In CTTH, in contrast to transformed migraine, most features of migraine are absent, as is prior or coexistent episodic migraine.

We propose several modifications to the current classification of CTTH. CTTH (IHS 2.2) requires head pain on at least 15 days a month for at least six months; patients often have daily headaches. Although the pain criteria are identical to ETTH, the IHS classification allows nausea, but not vomiting. There is a need for operational rules regarding nausea, photophobia and phonophobia, and for the decision regarding the prominence of these features.[7] It is possible that mild nausea or mild photophobia and phonophobia may prove to be compatible with the diagnosis of CTTH if better

● **Table 8.4** *Proposed diagnostic criteria for chronic tension-type headache (CTTH)*

2.2 Chronic tension-type headache

A   Average headache frequency >15 days/month (180 days/year) with average duration of >4 hours/day (if untreated) for 6 months fulfilling criteria (B–D) listed below

B   At least two of the following pain characteristics:
   1 Pressing/tightening quality
   2 Mild or moderate severity (may inhibit, but does not prohibit activities)
   3 Bilateral location
   4 No aggravation by walking stairs or similar routine physical activity

C   History of episodic tension-type headache in the past (needs to be tested)

D   History of evolutive headaches which gradually increased in frequency over at least a 3 month period (needs to be tested)

E   Both of the following:
   1 No vomiting
   2 No more than one of nausea, photophobia, or phonophobia (needs to be tested).

F   Does not meet criteria for hemicrania continua (4.8), new daily persistent headache (4.7) or transformed migraine (1.8).

G   At least one of the following:
   1 There is no suggestion of one of the disorders listed in groups 5–11
   2 Such a disorder is suggested, but it is ruled out by appropriate investigations.
   3 Such disorder is present, but first headache attacks do not occur in close temporal relation to the disorder.

Adapted from Silberstein et al.[3]

● **Table 8.5** *Proposed criteria for new daily persistent headache (NDPH)*

4.7 New daily persistent headache

A   Average headache frequency >15 days/month for >1 month

B   Average headache duration >4 hours/day (if untreated). Frequently constant without medication but may fluctuate

C   No history of tension-type headache or migraine which increases in frequency and decreases in severity in association with the onset of NDPH (over 3 months)

D   Acute onset (developing over <3 days) of constant unremitting headache

E   Headache is constant in location? (Needs to be tested)

F   Does not meet criteria for hemicrania continua (4.8)

G   At least one of the following:
   1 There is no suggestion of one of the disorders listed in groups 5–11.
   2 Such a disorder is suggested, but it is ruled out by appropriate investigations.
   3 Such disorder is present, but first headache attacks do not occur in close temporal relation to the disorder.

Adapted from Silberstein et al.[3]

measures of symptom severity are developed.[7,17] However, the need to include any of these migrainous features in the IHS definition of CTTH may be a result of including cases of transformed migraine under the rubric of CTTH.

CTTH evolving from ETTH requires a prior diagnosis of ETTH. Diagnostic confidence increases if ETTH increases in frequency until the criteria of CTTH are met. There are no explicit time durations of headache in the IHS definition of CTTH. CTTH criteria should be modified to include an average headache duration of >4 hours (Table 8.4). CTTH can exist in two varieties: headaches associated with (2.2.0.1) and not associated with (2.2.0.2) medication overuse. One could argue that CTTH could begin without preceding ETTH analogous to the situation in chronic cluster (i.e. unrelenting from onset). However, with cluster headache we are dealing with a series of episodic attacks, not a constant headache.

New daily persistent headache (Table 8.5)

NDPH is the abrupt development of a headache that does not remit.[21] It develops over <3 days and some patients remember the exact day or time the headache started. NDPH is likely to be a heterogeneous disorder. Some cases may reflect a postviral syndrome.[21] Patients with NDPH are generally younger than those with transformed migraine.[21]

We elected not to classify NDPH as a type of *de novo* CTTH, for it is not clear whether or not this condition is aetiologically related to TTH. Since NDPH and CTTH have similar characteristics, the disorders are distinguished by the presence or absence of a past history of headache. NDPH requires the absence of a history of evolution from migraine or ETTH. Excluding all patients with a history of ETTH is problematic, as almost 70% of men and 90% of women have had a TTH at some time in the past. We allow a diagnosis of NDPH in patients with migraine or ETTH if these disorders do not increase in frequency to give rise to NDPH. The constancy of location is uncertain and needs to be field tested. NDPH may or may not be associated with medication overuse (4.7.1, 4.7.2). A diagnosis of NDPH takes precedence over transformed migraine and CTTH.

Hemicrania continua (Table 8.6)

Hemicrania continua is a rare,[22] indomethacin-responsive headache disorder characterized by a continuous, moderately severe, unilateral headache that varies in intensity, waxing and waning without disappearing completely. It may rarely alternate sides.[23] It is frequently associated with jabs and jolts (idiopathic stabbing headache). Hemicrania continua is not triggered by neck movements but tender spots in the neck may be present. Exacerbations of pain are often associated with autonomic disturbances such as ptosis, miosis, tearing and sweating.[24] Some patients may have photophobia, phonophobia and nausea.

Case report

A 45-year-old woman[24] presented with a ten-year history of daily unilateral headache. In the remote past, she had occasional periods of left-sided headache lasting from one month to one year. At the time of presentation, she had a constant, widely distributed, left-sided hemicranial headache which waxed and waned in severity. The pain was usually mild to moderate but 8–20 times per month she experienced exacerbations which lasted up to 12 hours, characterized by more severe left periorbital and hemicrania pain accompanied by left-side miosis, ptosis and nasal congestion. The exacerbations were also associated with nausea and sensitivity to sensory stimuli. Her past medical history was unremarkable. General medical and neurological examinations and routine laboratory studies were unremarkable. Magnetic resonance imaging of the head was normal in the past.

She had been treated with several beta-blockers, calcium-channel blockers, tricyclic antidepressants, selective serotonin reuptake inhibitors (SSRI), methysergide and divalproex sodium without substantial relief. Inpatient treatment with dihydroergotamine did not improve her headaches. Acute treatment with several non-steroidal anti-inflammatory drugs (NSAID) and transnasal butorphanol and butalbital combination products were not helpful. Sumatriptan subcutaneously produced short-term relief during painful exacerbations.

Following a tentative diagnosis of hemicrania continua, she was started on indomethacin 50 mg t.d.s. Her daily headache resolved following each dose but recurred at the end of dosing intervals. Her regimen was gradually increased to a final dose of 75 mg t.d.s. with ranitidine (150 mg b.d.). Her other medications have been tapered and she is headache-free unless she skips a dose of indomethacin.

Although the disorder almost invariably has a prompt and enduring response to indomethacin, requiring a therapeutic response as a diagnostic criterion is problematic. It effectively excludes the diagnosis of hemicrania continua in patients never treated with indomethacin (perhaps because another agent helped) and in patients who failed to respond to indomethacin. Treatment response is generally not part of IHS case definitions of headache disorders. Cases have been described which did not respond to indomethacin but

Table 8.6 *Proposed criteria for hemicrania continua*

4.8 Hemicrania continua (HC)*	
A	Headache present for at least 1 month
B	Strictly unilateral headache
C	Pain has all of the following present: 1 Continuous but fluctuating 2 Moderate severity, at least some of the time 3 Lack of precipitating mechanisms
D	1 Absolute response to indomethacin, or 2 One of the following autonomic features with severe pain exacerbation: • Conjunctival infection • Lacrimation • Nasal congestion • Rhinorrhoea • Ptosis • Eyelid oedema
E	May have associated stabbing headaches
F	At least one of the following: 1 There is no suggestion of one of the disorders listed in groups 5–11. 2 Such a disorder is suggested, but it is ruled out by appropriate investigations. 3 Such disorder is present, but first headache attacks do not occur in close temporal relation to the disorder.

Adapted from Goadsby and Lipton[24]
* HC is usually non-remitting, but rare cases of remission have been reported.

meet the phenotype. For this reason we have provided an alternate means of diagnosis (Table 8.6).

Hemicrania continua exists in both continuous and remitting forms. In the continuous form, which must be differentiated from transformed migraine, headaches occur on a daily basis, sometimes for years. Many patients with this disorder overuse acute medication. In the remitting form, periods of daily headache alternate with pain-free remissions. Both forms meet the criteria in Table 8.6. Hemicrania continua takes precedence over the diagnosis of other types of primary CDH.

Clinical features

Newman and colleagues have classified hemicrania continua into three groups: a remitting form with distinct headache phases lasting weeks to months with prolonged pain-free remissions; an evolutive, unremitting form that arises from the remitting form; and an unremitting form characterized by continuous headache from the onset. Fifteen percent of patients have the remitting form, 32% have the evolutive form and 53% have the unremitting form. A chronic form evolving to a remitting form, a bilateral case, and a patient whose attacks alternated sides have all been described. Like the short-lived trigeminal autonomic cephalalgias (TACs), hemicrania continua is characterized by episodic attacks of head pain associated with ipsilateral autonomic features. Like the paroxysmal hemicranias, hemicrania continua is uniquely responsive to indomethacin, although a series of four patients who did not respond but fit the clinical phenotype have been described. A case responding to the piroxicam-β-cyclodextrin further suggests that while the NSAID response is of great interest, it points to, rather than expresses, the pathophysiology.

Hemicrania continua is differentiated from the other TACs primarily by continuous moderate pain without autonomic features between the painful exacerbations. Although there are no reports of secondary hemicrania continua, a C7 root irritation due to a disc herniation has been noted to aggravate the condition.[56] A case of a mesenchymal tumour in the sphenoid bone in which the response to indomethacin faded after two months has also been reported. These cases suggest that escalating doses or loss of indomethacin's efficacy should be treated with suspicion and the patient re-evaluated. The condition is seen in non-Caucasian populations.

Pathophysiological studies

The relative rarity of hemicrania continua has made it difficult to study its pathophysiology. Pain pressure thresholds are reduced in patients with hemicrania continua, as they are in CPH patients.[34] In contrast, orbital phlebography is relatively normal compared to patients with CPH,[47] although it should be observed that this area is controversial. Pupillometric studies have shown no clear abnormality in hemicrania continua, and studies of facial sweating have shown modest changes, similar to those seen in CPH.[36]

Drug overuse and rebound headache

Patients with frequent headaches often overuse narcotics, simple analgesics, ergotamine and sumatriptan (Figure 8.3). Medication overuse by headache-prone patients frequently produces CDH (drug-induced 'rebound headache') accompanied

DRUGS: A DOUBLE-EDGED SWORD

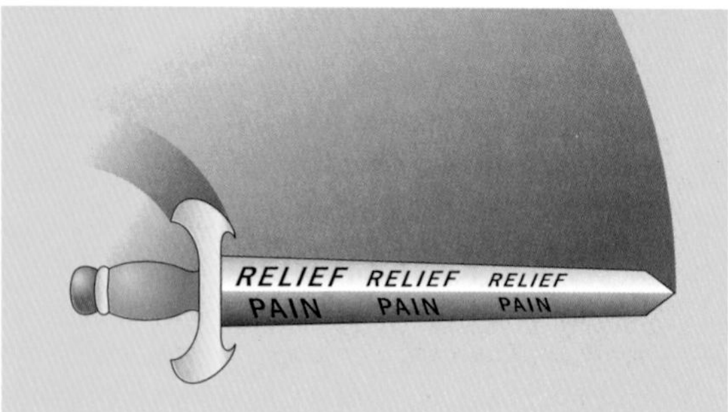

RELIEF RELIEF RELIEF
PAIN PAIN PAIN

● **Figure 8.3** *Overuse of medication by headache-prone patients frequently produces drug-induced CDH accompanied by dependence on symptomatic medication.*

by dependence on symptomatic medication. In addition, medication overuse can make headaches refractory to prophylactic medication.[20,25-29] Although stopping the symptomatic medication may result in withdrawal symptoms and a period of increased headache initially, the general rule is subsequent headache improvement.[29-33] Many CDH patients withdrawn from ergotamine and analgesics and given no further therapy stopped having daily headaches, although they often still had episodic migraine attacks.[34,35]

In subspecialty centres, most patients with drug-induced headache have a history of episodic migraine that has been converted into transformed migraine as a result of medication overuse.[18,20,25,29,35-38] Patients with TTH, hemicrania continua and NDPH may also overuse symptomatic medications. Drug-induced CDH, or, as Isler[39] has termed it, 'painkiller headache', has been reported since the 17th century, with occurrences reaching epidemic proportions in Switzerland after World War II.

The epidemiology of chronic drug-induced headache is uncertain since some headaches are drug-induced and some are just associated with drug overuse. In European headache centres, 5–10% of the patients have drug-induced headache. One series of 3000 consecutive headache patients reported that 4.3% had drug-induced headaches.[40] Experience in the United Kingdom suggests that drug-associated headache is more common in Europe than the literature suggests. In American specialty headache clinics, as many as 50–80% of patients who presented with CDH used analgesics on a daily or near-daily basis.[32] These differences may reflect the genuine influence of patterns of healthcare use. In the United States, over-the-counter analgesics are readily available and patients often consult multiple physicians who may not be aware of the other analgesics that the patient is taking.

Clinical features of rebound headache

Analgesic rebound headache has not been demonstrated in placebo-controlled trials. However, stopping daily low-dose caffeine frequently results in withdrawal headache.[41] In a controlled study of caffeine withdrawal, 64 normal adults (71% women) with low-to-moderate caffeine intake (the equivalent of about 2.5 cups of coffee a day) were given a two-day caffeine-free diet and either placebo or replacement caffeine. Under double-blind conditions, 50% of the patients who were given placebo had a headache by day 2, compared to 6% of those given caffeine. Nausea, depression, and flu-like symptoms were very common in the placebo group. This study is relevant since caffeine is frequently used by headache sufferers for pain relief, often in combination with analgesics or ergotamine. The study is a model for short-term caffeine withdrawal, but does not demonstrate the long-term consequences of detoxification.

The actual dose limits and time needed to develop rebound headaches have not been defined in rigorous studies. In addition, the relationship of drug half-life to the development of rebound is unknown. Our clinical knowledge is derived from observing patterns of medication use in patients who present with rebound headaches. Because there may be large individual differences in susceptibility to rebound headaches, anecdotal data must be generalized cautiously. It is believed that overuse occurs when patients take narcotics or ergotamine tartrate more often than two days a week, three or more simple analgesics a day more often than five days a week, or combination analgesics containing barbiturates or sedatives more often than three days a week (Figure 8.4).[20,25–28]

Specific limits are necessary to prevent analgesic, ergotamine and sumatriptan overuse. The frequency of days of ergotamine use (treatment days, events) is as important as, if not more important than, the total monthly dose.[19,30] Rebound can develop in patients taking as little as 0.5–1 mg of ergotamine three times a week.[27,28,33,42] Recently, sumatriptan, a selective 5-HT$_1$ agonist that is effective in acute migraine treatment, has been reported to induce rebound headache.[43] We recommend limiting the use of sumatriptan to three days a week or at least careful daily monitoring of drug use with frequent physician review when the headache frequency is two or more days a week.

Most daily headache patients overuse symptomatic medication[20] and may develop psychological dependence, tolerance and abstinence syndromes. Medication overuse may be responsible in part for the transformation of episodic migraine or ETTH into daily headache and for the perpetuation of the syndrome. However, medication overuse is not the *sine qua non* of transformed migraine or CTTH. Some patients develop transformed migraine or CTTH without overusing medication and others continue to have daily headaches long after the overused medication is discontinued. Medication overuse is usually motivated by a patient's desire to treat the headaches. However, some headache patients may overuse combination analgesics to treat their mood disturbance. Medication overuse rarely represents primary substance abuse.

In addition to exacerbating the headache disorder, drug overuse has other serious effects. The overuse of symptomatic drugs may interfere with the effectiveness of preventive headache medications. The extended use of large amounts of medication may cause renal or hepatic toxicity in addition to tolerance, habituation or dependence. ('Tolerance' refers to the decreased effectiveness of the same dose of an analgesic, often leading to the use of higher doses to achieve the same degree of effectiveness. 'Habituation' and dependence are, respectively, the psychological and physical need to repeatedly use drugs).

Psychiatric comorbidity

Anxiety, depression, and bipolar disease are more frequent in migraine patients than in non-migraine control subjects.[44,45] Since transformed migraine evolves from migraine, one would also expect psychiatric comorbidity in transformed migraine. In a clinic-based study of 630 patients with CDH, including patients with transformed migraine, CTTH, NDPH and post-traumatic headache, the Minnesota Multiphasic Personality Inventory was abnormal in 61%, compared with 12.2% of patients with episodic migraine. Zung and Beck Depression Scale scores were significantly higher in the CDH patients than in migraine controls.[46] In several subspecialty centre-based studies, depression occurred in about 80% of transformed migraine patients.[20,25,28] Clinical experience suggests that comorbid depression often improves when the cycle of daily head pain is broken.[47] The biological relationship of migraine vulnerability to rebound headache and psychiatric comorbidity remains to be clarified.

Pathophysiology

The source of pain in CDH is unknown. Chronic continuous pain is often due to ongoing peripheral activation of nociceptors (e.g. chronic inflammation), although at times chronic pain may occur in the absence of painful stimuli. Peripheral sensitization due to tissue damage or inflammation reduces the threshold of nociceptive afferent input at the injury site, resulting in local pain and tenderness. Central sensitization results

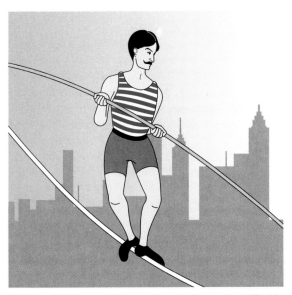

● *Figure 8.4* *Responsible use of analgesics can be difficult!*

from increased excitability of spinal neurons, producing an exaggerated response so that non-painful stimuli feel painful even outside the injured site. Although the pathophysiology of CDH is unknown, recent work suggests several mechanisms that could contribute to the process. CDH may be due to:

(I) abnormal excitation of peripheral nociceptive afferent fibres with peripheral sensitization (perhaps due to chronic neurogenic inflammation),
(ii) enhanced responsiveness of the nucleus caudalis neurons (central sensitization),
(iii) defective pain modulation,
(iv) spontaneous central pain,
(v) continuous activity of the 'migraine brainstem generation', or
(vi) a combination of these (see Chapter 5).

Drug-induced headache mechanisms

Overuse of analgesics, barbiturates or ergotamine-containing compounds may contribute to the transformation of episodic migraine into transformed migraine. Some believe that drug-induced CDH is due to a rebound effect wherein medication withdrawal triggers the next headache, which, in turn, leads to the consumption of more drug. This may produce a vicious cycle resulting in more frequent drug use and drug-induced CDH. Formulations of drugs that maintain sustained, non-fluctuating levels might avoid the development of drug-induced headache.[48]

The consequences of drug discontinuation depend on the type of therapeutic response it engenders. Discontinuation might be associated with relapse for several reasons:

(I) loss of therapeutic drug effects,
(ii) rebound changes caused by drug withdrawal, or
(iii) re-induction of the primary pathophysiological process with the occurrence of a new episode.[48,49]

Increased activity of the on-cells in the pain modulation system of the brainstem could enhance the response to any painful or non-painful stimuli and result in sensitization. The activity of this system is enhanced during narcotic withdrawal. A similar mechanism may occur during drug-induced headaches. Transformed migraine not associated with drug overuse may result from sensitization of nociceptors in the nucleus caudalis as a result of enhanced on-cell activity, which could be, in part, a problem of the network modulating pain from the head and face.

Continued high fluctuating doses of ergots, analgesics or narcotics could result in resetting of the pain control mechanisms in susceptible individuals, perhaps by enhancing on-

cell activity, enhancing central sensitization through N-methyl-D-aspartate receptors, or blocking adaptive antinociceptive changes. Compensatory adaptive changes associated with frequent headaches (if they occur) may not be enough to allow continued drug effectiveness. If tolerance has decreased drug effectiveness, a drug holiday could renew the response.[48] Drug overuse may, in part, prevent the occurrence of antinociceptive adaptive changes.

The transformation of episodic to chronic headache or the development of de novo CDH probably is a result of sensitization in the pathways of the trigeminal system. This could result from a painful peripheral receptor stimulus (other painful disorders in the trigeminal or cervical territory), from stressful events which could enhance pain perception, or from neurochemical or hormonal changes. Increased on-cell activity, decreased central pain inhibition, and activation of the peripheral nociceptor may act together to produce CDH. It is not known for certain whether there are increases in kindling, N-methyl-D-aspartate receptor activity, or nerve growth factor (NGF) and NGF mast cell activation, but these theoretical possibilities suggest potential therapy. In addition, the phenomena of contigent tolerance (see Chapter 5) may be at work.

Clinical strategies based on these concepts might be used to reverse tolerance in the long-term treatment of migraine or transformed migraine. Switching a patient to a drug that has a different mechanism of action and does not show cross-tolerance or discontinuing the ineffective drug and re-introducing it later may be effective in some migraine or transformed migraine patients.

Treatment

Overview (Figures 8.5–8.7)

It can be difficult to treat patients suffering from CDH especially when it is complicated by medication overuse and comorbid depression.[18,28] Effective management requires the following steps. First, exclude secondary headache disorders; second, diagnose the specific long duration primary CDH disorder (i.e. transformed migraine, hemicrania continua, NDPH or CTTH); and third, identify comorbid medical and psychiatric conditions and exacerbating factors, especially medication overuse. Limit all symptomatic medications (with the possible exception of the long-acting NSAID). For outpatients, we gradually taper the overused medications, at a rate of 10% a week, often replacing them with NSAID. Patients should be started on a programme of preventive medication (to decrease reliance on symptomatic medication), with the explicit understanding that the drugs may not become fully effective until medication overuse has been eliminated and the washout period completed.[50] Patients

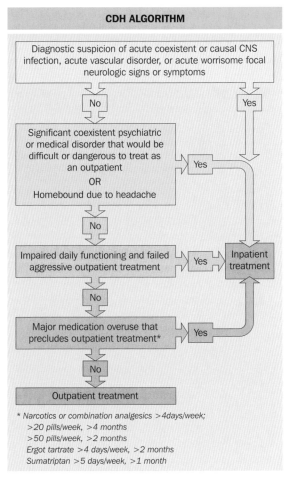

● **Figure 8.5** *CDH treatment algorithm.*

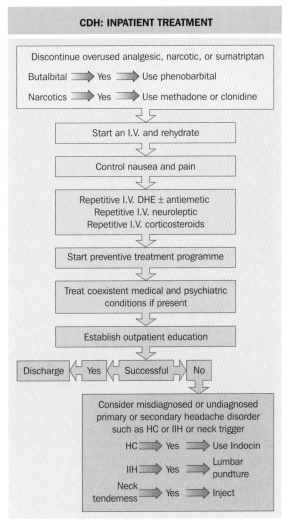

● **Figure 8.6** *CDH inpatient treatment algorithm.*

need education and continuous support during the detoxification period, which may require one to several months.

If outpatient detoxification proves difficult or is dangerous, hospitalization may be required. The detoxification process can last from two to ten weeks after medication overuse is eliminated. Withdrawal symptoms include severely exacerbated headache accompanied by nausea, vomiting, agitation, restlessness, sleep disorder and (rarely) seizures. Barbiturates and benzodiazepines must be tapered gradually to avoid a serious withdrawal syndrome. The washout period may last three to eight weeks; once it is over, there is frequently considerable headache improvement.[13,18,33,51] Inpatient and outpatient detoxification options are available. A recent consensus paper by the German Migraine Society recommends outpatient withdrawal for highly motivated patients who do not take barbiturates or tranquillizers with their analgesics. Inpatient treatment is recommended for patients who fail outpatient treatment, have high depression scores, or take tranquillizers, codeine or barbiturates.[52]

Disturbances in mood and function are common and require management with behavioural methods of pain management and supportive psychotherapy (including biofeedback, stress management and cognitive behavioural therapy). Treatment of the comorbid psychiatric illness is often necessary before the CDH comes under control.

Psychophysiological therapy involves reassurance, counselling, stress management, relaxation therapy and biofeedback. The use of traditional acupuncture is controversial, and has not proved more effective than placebo.[53] Physical therapy consists of modality treatments (heat, cold packs, ultrasound and electrical stimulation), improvement of posture through stretching, exercise, and traction, trigger point injections, occipital nerve blocks, and a programme of regular exercise, stretching, balanced meals and adequate sleep.[54]

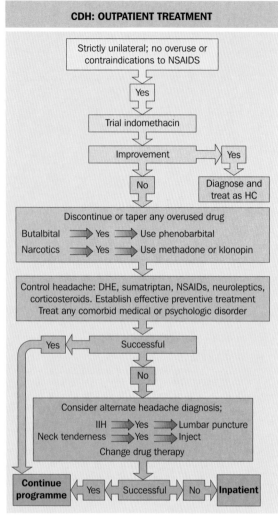

CDH: OUTPATIENT TREATMENT

Strictly unilateral; no overuse or contraindications to NSAIDS

↓ Yes

Trial indomethacin

↓

Improvement → Yes

No ↓ ↓

Diagnose and treat as HC

Discontinue or taper any overused drug

Butalbital ⇒ Yes ⇒ Use phenobarbital

Narcotics ⇒ Yes ⇒ Use methadone or klonopin

Control headache: DHE, sumatriptan, NSAIDs, neuroleptics, corticosteroids. Establish effective preventive treatment Treat any comorbid medical or psychologic disorder

Yes ← Successful

↓ No

Consider alternate headache diagnosis;

IIH ⇒ Yes ⇒ Lumbar puncture
Neck tenderness ⇒ Yes ⇒ Inject
Change drug therapy

Continue programme ⇐ Yes ⇐ Successful ⇒ No ⇒ **Inpatient**

● *Figure 8.7* *CDH outpatient treatment algorithm.*

It has been our experience that treating painful trigger areas in the neck can result in the improvement of intractable CDH.

Acute pharmacotherapy

Patients who do not overuse symptomatic medication can treat acute severe headache exacerbations with antimigraine drugs including sumatriptan, dihydroergotamine, and ergotamine, as well as narcotics. These drugs must be strictly limited to prevent the development of superimposed rebound headache that will complicate treatment and require detoxification. The risk of rebound is much lower for dihydroergotamine and sumatriptan than for analgesics, narcotics and ergotamine. In our experience rebound hardly, if ever, occurs with dihydroergotamine, but can occur with daily use of sumatriptan.

Preventive pharmacotherapy

Patients with daily headaches should be treated primarily with preventive medications, with the explicit understanding that medications may not become fully effective until the overused medication has been eliminated. It may take three to six weeks for treatment effects to develop.

The following principles guide the use of preventive treatment:[55]

- from among the first-line drugs, choose preventive agents based on their side-effect profiles, comorbid conditions and specific indications (e.g. indomethacin for hemicrania continua);
- start at a low dose;
- gradually increase the dose until you achieve efficacy, until the patient develops side effects, or until the ceiling dose for the drug in question is reached;
- treatment effects develop over weeks and treatment may not become fully effective until rebound is eliminated;
- if one agent fails and if all other things are equal, choose an agent from another therapeutic class;
- prefer monotherapy, but be willing to use combination therapy;
- communicate realistic expectations.

Most preventive agents used for CDH have not been examined in well-designed double-blind studies. Table 8.7 summarizes an assessment of the efficacy, safety and evidence for a number of agents.[50]

Antidepressants are attractive agents for use in CDH (transformed migraine, CTTH, NDPH), since many patients have comorbid depression and anxiety. The most widely used antidepressant are the tricyclic antidepressants which include nortriptyline (Aventyl, Pamelor), amitriptyline[56-65] (Elavil) and doxepin[66] (Sinequan) (start at 10–25 mg at bedtime and gradually increase). Fluoxetine (Prozac), a SSRI, is coming into wider use for daily headaches; evidence from a double-blind study demonstrates its efficacy in CDH.[56,67] Fluvoxamine appears to be effective[68] and may have analgesic properties.[69] Other SSRI, the new selective norepinephrine- and serotonin-re-uptake inhibitors such as venlafaxine, and monoamine oxidase inhibitors, may have a therapeutic role, but this has not been proven to date.[70]

Beta-blockers (propranolol, nadolol) remain a mainstay of therapy for migraine[50] and are used for CDH.[63,71] Though clinicians fear that beta-blockers may exacerbate depression, this is controversial.[72] For this reason they are often used in combination with antidepressants. Beta-blockers are relatively contraindicated in patients with asthma and Raynaud's disease.

● **Table 8.7** *Summary of prophylactic drugs for use in chronic daily headache*

Drug	Clinical efficacy	Side effects	Clinical evidence*
Antidepressants			
Amitriptyline	+++	++	+++
Doxepin	+++	++	++
Fluoxetine	++	+	+++
Anticonvulsants			
Divalproex	+++	++	++
Beta-blockers			
Propranolol, nadolol, etc.	++	+	+
Calcium-channel blockers			
Verapamil	++	+	+
Miscellaneous			
Methysergide	+++	+++	+

Modified from Tfelt-Hansen and Welch[84]
All categories are rated from + to ++++ based on a combination of published literature and clinical experience.
*Ratings of +++ for clinical evidence indicate at least one double-blind, placebo-controlled study. A rating of ++ indicates open well-designed studies and + indicates ratings based on clinical experience. A rating of ++++ requires at least two double-blind placebo-controlled trials.

Calcium-channel blockers are well tolerated;[50] however, the only evidence that supports their use for transformed migraine is anecdotal. Verapamil (Calan) is the most widely prescribed agent in this family. Diltiazem (Cardizem) and nifedipine (Procardia) are of unproven efficacy. Flunarazine[47,50] is effective and widely used in Canada, Europe, and South-east Asia, but is not available in the United States.

The anticonvulsant, divalproex sodium (Depakote),[73] is an important drug for use in CDH, even in patients who have failed other agents. Four double-blind placebo-controlled studies demonstrate its efficacy in migraine.[73-76] Smaller open studies support its utility in transformed migraine.[77] Doses lower than those used in epilepsy (250 mg two to three times a day) may be sufficient. Divalproex sodium is an especially useful agent in patients with comorbid epilepsy and manic-depressive illness and, possibly, anxiety disorders.

The ergot derivative, methysergide,[50] is the first Food and Drug Agency-approved migraine prophylactic drug, and one that is sometimes unreasonably feared. It is an effective migraine preventive agent and can be safely combined with tricyclic antidepressants, SSRI, or calcium-channel blockers. The usual initial dose of methysergide is 2 mg twice a day. It can be increased to a maximum of 8 mg/day (2 mg four times a day); higher doses, though not recommended by the *Physicians' Desk Reference*, are sometimes useful.

The NSAID can be used for both symptomatic and preventive headache treatment. Naproxen sodium is effective in prevention at a dose of one or two 275 mg tablets twice a day.[78] Other effective NSAID include tolfenamic acid, ketoprofen, mefenamic acid, fenoprofen and ibuprofen.[79,80] Aspirin was found to be effective in one study[81] and equal to placebo in another.[82] The short-acting NSAID such as ibuprofen and aspirin may cause rebound and their use should be limited. It is uncertain about the other NSAID. Indomethacin is the drug of choice for hemicrania continua, and the response to this medication contributes to the definition of the disorder. We give indomethacin a therapeutic trial (up to 150–225 mg/day for one week) to rule out hemicrania continua, but otherwise limit the use of other NSAID.

Although monotherapy is preferred, it is sometimes necessary to combine preventive medications. Antidepressants are often used with beta-blockers or calcium-channel blockers and divalproex sodium may be used in combination with any of these medications.

Detoxification

Outpatient

There are two general outpatient strategies. One approach is to taper the overused medication, gradually substituting a long-acting NSAID as effective preventive therapy is established. The alternative strategy is to abruptly discontinue the overused drug and either substitute an NSAID or use intramuscular dihydroergotamine or corticosteroids. Serious withdrawal syndromes that can be produced by the overused drug must be prevented. For example, if high doses of a butalbital-containing analgesic combination are abruptly discontinued, phenobarbital should be used to prevent barbiturate withdrawal. Similarly, benzodiazepines must be gradually tapered. Outpatient treatment, while preferred for motivated patients, is not always safe or effective.

Inpatient

If outpatient treatment fails or is not safe, or if there is significant medical or psychiatric comorbidity present, inpatient treatment may be needed.[50] The goals of inpatient treatment include:

(I) detoxification and rehydration,
(ii) pain control with parenteral therapy,
(iii) establishment of effective prophylaxis,
(iv) interruption of the cycle of pain,
(v) patient education, and
(vi) establishment of outpatient methods of pain control.[50]

The detoxification process can be enhanced and shortened and the patient's symptoms made more tolerable by the use

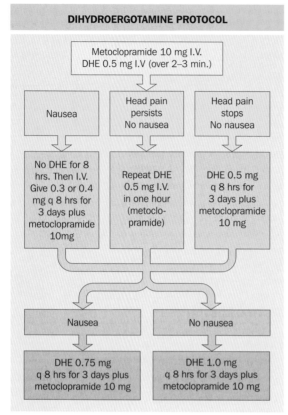

DIHYDROERGOTAMINE PROTOCOL

Metoclopramide 10 mg I.V.
DHE 0.5 mg I.V (over 2–3 min.)

Nausea

Head pain persists
No nausea

Head pain stops
No nausea

No DHE for 8 hrs. Then I.V. Give 0.3 or 0.4 mg q 8 hrs for 3 days plus metoclopramide 10mg

Repeat DHE 0.5 mg I.V. in one hour (metoclopramide)

DHE 0.5 mg q 8 hrs for 3 days plus metoclopramide 10 mg

Nausea

No nausea

DHE 0.75 mg q 8 hrs for 3 days plus metoclopramide 10 mg

DHE 1.0 mg q 8 hrs for 3 days plus metoclopramide 10 mg

● *Figure 8.8* Dihydroergotamine treatment protocol. After Raskin.[51]

● **Table 8.8** Why treatment fails

The diagnosis is incomplete or incorrect

An undiagnosed secondary headache disorder is present

A primary headache disorder is misdiagnosed

Two or more different headache disorders are present

Important exacerbating factors may have been missed

Medication overuse (including OTCs)

Caffeine overuse

Dietary or lifestyle triggers

Hormonal triggers

Psychosocial factors

Other medications which trigger headaches

Pharmacotherapy has been inadequate

Ineffective drug

Excessive initial doses

Inadequate final doses

Inadequate duration of treatment

Other factors

Unrealistic expectations

Cormorbid conditions complicate therapy

Inpatient treatment required

of repetitive intravenous dihydroergotamine coadministered with metoclopramide or domperidone (Figure 8.8),[51] which helps control nausea. Following 10 mg i.v. metoclopramide or a domperidone suppository, dihydroergotamine 0.5 mg is administered intravenously. Subsequent doses are adjusted based on pain relief and side effects. Patients who are not candidates for dihydroergotamine or are truly intolerant of the drug may require repetitive intravenous neuroleptics, such as chlorpromazine, prochlorperazine and/or corticosteroids. These agents may also supplement repetitive intravenous dihydroergotamine in refractory patients.[13] Hospitalization is also used as a time for patient education, for introducing behavioural methods of pain control, and for adjusting an outpatient programme of preventive and acute therapy. In our experience[13] repetitive intravenous dihydroergotamine is a safe and effective means of rapidly controlling intractable headache.

Prognosis

The 'natural history' of CDH disorders, and of rebound headache in particular, have never been studied and probably never will be for ethical and technical reasons. Recognition of the rebound process probably is itself therapeutic and could affect the patient's behaviour or the physician's approach. Retrospective analysis suggests that there may be periods of stable drug consumption and phases of accelerated medication use. Patients treated aggressively generally improve. There are no literature reports of spontaneous improvement of rebound headache, although this may happen. We performed follow-up evaluations on 50 hospitalized CDH drug overuse patients who were treated with repetitive intravenous dihydroergotamine and became headache-free.[83] Once detoxified, treated and discharged, most patients did not resume daily analgesic or ergotamine use. Seventy-two percent continued to show significant improvement at three months and 87% continued to show significant improvement after two years. Patients with drug-induced CDH, while difficult to treat, often return to a state of intermittent episodic headache after detoxification and treatment with a preventive medication. Our two-year success rate of 87% is consistent with the long-term success rates reported in the literature.[83]

Why treatment fails (Table 8.8)

When patients fail to respond to therapy or announce at the first consultation that they have already tried everything and that nothing will work, it is important to try to identify the reason or reasons that treatment has failed. The cause of treatment failure may be an incomplete or incorrect diagnosis. For example:

(I) an undiagnosed secondary headache disorder is the major source of the head pain,

(ii) a misdiagnosed primary headache disorder is present (i.e. hemicrania continua is mistaken for transformed migraine, episodic paroxysmal hemicrania or hypnic headache is mistaken for cluster), and

(iii) two or more different headache disorders are present. In addition, important exacerbating factors such as medication overuse may have been missed or pharmacotherapy may have been inadequate. Other factors may also be present.

Prevention

Headache sufferers often do not realize that excessive or frequent self-treatment may perpetuate or exacerbate their headaches. Since most headache sufferers do not seek medical advice until and unless the pain becomes frequent or intense, the opportunity for diagnosis and physician intervention to halt the cycle is often missed. Physicians need to screen CDH patients for analgesic overuse. Headache patients must be informed about the risks of analgesic overuse and rebound headache. Yet, even when patients are aware of the risks, they may still overmedicate. This requires continued vigilance on the part of the treating physician.

Patients who overuse medication may feel ashamed and out of control, and unable to provide an accurate history of drug use. To facilitate this process, the condition of medication rebound should be explained as a part of the natural history of migraine. Even if the patient is not rebounding at the time, doses of all symptomatic headache medications, with the possible exception of the long-acting NSAID, need to be limited.

References

1. Newman LC, Lipton RB, Solomon S, Stewart WF. Daily headache in a population sample: results from the American Migraine Study. *Headache* 1994; 34(1): 295.

2. Rasmussen BK. Migraine and tension-type headache in a general population: psychosocial factors. *Int J Epidemiol* 1992; 21: 1138–43.

3. Silberstein SD, Lipton R, Solomon S, Mathew N. Classification of daily and near daily headaches: proposed revisions to the IHS classification. *Headache* 1994; 34: 17.

4. Solomon S, Lipton RB, Newman LC. Evaluation of chronic daily headache comparison to criteria for chronic tension-type headache. *Cephalalgia* 1992; 12: 365–8.

5. Sanin LC, Mathew NT, Bellmyer LR, Ali S. The International Headache Society (IHS) headache classification as applied to a headache clinic population. *Cephalalgia* 1994; 14: 443–6.

6. Messinger HB, Spierings ELH, Vincent AJP. Overlap of migraine and tension-type headache in the International Headache Society classification. *Cephalalgia* 1991; 11: 233–7.

7. Pfaffenrath V, Isler H. Evaluation of the nosology of chronic tension-type headache. *Cephalalgia* 1993; 13(12): 60–2.

8. Sjaastad O, Saumte C, Hovdahl H *et al*. Cervicogenic headache, an hypothesis. *Cephalalgia* 1983; 3: 249–256.

9. Sjaastad O. The headache challenge in our time: cervicogenic headache. *Funct Neurology* 1990; 5: 155–8.

10. Pfaffenrath V, Kaube H. Diagnostics of cervicogenic headache. *Funct Neurology* 1990; 5: 159–64.

11. Edmeads J. The cervical spine and headache. *Neurology* 1988; 38: 1874–8.

12. Brain WR. Some unsolved problems of cervical spondylosis. *BMJ* 1963; 1: 771–7.

13. Silberstein SD, Schulman EA, Hopkins MM. Repetitive intravenous DHE in the treatment of refractory headache. *Headache* 1990; 30: 334–9.

14. Silberstein SD, Lipton RB, Sliwinski M. Classification of daily and near-daily headaches: field trial of revised IHS criteria. *Neurology* 1996; 47 871–5.

15. Mathew NT. Transformed migraine. *Cephalalgia* 1993; 13(Suppl. 12): 78–83.

16. Saper JR, Silberstein SD, Gordon CD, Hamel RL. *Handbook of Headache Management*. Baltimore: Williams & Wilkins, 1993.

17. Mathew NT, Stubits E, Nigam MR. Transformation of episodic migraine into daily headache: analysis of factors. *Headache* 1982; 22: 66–8.

18. Mathew NT, Reuveni U, Perez F. Transformed or evolutive migraine. *Headache* 1987;27:102–6.

19. Saper JR. Headache disorders: current concepts in treatment strategies. Massachusetts: Wright-PSG, 1983.

20. Mathew NT, Kurman R, Perez F. Drug induced refractory headache — clinical features and management. *Headache* 1990; 30: 634–8.

21. Vanast WJ. New daily persistent headaches: definition of a benign syndrome. *Headache* 1986; 26: 317.

22. Newman LC, Lipton RB, Solomon S. Hemicrania continua: 7 new cases and a literature review. *Headache* 1993; 32: 267.

23. Bordini C, Antonaci F, Stovner LJ, Schrader H, Sjaastad O. 'Hemicrania continua' — a clinical review. *Headache* 1991; 31: 20–6.

24. Goadsby PJ, Lipton RB. A review of paroxysmal hemicranias, SUNCT syndrome, and other short-lasting headaches with autonomic features, including new cases. *Brain* 1997; 120: 193–209.

25. Mathew NT. Drug-induced headache. *Neurol Clin* 1990; 8: 903–12.

26. Diamond S, Dalessio DJ. Drug abuse in headache. In: *The Practicing Physician's Approach to Headache*. 3rd edition.Baltimore: Williams & Wilkins, 1982: 114–21.

27. Wilkinson M. Introduction. In: Diener HC, Wilkinson M (eds). *Drug-Induced Headache*. Berlin: Springer-Verlag. 1988: 12.

28. Saper JR. Ergotamine dependence — a review. *Headache* 1987; 27: 435–8.

29. Saper JR. Chronic headache syndromes. *Neurol Clin* 1989; 7: 387–412.

30. Saper JR, Jones JM. Ergotamine tartrate dependency: features and possible mechanisms. *Clin Neuropharmacol* 1986; 9: 244–56.

31. Andersson PG. Ergotism — the clinical picture. In: Diener H-C, Wilkinson M (eds). *Drug-Induced Headache*. Berlin: Springer-Verlag, 1988: 1619.

32. Rapoport AM, Weeks RE, Sheftell FD, Baskin SM, Verdi J. The 'analgesic washout period': a critical variable evaluation in the evaluation of headache treatment efficacy. *Neurology* 1986; 36(Suppl.1): 100–101.

33. Baumgartner C, Wessely P, Bingol C, Maly J, Holzner F. Long-term prognosis of analgesic withdrawal in patients with drug-induced headaches. *Headache* 1989; 29: 510–14.

34. Dichgans J, Diener HC, Gerber WD, Verspohl EJ, Kukiolka H, Kluck M. Analgetika induzierter Dauerkopfschmerz. *Dtsch Med Wschr* 1984; 109: 369–73.

35. Rapoport AM. Analgesic rebound headache. *Headache* 1988; 28: 662–5.

36. Kudrow L. Paradoxical effects of frequent analgesic use. *Adv Neurol* 1982; 33: 335–41.

37. Diener HC, Dichgans J, Scholz E, Geiselhart S, Gerber WD, Bille A. Analgesic-induced chronic headache: long-term results of withdrawal therapy. *J Neurol* 1989; 236: 914.

38. Rasmussen BK, Jensen R, Olesen J. Impact of headache on sickness absence and utilization of medical services: a Danish population study. *J Epidemiol Community Health* 1992; 46: 443–6.

39. Isler H. Headache drugs provoking chronic headache: historical aspects and common misunderstandings. In: Diener H-C, Wilkinson M (eds). *Drug-Induced Headache.* Berlin: Springer-Verlag, 1988: 87–94.

40. Micieli G, Manzoni GC, Granella F, Martignoni E, Malferrari G, Nappi G. Clinical and epidemiological observations on drug abuse in headache patients. In: Diener H-C, Wilkinson M (eds). *Drug-Induced Headache.* Berlin: Springer-Verlag, 1988: 20–8.

41. Silverman K, Evans SM, Strain EC, Griffiths RR. Withdrawal syndrome after the double-blind cessation of caffeine consumption. *New Engl J Med* 1992; 327(16): 1109–14.

42. Silberstein SD. Chronic daily headache and tension-type headache. *Neurology* 1993; 43: 1644–9.

43. Catarci T, Fiacco F, Argentino C *et al.* Ergotamine-induced headache can be sustained by sumatriptan daily intake. *Cephalalgia* 1994; 14: 374–5.

44. Merikangas KR, Angst J, Isler H. Migraine and psychopathology: results of the Zurich cohort study of young adults. *Arch Gen Psychiatry* 1990; 47: 849–53.

45. Breslau N, Davis GC. Migraine, physical health and psychiatric disorders: a prospective epidemiologic study of young adults. *J Psychiatric Res* 1993; 27(2): 211–21.

46. Mathew NT. Chronic daily headache: clinical features and natural history. In: Nappi G, Bono G, Sandrini G, Martignoni E, Micieli G (eds). *Headache and Depression: Serotonin Pathways as a Common Clue.* New York: Raven Press, 1991: 49–58.

47. Lake AE, Saper JR, Madden SF, Kreeger C. Comprehensive inpatient treatment for intractable migraine: a prospective long-term outcome study. *Headache* 1993; 33: 55–62.

48. Post RM, Silberstein SD. Shared mechanisms in affective illness, epilepsy, and migraine. *Neurology* 1994; 44(7): S37–47.

49. Isler H. Migraine treatment as a cause of chronic migraine. In: Rose FC (ed.). *Advances in Migraine Research and Therapy.* New York: Raven Press, 1982: 159–64.

50. Silberstein SD, Saper J. Migraine: diagnosis and treatment. In: Dalessio D, Silberstein SD (eds). *Wolff's Headache and Other Head Pain.* 6th edition. New York: Oxford University Press, 1993: 961–70.

51. Raskin NH. Repetitive intravenous dihydroergotamine as therapy for intractable migraine. *Neurology* 1986; 36: 995–7.

52. Diener HC, Pfaffenrath V, Soyka D, Gerber WD. Therapie des medikamenten induzierten dauerkopfschmerzes. *Münch Med Wschr* 1992; 134: 159–62.

53. Tavola T, Gala C, Conte G, Invernizzi G. Traditional Chinese acupuncture in tension type headache: a controlled study. *Pain* 1992; 48: 325–9.

54. Silberstein SD. Treatment of headache in primary care practice. *Am J Med* 1984; 77(3A): 65–72.

55. Silberstein SD, Lipton RB. Overview of diagnosis and treatment of migraine. *Neurology* 1994; 44(7): S6–16.

56. Bussone G, Sandrini G, Patruno G *et al.* Effectiveness of fluoxetine on pain and depression in chronic headache disorders. In: Nappi G, Bono G, Sandrini G, Martignoni E, Micieli G (eds). *Headache and Depression: Serotonin Pathways as a Common Clue.* New York: Raven Press, 1991: 265–72.

57. Couch JR, Ziegler DK, Hassainein R. Amitriptyline in the prophylaxis of migraine. *Arch Neurol* 1976; 26: 121–7.

58. Diamond S, Baltes B. Chronic tension headache treated with amitriptyline: a double blind study. *Headache* 1971; 11: 110–16.

59. Holland J, Holland C, Kudrow L. Low-dose amitriptyline prophylaxis in chronic scalp muscle contraction headache. In: *Proceedings of the First International Headache Congress.* Munich, September 1983.

60. Lance JW, Curran DA. Treatment of chronic tension headache. *Lancet* 1964; 1: 1236–9.

61. Pluvinage R. Le traitement des migraines et des cephalees psychogenes par l'amitriptyline. *Sem Hop* 1978;54:713–716.

62. Pfaffenrath V, Diener HC, Isler H *et al.* Efficacy and tolerability of amitriptylinoxide in the treatment of chronic tension-type headache: a multicentre controlled study. *Cephalalgia* 1994;14:149–155.

63. Pfaffenrath V, Kellhammer U, Pollmann W. Combination headache: practical experience with a combination of a beta-blocker and an antidepressive. *Cephalalgia* 1986;6(5):25–32.

64. Holroyd KA, Nash JM, Pingel JD. A comparison of pharmacologic (amitriptyline Hcl) and nonpharmacologic (cognitive-behavioral) therapies for chronic tension headaches. *J Consult Clin Psychol* 1991; 59: 387–93.

65. Gobel H, Hamouz V, Hansen C *et al.* Chronic tension-type headache: amitriptyline reduces clinical headache-duration and experimental pain sensitivity but does not alter pericranial muscle activity readings. *Pain* 1994; 59: 241–6.

66. Morland TJ, Storli OV, Mogstad TE. Doxepin in the prophylactic treatment of mixed 'vascular' and tension headache. *Headache* 1979; 19: 382–3.

67. Saper JR, Silberstein SD, Lake AE, Winters ME. Double-blind trial of fluoxetine: chronic daily headache and migraine. *Headache* 1994; 34: 497–502.

68. Manna V, Bolino F, DiCicco L. Chronic tension-type headache, mood depression and serotonin: therapeutic effects of fluvoxamine and mianserine. *Headache* 1994; 34: 44–49.

69. Palmer KJ, Benfield P. Fluvoxamine: an overview of its pharmacologic properties and a review of its use in nondepressive disorders. *CNS Drugs* 1994; 1: 57–87.

70. Langemark M, Olesen J. Sulpiride and paroxetine in the treatment of chronic tension type headache. An explanatory double-blind trial. *Headache* 1994; 34: 20–4.

71. Mathew NT. Prophylaxis of migraine and mixed headache. A randomized controlled study. *Headache* 1981; 21: 105–9.

72. Bright RA, Everitt DE. Beta-blockers and depression: evidence against an association. *JAMA* 1992; 267(13): 1783–7.

73. Jensen R, Brinck T, Olesen J. Sodium valproate has a prophylactic effect in migraine without aura. *Neurology* 1994; 44: 647–51.

74. Mathew NT, Saper JR, Silberstein SD *et al.* Migraine prophylaxis with divalproex. *Arch Neurol* 1995;52;281–286.

75. Hering R, Kuritzky A. Sodium valproate in the prophylactic treatment of migraine: a double-blind study versus placebo. *Cephalalgia* 1992; 12: 81–84.

76. Klapper J. Divalproex sodium in the prophylactic treatment of migraine (abstr). *Headache* 1995; 35: 290.

77. Mathew NT, Ali S. Valproate in the treatment of persistent chronic daily headache. An open label study. *Headache* 1991; 31: 71–74.

78. Miller DS, Talbot CA, Simpson W, Korey A. A comparison of naproxen sodium acetaminophen and placebo in the treatment of muscle contraction headache. *Headache* 1987; 27: 392–396.

79. Johnson ES, Tfelt-Hansen P. Nonsteroidal antiinflammatory drugs. In: Olesen J, Tfelt Hansen P, Welch KMA (eds). *The Headaches.* New York: Raven Press, 1993: 397–402.

80. Mylecharane EJ, Tfelt-Hansen P. Miscellaneous drugs. In: Olesen J, Tfelt-Hansen P, Welch KMA (eds). *The Headaches.* New York: Raven Press, 1993: 397–402.

81. Kangasniemi PJ, Nyrke T, Lang AH, Petersen E. Femoxetine — a new 5-HT uptake inhibitor — and propranolol in the prophylactic treatment of migraine. *Acta Neurol Scand* 1983; 68: 262–7.

82. Scholz E, Gerber WD, Diener HC, Langohr HD *et al.* Dihydroergotamine vs. flunarizine vs. nifedipine vs. metoprolol vs. propranolol in migraine prophylaxis: a comparative study based on time series analysis. In: Rose CF (ed.). *Advances in Headache Research.* London: John Libbey & Co., 1987: 139–45.

83. Silberstein SD, Silberstein JR. Chronic daily headache: long-term prognosis following inpatient treatment with repetitive IV DHE. *Headache* 1992; 32: 439–45.

84. Tfelt-Hansen P, Welch KMA. Prioritizing prophylactic treatment. In: Olesen J, Tfelt Hansen P, Welch KMA (eds). *The Headaches.* New York: Raven Press, Ltd. 1993: 403–5.

chapter 9

Cluster headache: diagnosis and treatment

Cluster headache is a distinct, although rare, clinical and epidemiological entity, named by Friedman and Mikropoulos in 1958.[1] Its importance as a primary headache derives from its extraordinary morbidity. The pain is devastating and the syndrome so unique and rewarding to manage that physicians with an interest in head pain must be acquainted with the condition. Related short-lasting headaches with autonomic symptoms may be confused with cluster headache. These other disorders are less common than cluster headache. They do not respond to cluster headache treatments in the same robust manner and must be differentiated from cluster headache. These unusual syndromes may be substantially under-recognized. Their curious associated features may help us to better understand the mechanisms of the more common primary headaches. These syndromes are best classified together as trigeminal autonomic cephalgias (TACs).[2] We have divided them into cluster headache and other TACs for convenience.

Cluster headache is a relatively well-characterized syndrome whose description dates back hundreds of years. Isler provides a very interesting description by Gerhard van Swieten in 1745.[3]

> A healthy, robust man of middle age (was suffering from) trouble-some pain which came on every day at the same hour at the same spot above the orbit of the left eye, where the nerve emerges from the opening of the frontal bone; after a short time the left eye began to redden, and to overflow with tears; then he felt as if his eye was slowly forced out of its orbit with so much pain, that he nearly went mad. After a few hours all these evils ceased, and nothing in the eye appeared at all changed.

The historical aspects have been dealt with by Sjaastad[4] and there are excellent complete texts on the subject.[4,5]

The clear descriptions of this syndrome can be dated to this century, with the watermarks being Ekbom's description of its periodicity[6] and Kunkle's recognition of the very important feature of *clustering*.[7] Many creative terms have been used for the disorder, which is a reflection of the curiosity it has created amongst medical practitioners.[8] The names have very often revealed accurate views about some of the pathophysiology of the condition (Table 9.1).

Clinical features

The image of the tortured sufferer rocking or pacing in the dark, with tears streaming from one eye and face contorted in exquisite pain, is distinct and unique in medicine. Attacks occur in series lasting for weeks or months (cluster periods), with the attack frequency ranging from one every other day to eight a day. The cluster periods are separated by remission that usually last months or years. About 10% of patients have chronic symptoms with no remission periods. The International Headache Society (IHS) Criteria[9] for cluster require at least five attacks of severe, unilateral, orbital, sub-orbital and/or temporal pain lasting 15–180 min if untreated, and associated with at least one of the following: conjunctival injection; lacrimation; nasal congestion; rhinorrhoea; forehead and facial sweating; miosis; ptosis; or eyelid oedema.

The IHS[9] further subdivided episodic cluster headache based on whether or not the periodicity was determined. It subdivided chronic cluster headache depending on whether or not the current chronic bout had been preceded by episodic cluster headache. Such distinctions may be helpful with prognostication. Chronic cluster headache can be a dreadful problem that drives otherwise normal people to extraordinary acts.

Cluster headache attacks are stereotypical. They are generally shorter than migraine, lasting from 15–30 min up to two to three hours. They are almost invariably unilateral and very severe. Patients who have both cluster headache and migraine state that their cluster headache attacks are more severe than their migraines. Cluster headache patients who have had other painful experiences, such as kidney stones or

● **Table 9.1** *Some terms used for cluster headache*

- Migrainous neuralgia
- Histamine cephalagia
- Petrosal neuralgia
- Sphenopalatine neuralgia
- Hemicrania periodic neuralgiforms
- Vidian neuralgia
- Sluder's neuralgia
- Erthroprosopalgia of Bing
- Horton's headache
- 'A particular variety of headache'(Symonds)

childbirth, readily admit that cluster headache pain is worse. The pain is usually located around the orbit or over the temporal regions. The attack frequency is from one a day or every second day to two or more a day. It is usually said that eight per day is a maximum; certainly such a frequency begins to make one think of the other TACs (see Chapter 10). The signature feature of cluster headache, and indeed the entire array of the TACs, is the association with autonomic symptoms. These features include lacrimation and nasal congestion, suggestive of cranial parasympathetic activation, and miosis and ptosis, suggestive of a Horner's syndrome (Table 9.2). The IHS system requires, and indeed good clinical practice would dictate, that the syndrome is diagnosed when there is no other intercurrent illness that could be responsible.

Differential diagnosis

Before the diagnosis of cluster can be made, other paroxysmal unilateral primary headache disorders and secondary headache disorders that mimic cluster headache need to be excluded (Table 9.3). Most patients with the typical syndrome have no organic cause, but a few patients have been described with lesions responsible for their headaches. Cluster headache must first be differentiated from the other TACs (see Chapter 10), particularly paroxysmal hemicrania when the attacks are relatively prolonged and the frequency is not too great. It is often wise to err on the side of a trial of indomethacin in doses suitable for paroxysmal hemicrania if one encounters attacks that are abnormal or particularly if they are unresponsive to the conventional treatments outlined below. A few case reports of secondary cluster headache exist in the literature. This requires consideration,

or at least awareness, of the types of lesions that have been reported. One series followed 11 patients with facial trauma with soft-tissue injury.[10] In all but one patient, the injury involved the trigeminal territory. Although the attacks had the clinical appearance of cluster headache, with ipsilateral autonomic features, they were refractory to treatment and did not show the usual periodicity or remissions. In our experience the trauma is usually in the ophthalmic division of the trigeminal nerve. Cluster-like headaches have also been reported to occur in patients with an arteriovenous malformation in the occipital lobe[11], a pituitary adenoma[12], upper cervical meningioma[13], vertebral artery aneurysm[14], and dissection[15] with ipsilateral pain. Koenigsberg[16] reported cluster headaches in association with a pseudoaneurysm of the intracavernous carotid artery. The headaches resolved when the aneurysm was clipped. The authors postulated that the aneurysm irritated the C_1 and C_2 fibres that innervate the dura mater. Their experience supports the generally held view that the cavernous sinus may be a key locus of pathology in cluster headaches, with a convergence of fibres from the first two divisions of the trigeminal nerve, as well as both sympathetic and parasympathetic fibers. However, recent positron emission tomography data suggests that cavernous sinus involvement may be a general feature of ophthalmic division pain and not specific for cluster headache.[17]

Epidemiology

Ekbom et al.[18] studied 18-year-old Swedish army recruits and found the prevalence of cluster headache to be 0.09%. Kudrow extrapolated these results to distribution of age at onset obtained from headache clinic data to yield a rate of approximately 0.4%.[19] In Minnesota, the age-adjusted incidence of cluster headache was 15.6 per 100 000 person-years for men and 4.0 per 100 000 person-years for women.

● **Table 9.2** *Diagnostic features of cluster headache (after IHS)*

A	At least 5 attacks fulfilling B–D
B	Severe unilateral orbital, supraorbital and/or temporal pain lasting 15–180 minutes untreated
C	Headache associated with at least one of the following signs which have to be present on the pain side:
	1 Conjunctival injection
	2 Lacrimation
	3 Nasal congestion
	4 Rhinorrhoea
	5 Forehead and facial sweating
	6 Miosis
	7 Ptosis
	8 Eyelid oedema
D	Frequency of attacks: from 1 every other day to 8 per day

● **Table 9.3** *Differential diagnosis of cluster headache*

Primary syndromes	Secondary syndromes
Cluster headache	Maxillary sinusitis
Cluster migraine	Tolosa–Hunt syndrome
Cluster–tic syndrome	Temporal arteritis
Paroxysmal hemicrania	Raeder's paratrigeminal neuralgia
SUNCT syndrome*	Meningioma of wing of lessor sphenoid
	Facial trauma
	Occipital AVM
	Pituitary adenoma
	Upper cervical meningioma
	Vertebral artery aneurysm or dissection

SUNCT = short-lasting unilateral neuralgiform pains with conjunctival injection and tearing

Cluster headache affects men more frequently than women, with a ratio of 4.5–6.7:1. The mean age of onset is 27 to 31 years,[5,20,21] approximately 10 years later than that of migraine. Kudrow[5] found cluster headache, in his clinic, to be disproportionately more prevalent among black than white patients, and particularly so among black women, where the male:female ratio was 3:1.

Kudrow studied 200 women with cluster headache, of whom 24 (12%) were found to have at least one affected first-degree relative. Cluster headache was found in seven of 24 kindreds (29.2%) in three generations. Of 1652 first-degree relatives of 300 men and women, 3.45% had cluster headache, 13 times the expected population frequency. These findings were recently corroborated by Russel *et al.*[22], who reported a 14-fold increase in the risk of cluster headache among first-degree relatives.

Pathophysiology

The aetiology and pathophysiology of cluster headache is unknown. Some of the features of cluster headache overlap with those of other primary vascular headaches, such as migraine, and have a similar neurobiology, which is covered in Chapter 5. Pain is usually centered about the eye and is reported as retro-orbital or temporal. This implies involvement of the ophthalmic (first) division of the trigeminal nerve. The pain may be referred to the first division by an intracranial process. It has been suggested, on anatomical grounds, that this may be an inflammatory or vasculitic process in or around the cavernous sinus. The cavernous sinus is a point of intersection of the first division of the trigeminal nerve and the cranial sympathetic and cranial parasympathetic nerves (Figure 9.1). Given the pain (trigeminal nerve), the signs of sympathetic dysfunction, the Horner's syndrome of miosis and ptosis, and the parasympathetic overactivity, lacrimation, nasal congestion, and injection of the eye, the cavernous sinus site is attractive. Few investigators have managed to image the cavernous sinus of a patient having an acute cluster headache save the celebrated case reported by Ekbom, in which angiography showed carotid narrowing.[23] Given the availability of modern imaging with magnetic resonance angiography, these observations should be repeated and extended.[24] Although this site is a convenient one to provide an explanation for many of the clinical features of the disorder, positron emission tomographic data now suggest that blood flow changes in the region of the cavernous sinus may not be limited to cluster headache. Indeed it has been shown that after supraorbital injection of capsaicin, flow in the cavernous sinus is increased[17], implying that

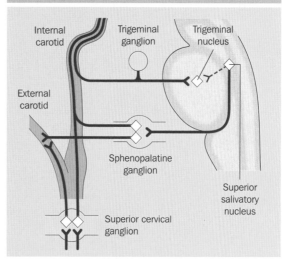

NEURAL INNERVATION OF THE CRANIAL CIRCULATION

● *Figure 9.1* *Neural innervation of the carotid arteries relevant to cluster headache. Sympathetic fibres arise in the superior cervical ganglion (SCG) and follow the external (EC) and internal (IC) carotid arteries. The parasympathetic fibres arise in the superior salivatory nucleus in the pons and project to the sphenopalatine (SPG, pterygopalatine in humans) ganglion, as well as the otic and some carotid miniganglia. There is a reflex loop between the trigeminal innervation, that arises in the trigeminal ganglion (VG), which activates the parasympathetic fibres.*

extreme ophthalmic division pain of many types can trigger flow changes in the cavernous sinus as part of the trigeminal-parasympathetic reflex so well described in experimental animals.[25] The flow changes observed are then a response to the pain and do not primarily generate the disorder. This raises the possibility that the pathophysiology is driven partially or entirely from the central nervous system (Figure 9.2).

The key pathophysiological process that takes place in cluster headache must be central. The most curious feature of the disorder is its episodic nature from which the very apt name is derived. Patients have their headaches turn on and off like clock work, respecting some daily (circadian) rhythm that has the stamp of the biological clock. Moreover, the remarkable half-yearly, yearly or even biennial cycling of the bouts is one of the most fascinating cycling processes of human biology. These processes implicate involvement of at least the suprachiasmatic region, and the unravelling of their neurobiology will tell us much about human biological clocks. The increase in bouts that is associated with the summer and winter solstice and the relative reduction around the equinoxes, which may be related to many Western countries shifting clocks for daylight savings time, is truly remarkable. It is entirely plausible that some central permissive process

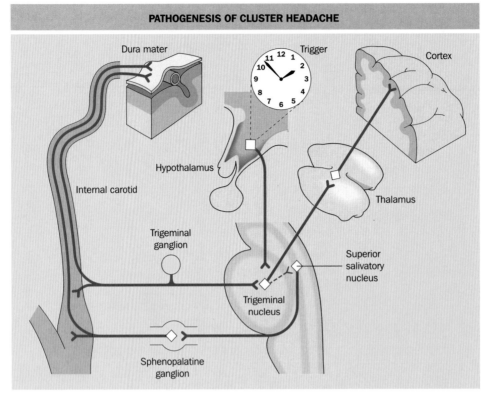

PATHOGENESIS OF CLUSTER HEADACHE

Dura mater

Trigger

Cortex

Internal carotid

Hypothalamus

Thalamus

Trigeminal ganglion

Superior salivatory nucleus

Trigeminal nucleus

Sphenopalatine ganglion

● **Figure 9.2**
Illustration of the major areas likely to be involved in the pathogenesis and expression of cluster headache. The hypothalamic grey is likely from PET studies to be the basic site of dysfunction which interacts with the trigemino-parasympathetic pathways to produce the pain and autonomic symptomatology.

entrains or releases the trigeminovascular pain system. Given recent imaging using PET of nine patients in acute attacks of cluster headache that have demonstrated unilateral activation in the hypothalamic grey ipsilateral to the headache side only during the pain (May, Bahra, Buchel, Frackowiak and Goadsby, submitted for publication) it is highly likely that the fundamental driving process arises in the diencephalic pace-makers. While migraine and cluster headache share much in the expression of the pain, their underlying generation distinguishes them. It is the central nervous system triggering or driving process that ultimately characterize many of the primary syndromes.

Treatment

Pharmacological treatment for cluster headache can be abortive (acute; Table 9.4), prophylactic (preventive; Table 9.5), or a combination of both methods. Abortive treatment is directed at managing the individual attack. Preventive treatment is directed at shortening the bouts of episodic cluster and controlling the frequency of attacks in both the episodic and chronic forms of the disorder. General advice about avoiding triggers may be offered and such things as alcohol, nitrates or organic solvents might be identified.

Management of acute attacks (Table 9.4)

Treatments for the sudden-onset, short-duration, acute attacks of cluster headache include oxygen inhalation, sumatriptan, ergotamine, dihydroergotamine (DHE), and local anaesthetics. There is such a short latency to the peak of the pain that parenteral or pulmonary drug administration is

● **Table 9.4** *Abortive treatment*

- 100% oxygen at 7–10 l/min for 15 min
- Sumatriptan 6 mg S.C.
- DHE 1.0 mg I.M. or I.V.
- Nasal lidocaine (4–6%)

● **Table 9.5** *Prophylactic treatment*

Episodic cluster headache	Chronic cluster headache
Verapamil 120–480 mg/day	Verapamil
Ergotamine tartrate 3–4 mg/day	Lithium carbonate
Lithium carbonate	Methysergide
Methysergide	Valproate
Valproate	Pizotifen
Prednisone	?Gabapentin
Pizotifen 2–3 mg/day	

highly beneficial. The fastest relief is afforded by oxygen inhalation[26], subcutaneous sumatriptan[27,28], and dihydroergotamine. Local intranasal anaesthetic agents (cocaine, lidocaine[29]) have occasionally been effective. Most ergotamine preparations, with the exception of parenteral dihydroergotamine, are too slowly absorbed to be rapidly effective.

Oxygen

Oxygen inhalation, a standard abortive treatment for cluster headache, was first used by Horton.[30] Given via a non-rebreathing mask at a flow rate of 7–10 l/min for 15 min, it is effective in approximately 70% of patients, usually within 5 min.[26,31] In some patients, oxygen may delay rather than abort the attack, and pain may return. Oxygen's effectiveness may depend on the timing of its administration: it may be most effective when given at the maximum intensity of the pain.[32] High flow, high oxygen percentage and allowing a reasonable time period of inhalation are all key elements in the success of the treatment. In most countries small portable cylinders are available. These can be taken in the car to work or kept at the bedside for nighttime attacks.

In a placebo-controlled study, hyperbaric oxygen (2 atm) for 30 min aborted an acute attack of cluster within 5–13 min in six of seven patients, while none of the placebo group had relief. Long-term, three patients reported complete and three patients partial interruption of their cluster cycle.[33] Other authors have reported similar benefit of hyperbaric oxygen.[34,35]

Sumatriptan

Sumatriptan, a $5\text{-HT}_{1B/1D}$ agonist, is available as a 6 mg subcutaneous injection, a 20 mg nasal spray and 25 mg, 50 mg and 100 mg oral tablets depending on availability in various countries. In a double-blind, placebo-controlled study, sumatriptan (6 mg S.C.) was more effective than placebo. A response was noted by 10 min and 74% of treated patients were pain-free by 15 min.[27] Sumatriptan may continue to be effective after continued use for several months.[28] While generally well tolerated, sumatriptan is contraindicated in patients with ischaemic heart disease or uncontrolled hypertension. Sumatriptan given as a 6 mg S.C. injection is a remarkably effective treatment.[27,28,36] It works rapidly and efficiently to often produce benefit in 5–7 min after administration.[37] The current injector devices are easy to use and patients seem not to develop tachyphylaxis even over long bouts of cluster headache.[38] The mechanisms of action of sumatriptan in cluster headache is likely to be similar to what is described in migraine (see Chapter 5) and the peripheral and central sites of action of the class are illustrated in Figure 9.3.

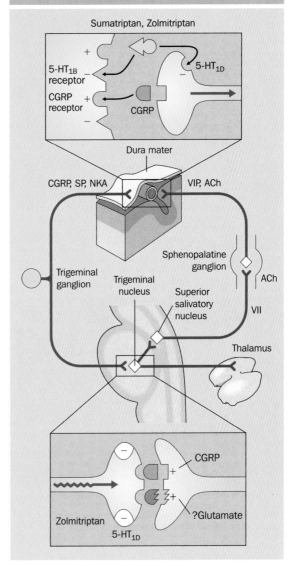

SITES OF ACTION OF THE TRIPTANS

● **Figure 9.3** *Illustration of the possible sites of action of the triptans both peripherally and within the central nervous system.*

Dihydroergotamine

Dihydroergotamine (DHE), available in injectable and intranasal forms, is effective in relieving acute attacks of cluster headache. Intravenous injection gives more rapid relief than intramuscular injection, with benefit in less than 10 min. DHE nasal spray, available in some countries, has just been approved by the Food and Drug Administration in the United States for the treatment of migraine.

Andersson and Jespersen[39] conducted a double-blind comparative trial of DHE nasal spray (1 mg; half the recommended dose for migraine). DHE did not change the duration or frequency of the attacks, but it did decrease pain intensity. Since DHE as a nasal spray has a 40% bioavailability, administration of a higher dose may be more effective for the treatment of cluster headache.

Ergotamine

Ergotamine tartrate (available as a tablet, suppository or in some countries, as an inhalant) may only partially ameliorate an acute cluster attack because of the pharmacokinetics of the preparation. Curiously, some patients may respond to rectal ergotamine.

Topical local anaesthetics

Local intranasal anaesthetic agents, such as cocaine[40] or lidocaine[29,41], have been reported to be effective. Cocaine, because of its addictive potential, is not preferentially utilized. Lidocaine 4–6% nasal drops (1 cc) may be used and repeated once after 15 min.[41]

Analgesics and narcotics

Non-parenteral analgesics and narcotics have little role in the treatment of cluster headache. The opiate butorphanol can be administered by a nasal spray and would be a useful strategy should it prove effective. Although this compound is a sedative as well as analgesic, this can be a useful combination in patients with attacks of cluster headache that wake them from sleep, and, in that setting, can be a very useful option. It has no cardiovascular risks and is thus a medically safe option in patients in whom vasoconstrictor compounds are contraindicated or oxygen has failed to be useful. There is no clinical experience at this time with nasal administration of sumatriptan or its analogues although studies have commenced.

Prophylactic pharmacotherapy of cluster headache

Preventive treatment in cluster headache is aimed at both shortening bouts[42] and controlling attack frequency. All the treatments are largely empirical and but many are very effective. Most cluster patients require prophylactic therapy at some point since:

(1) attacks are frequent, severe, of rapid onset and often too short-lived for abortive medication to take effect;

(2) abortive treatment may only postpone the attack;

(3) treating frequent attacks abortively may result in overmedication; and

(4) failing to stop the cluster period early may prolong the suffering for months.[43]

Medications generally accepted as effective in the prophylactic treatment of cluster include ergotamine, methysergide, corticosteroids, verapamil, lithium carbonate, valproic acid, and, occasionally, indomethacin. Chlorpromazine, although it has been reported to be effective[44], β-blockers, antidepressants and histamine desensitization are probably ineffective as prophylaxis, and corticosteroids are not recommended for the treatment of chronic cluster. The goal of prophylactic therapy is to produce a rapid remission of headaches and to maintain that remission with minimal side effects until the cluster period is over. Recent open studies suggest gabapentin may be useful in cluster headache.

The principles of prophylactic pharmacotherapy are as follows:

(1) start medications early in the cluster period;

(2) continue the drugs until the patient is headache-free for at least two weeks;

(3) taper the drugs rather than abruptly withdrawing them; and

(4) restart the drugs at the beginning of the next cluster period.[43]

If an acute attack occurs despite preventive treatment, abortive agents such as oxygen, sumatriptan, DHE, or intranasal lidocaine can be used.

The medication choice will depend on:

(1) previous drug response;

(2) prior adverse drug reactions;

(3) contraindications to drug use;

(4) type of cluster (episodic or chronic);

(5) frequency and timing of attacks (nocturnal versus diurnal);

(6) expected length of cluster period: and

(7) age and lifestyle of the patient.

Combinations of two or more drugs may be necessary.

Ergotamine derivative

Ergotamine tartrate, like DHE[45], is an agonist at 5-HT$_{1B/1D}$ receptors as is sumatriptan and shares many of its pre-clinical actions.[46] Ergotamine tartrate, up to 4 mg (in divided doses), is effective and probably poses no risk of rebound headache, unlike when it is used for migraine. Ergotamine is particularly useful in controlling nocturnal attacks when taken at bedtime.[6,47,48]

Methysergide maleate

Methysergide maleate is a congener of methylergonovine and lysergic acid diethylamide. It is widely distributed throughout the body, crosses the blood–brain barrier, and binds to serotonin receptors in the brain. It has affinity for $5-HT_1$ and $5-HT_2$ receptors and, when given chronically, blocks the development of neurogenic inflammation.[49]

Methysergide is effective in 65–69% of patients who have episodic cluster headache[5,50]. Response rates are lower in chronic cluster. This drug is indicated in younger patients, who are without the potential risk of arthrosclerotic heart disease. Side effects include muscle cramps, nausea, diarrhoea and abdominal discomfort; these often occur initially, but usually subside over several days. Prolonged treatment has been associated with fibrotic reactions (retroperitoneal, pleural, pulmonary and cardiac valvular), although it is rare. Since the duration of episodic cluster headache is usually less than four months, methysergide use in general does not cause this complication. In chronic cluster, however, methysergide has to be used with caution, with provision made for a one-month drug holiday between six-month treatment periods. If methysergide use is prolonged and a drug holiday is omitted, periodic chest X-ray, echocardiogram and magnetic resonance imaging of the abdomen must be performed.

Calcium-channel blockers

The calcium antagonists are a group of chemically heterogeneous drugs developed as cardiovascular agents. They interact with the L-type voltage-gated calcium channel although flunarizine can interact with the P/Q channel that has been implicated in familial hemiplegic migraine.

Nimodipine

Nimodipine, in a dose of 30 mg q.i.d., has been found to be effective in several open trials, but is not widely used.[51,52]

Verapamil

Verapamil has been studied in the treatment of cluster headache, and many believe it is the prophylactic drug of choice in both the episodic and chronic varieties.[52–54] Doses range between 120 and 480 mg, but much higher doses have been used. Constipation is the most common side effect. Other symptoms include oedema, dizziness, nausea, hypotension and fatigue. Verapamil can be combined with ergotamine or lithium. When verapamil and lithium are used together, there may be an increased sensitivity to lithium.[55] In one double-blind trial verapamil was found to be as effective as lithium.[56]

Lithium carbonate

Lithium's mode of action in cluster headache (and in manic-depressive illness) is unknown. It alters circadian rhythms and dampens random eye movement sleep. It has been suggested that the lithium-induced depletion of inositol results

in a decrease of inositol triphosphate (a second messenger) production, dampening neuronal activity. It is rapidly and almost completely absorbed.

Lithium carbonate is more effective in chronic than in episodic cluster headache.[56,57] Seventy-eight percent of patients with chronic and 63% of patients with episodic cluster headache respond. The usual initial dose of lithium is 300 mg b.i.d., but higher doses may be required. Lithium has a long half-life (24 hours) and takes about one week to reach steady-state levels, at which time a lithium level should be obtained (and periodically thereafter). Lithium is often effective at a blood level of 0.4–0.8 mEq/l, (less than the usual therapeutic dose for mania). A therapeutic response is often seen within one week. Approximately 20% of chronic cluster headache may become episodic on lithium treatment, and many patients may require an additional agent, such as ergotamine or verapamil, along with lithium. Some patients eventually become resistant to lithium.

Side effects of lithium include slight weakness, mild nausea, and thirst, which usually subsides (tremor, lethargy, slurred speech and blurred vision). Toxicity is manifested by nausea, vomiting, anorexia, diarrhoea, and neurological signs of confusion, nystagmus, ataxia, extrapyramidal signs and seizures. Concomitant use of sodium-depleting diuretics should be avoided, as sodium depletion will result in high lithium levels and neurotoxicity. Hypothyroidism and polyuria (nephrogenic diabetes insipidus) can occur with long-term use. Polymorphonuclear leukocytosis may occur and be mistaken for occult infection.

Corticosteroids

The mechanism of action of corticosteroids in cluster headache is uncertain. Corticosteroids (prednisone and dexamethasone) are the most rapid-acting of the prophylactic drugs used in the treatment of cluster headache and are frequently used short term (two to three weeks in tapering doses) as initial therapy to induce remission. This may break the headache cycle while waiting for other drugs to become effective. Prednisone produced relief in 77% of cluster headache patients, partial improvement in another 12%, and total relief in up to 50%.[58] Dexamethasone (4 mg b.i.d. for two weeks, 4 mg/day for one week) is also effective.[59] Corticosteroids are also useful in chronic cluster headache; however, as in episodic cluster, when the medication is tapered, the headache recurs. Since the side effects of steroids increase with long-term use, their use is limited to inducing remission and in occasional patients with refractory chronic cluster. Adverse effects include insomnia, restlessness, personality changes, hyponatraemia, oedema, hyperglycaemia, osteoporosis, myopathy, and gastric ulcers. Recently, necrosis of the hip has been reported and this is an important side effect to consider and warn patients about.

Sodium valproate

Sodium valproate (200–1000 mg/day b.i.d.) has been reported to be effective in cluster headache.[60] Treatment was well-tolerated with only nausea reported. Lethargy, tremour, weight gain and hair loss are some of the common side effects. With valproate use, pancreatitis and liver function abnormalities are rarer but more severe adverse events. The valproate level should be maintained between 50 and 120 mg/ml (400 to 600 mmol). Liver-function studies and blood counts should be obtained prior to initiating treatment and during follow-up if the patient is symptomatic. Valproate should not be used in patients with liver disease.

Pizotifen

Pizotifen, in open trials, has been reported to be of benefit in cluster.[61–63] While widely used in England and Canada for migraine, it is not available in the United States and is generally not held to be very useful in cluster headache.

Capsaicin

Capsaicin desensitizes sensory neurons by depleting substance P. In a double-blind, placebo-controlled study using capsaicin (0.025% cream b.i.d.) applied intranasally via a cotton tipped applicator on the side of headache for seven days, patients who received the active drug had significantly less frequent and less severe attacks.[64]

Indomethacin

Indomethacin is particularly useful in the treatment of both the chronic and episodic varieties of paroxysmal hemicrania and although some cluster headache patients respond to it the significance of this is unknown (see Chapter 10). While the responsiveness to indomethacin is absolute in paroxysmal hemicrania and hemicrania continua, it is only partial in the other entities, including cluster headache.

Some treatment protocols

Treatment and dosage must be individualized. Many clinicians start treatment of episodic cluster headache with verapamil 120–480 mg/day. Other clinicians start with ergotamine tartrate 1–4 mg/day, particularly in patients with nocturnal attacks, in which a dose is given at bedtime. Ergotamine can be used alone or in combination with verapamil. Methysergide 1–2 mg three to four times a day is an effective alternative, especially in younger patients. Methysergide should not be combined with ergotamine. Lithium or valproate can be used next, alone or in combination with verapamil. Pizotifen is preferred by some, when it is available, before verapamil, but this would not be our approach. Corticosteroids may be used to break the cycle of headache or to treat severe exacerbations.

Chronic cluster can be treated with verapamil or lithium, alone or in combination. In resistant cases, triple therapy using ergotamine, verapamil and lithium or methysergide, verapamil, and lithium may be considered. Valproate can be used alone or in combination with verapamil or methysergide.

Sumatriptan has been formally studied as a preventive in cluster headache. It was administered at a dose of 100 mg three times daily and no change in frequency of attacks was observed over the placebo.[65] Acetazolamide may be a useful pretreatment for patients whose attacks are triggered by altitude such as a ski trip. Kudrow suggests 250 mg twice daily for four days commencing two days prior to reaching the heights. Acetazolamide may also be useful in some patients with familial hemiplegic migraine, a condition suggested to be a channelopathy of voltage-gated calcium channels (see Chapter 5).

The treatment-resistant patient and options for surgical procedures

The patient with episodic cluster may become resistant to a previously successful prophylactic medication. The chronic cluster patient may require polypharmacy and eventually an ablative neurosurgical procedure. Treatment of these refractory cases can be very difficult. DHE given repetitively intravenously every eight hours in an inpatient setting is an effective treatment for intractable cluster, rendering most patients headache-free during treatment. Most had received multiple medications including ergotamine (oral and suppository), steroids, and even intramuscular DHE, and remained refractory until intravenous dihydroergotamine therapy was initiated.[66]

Histamine desensitization has been used to treat patients with intractable cluster with mixed results.[67]

Local steroid injection of the ipsilateral occipital nerve has been advocated, with headache relief for 5 to 73 days.[68] Many patients required more than one injection. In our experience, and that of others, local steroid injection is occasionally effective, but usually for a brief period.

If repetitive intravenous dihydroergotamine fails or is the only option available to control cluster, then other options may have to be considered. Approximately 10% of patients with cluster headaches do not respond to prophylactic pharmacotherapy or have significant contraindications to effective prophylactic agents. These patients are candidates for surgical consideration. Indications for surgical treatment include:

(1) strictly unilateral headache,
(2) total resistance to medical therapy or significant contraindications to effective medical therapy, and
(3) a stable personality profile with no addictive potential.

When sphenopalatine ganglionectomy[69] was attempted in 13 patients with severe intractable cluster headaches, only 2 patients had complete relief at one year follow-up, and 7 patients had little relief. This procedure has been replaced with trigeminal surgery.

The procedure of choice is radiofrequency thermocoagulation of the trigeminal ganglion.[70,71] The overall results have been encouraging, with almost 75% of patients becoming free of cluster headache attacks. Complications include anaesthesia dolorosa, transient corneal infection, transient diplopia, and recurrent sty. Recurrence of pain is possible after a number of years, and repeat surgery may be necessary. Recently, glycerol injection has been proposed for the treatment of intractable cluster headache with significant pain relief and corneal safety.[72] The main problem with this approach is control of the lesion size and inadvertent spread of the glycerol intracranially.

References

1. Friedman AP, Mikropoulos HE. Cluster headache. *Neurology* 1958; 8: 653.
2. Goadsby PJ, Lipton RB. A review of paroxysmal hemicranias, SUNCT syndrome and other short-lasting headaches with autonomic features, including new cases. *Brain* 1997; 120: 193–209.
3. Isler H. Episodic cluster headache from a textbook of 1745: Van Swieten's classic description. *Cephalalgia* 1993; 13: 172–4.
4. Sjaastad O. *Cluster Headache Syndrome*. London: Saunders, 1992.
5. Kudrow L. *Cluster headache: mechanisms and management*. Oxford: Oxford University Press, 1980.
6. Ekbom K. Ergotamine tartrate orally in Horton's 'histaminic cephalalgia' (also called Harris's cilary neuralgia). *Acta Psychiatrica Scandinavia* 1947; 46: 106.
7. Kunkle EC, J. B. Pfieffer J, Wilhoit WM, L. W. Hamrick J. Recurrent brief headache in cluster pattern. *Trans. of the Am. Neurological Assoc.* 1952; 27: 240–3.
8. Horton BT, MacLean AR, Craig WM. A new syndrome of vascular headache; results of treatment with histamine; a preliminary report. *Proc. of the Mayo Clinic* 1939; 14: 250–7.
9. Headache Classification Committee of The International Headache Society. Classification and diagnostic criteria for headache disorders, cranial neuralgias and facial pain. *Cephalalgia* 1988; 8 (suppl 7): 1–96.
10. Mathew NT, Rueveni U. Cluster-like headache following head trauma. *Headache* 1988; 28: 297.
11. Mani S, Deeter J. Arteriovenous malformation of the brain presenting as a cluster headache — a case report. *Headache* 1982; 22: 184–5.
12. Tfelt-Hansen P, Paulson OB, Krabbe AE. Invasive adenoma of the pituitary gland and chronic migrainous neuralgia. A rare coincidence or a causal relationship? *Cephalalgia* 1982; 2: 25–8.

13. Kuritzky A. Cluster headache-like pain caused by an upper cervical meningioma. *Cephalalgia* 1984; 4: 185–6.
14. West P, Todman D. Chronic cluster headache associated with a vertebral artery aneurysm. *Headache* 1991; 31: 210–12.
15. Cremer P, Halmagyi GM, Goadsby PJ. Secondary cluster headache responsive to sumatriptan. *J. Neurol. Neurosurg. Psychiatry* 1995; 59: 633–4.
16. Koenigsberg AD, Solomon GD, Kosmorsky DO. Pseudoaneurysm within the cavernous sinus presenting as cluster headache. *Headache* 1994; 34: 111–13.
17. May A, Kaube H, Buchel C, Rijntjes M, Weiller C, Diener HC. Trigeminal transmitted pain using capsaicin: a PET-study. *Cephalalgia* 1997; 17: 377.
18. Ebom K, Ahlborg B, Schele R. Prevalence of migraine and cluster headache in Swedish men of 18. *Headache* 1978; 18: 9.
19. Kudrow L. Cluster headache. In: Blau JN, ed. *Headache: Clinical, Therapeutic, Conceptual and Research Aspects*. London: Chapman and Hall, 1987.
20. Ekbom K. A clinical comparison of cluster headache and migraine. *Acta Neurol. Scand.* 1970; 46 (Suppl 41): 1.
21. Lance JW. *Mechanism and management of headache (5th edition)*. London: Butterworth Scientific, 1993.
22. Russell MB, Andersson PG, Thomsen LL, Iselius L. Cluster headache is an autosomal dominantly inherited disorder in some families: a complex segregation analysis. *J. of Medical Genetics* 1995; 32: 954–6.
23. Ekbom K, Greitz T. Carotid angiography in cluster headache. *Acta Radiologica* 1970; 10: 177–86.
24. Waldenlind E, Ekbom K, Torhall J. MR-Angiography during spontaneous attacks of cluster headache: a case report. *Headache* 1993; 33: 291–5.
25. Goadsby PJ, Duckworth JW. Effect of

stimulation of trigeminal ganglion on regional cerebral blood flow in cats. *Am. J. Physiol.* 1987; 253: R270–4.
26. Kudrow L. Response of cluster headache attacks to oxygen inhalation. *Headache* 1981; 21: 1–4.
27. Ekbom K. Treatment of acute cluster headache with sumatriptan. *N. Eng. J. Med.* 1991; 325: 322–6.
28. Ekbom K, Cole JA. Subcutaneous sumatriptan in the acute treatment of cluster headache attacks. *Can. J. of Neurological Sciences* 1993; 20 (Suppl 4): 61.
29. Robbins L. Intranasal lidocaine for cluster headache. *Headache* 1995; 35: 83–4.
30. Horton BT. Histaminic cephalalgia: differential diagnosis and treatment. *Proc. of the Mayo Clinic* 1956; 31: 325–33.
31. Fogan L. Treatment of cluster headache: a double blind comparison of oxygen vs air inhalation. *Arch. Neurol.* 1985; 42: 362–3.
32. Igarashi H, Sakai F, Tazaki Y. The mechanism by which oxygen interrupts cluster headache. *Cephalalgia* 1991; 11(Suppl 11): 238–9.
33. Di Sabato F, Fusco BM, Pelaia P, Giacovazzo M. Hyperbaric oxygen therapy in cluster headache. *Pain* 1993; 52: 243–5.
34. Weiss LD. Treatment of a cluster headache patient in a hyperbaric chamber. *Headache* 1989; 29: 109–10.
35. Porta M, Granella F, Coppola A, Longoni C, Manzoni GC. Treatment of cluster headaches with hyperbaric oxygen. *Cephalalgia* 1991; 11(Suppl 11): 236–7.
36. Ekbom K, Monstad I, Prusinski A, Cole JA, Pilgrim AJ, Noronha D. Subcutaneous sumatriptan in the acute treatment of cluster headache: a dose comparison study. *Acta Neurol. Scand.* 1993; 88: 63–9.
37. Goadsby PJ. Cluster headache and the clinical profile of sumatriptan. *Eur. Neurol.* 1994; 34 (Suppl): 35–9.

38. Ekbom K, Waldenlind E, Cole JA, Pilgrim AJ, Kirkham A. Sumatriptan in chronic cluster headache: results of continuous treatment for eleven months. *Cephalalgia* 1992 ; 12: 254–6.

39. Andersson PG, L. T J. Dihydroergotamine nasal spray in the treatment of attacks of cluster headache. *Cephalalgia* 1986; 6: 51–4.

40. Barre F. Cocaine as an abortive agent in cluster headache. *Headache* 1982; 22: 69–73.

41. Kitelle JP, Grouse DS, Seyboro ME. Cluster headache: local anesthetic abortive agents. *Arch. Neurol.* 1985; 42: 496–98.

42. Carolis Pd, Capoa Dd, Agati R, Baldratti A, Sacqnegna T. Episodic cluster headache: short and long term results of prophylactic treatment. *Headache* 1988; 28: 475–6.

43. Mathew NT. Cluster headache. *Neurology* 1992; 42(Suppl 2): 32–6.

44. Caviness VS, O'Brien P. Cluster headache: response to chlorpromazine. *Headache* 1980; 20 : 128–31.

45. Berde B, Schild HO. Ergot alkaloids and related compounds. In: Born GVR, Eichler O, Farah A, Herken H, Welch AD, eds. *Handbook of Experimental Pharmacology; vol 49.* Berlin: Springer-Verlag, 1978.

46. Goadsby PJ. Current concepts of the pathophysiology of migraine. In: Mathew NT, ed. *Neurologic Clinics of North America; vol.15.* Philadelphia: W.B. Saunders, 1997: 27–41.

47. Symonds C. Migrainous variants. *Trans. of the Med. Soc. of London* 1952; 67: 237–50.

48. Horton BT. Histaminic cephalalgia. *Lancet* 1952; II: 92–8.

49. Goadsby PJ, Silberstein SD. *Headache.* New York: Butterworth-Heinemann, 1997.

50. Curran DA, Hinterberger H, Lance JW. Methysergide. *Res. and Clin. Studies in Headache* 1967; 1: 74–122.

51. de Carolis P, Baldrati A, Agati R, de Capoa D, D'Alessandro R, Sacquegna T. Nimodipine in episodic cluster headache: results and methodological considerations. *Headache* 1987; 27: 397–9.

52. Meyer JS, Hardenberg J. Clinical effectiveness of calcium entry blockers in prophylactic treatment of migraine and cluster headache. *Headache* 1983; 23: 266–77.

53. Bussone G, Leone M, Peccarisi C, *et al.* Double blind comparison of lithium and verapamil in cluster headache prophylaxis. *Headache* 1990; 30: 411–17.

54. Gabai IJ, Spierings ELH. Prophylactic treatment of cluster headache with verapamil. *Headache* 1989; 29: 167–8.

55. Solomon SD, Lipton RB, Newman LC. Prophylactic therapy of cluster headaches. *Clin. Neuropharmacology* 1991; 14: 116–30.

56. Mathew NT. Clinical subtypes of cluster headache and response to lithium therapy. *Headache* 1978; 18: 26–30.

57. Ekbom K. Lithium for cluster headache: review of the literature and preliminary results of long-term treatment. *Headache* 1981; 21: 132–9.

58. Prusinski A, Kozubski W, Szulc-Kuberska J. Steriod treatment in the interruption of clusters in cluster headache patients. *Cephalalgia* 1987; 7(Suppl 6): 332–3.

59. Anthony M, Draher BN. Mechanism of action of steriods in cluster headache. In: Rose FC, ed. *New Advances in Headache Research-2.* London: Smith-Gordon, 1992: 271–4.

60. Hering R, Kuritzky A. Sodium valproate in the treatment of cluster headache: an open clinical trial. *Cephalalgia* 1989; 9: 195–8.

61. Sicuteri F, Franchi G, Del Bianco PL. An antaminic drug, BC 105, in the prophylaxis of migraine. *International Archives of Allergy* 1967; 31: 78–93.

62. Speight TM, Avery GS. Pizotifen (BC-105): a review of its pharmacological properties and its therapeutic efficacy in vascular headaches. *Am. J. Med. Sci.* 1972; 240: 327–31.

63. Ekbom K. Prophylactic treatment of cluster headache with the new serotonin agonist, BC-105. *Acta Neurol. Scand.* 1969; 45: 601–10.

64. Marks DR, Rapoport A, Padla D. A double-blind placebo-controlled trial of intra-nasal capsaicin for cluster headache. *Cephalalgia* 1993; 13: 114–16.

65. Monstad I, Krabbe A, Micieli G, *et al.* Preemptive oral treatment with sumatriptan during a cluster period. *Headache* 1995; 35: 607–13.

66. Mather P, Silberstein SD, Schulman E, Hopkins MM. The treatment of cluster headache with reptitive intravenous dihydroergotamine. *Headache* 1991; 31: 525–32.

67. Diamond S, Freitag FG, Prager J. Treatment of intractable cluster headache. *Headache* 1986; 26: 42–6.

68. Anthony M. The role of the occipital nerve in unilateral headache. In: Rose FC, ed. *Current Problems in Neurology: 4 Advances in Headache Research.* London: John Libbey, 1987: 257–62.

69. Meyer JS, Binns PM, Ericsson AD, Vulpe M. Sphenopalatine ganglionectomy for cluster headache. *Arch Otolaryngology* 1970; 92: 475–84.

70. Mathew NT, Hurt W. Percutaneous radiofrequency trigeminal gangliorhizolysis in intractable cluster headace. *Headache* 1988; 28: 328–31.

71. Onofrio BM, Campbell JK. Surgical treatment of chronic cluster headache. *Proc. of the Mayo Clinic* 1986; 61: 537–41.

72. Hassenbusch SJ, Kunkel RS, Kosmorsky GS, Covington EC, Pillay PK. Trigeminal cisternal injection of glycerol for treatment of chronic intractable cluster headaches. *Neurosurg.* 1991; 29: 504–8.

chapter 10

Short-lasting and related headaches:

paroxysmal hemicranias, short-lasting unilateral neuralgiform headache with conjunctival injection and tearing and hemicrania continua

Introduction

This chapter is devoted to a curious group of primary headache disorders characterized by short-lived unilateral pain and ipsilateral autonomic features (Table 10.1). Some short-lived headaches have serious underlying causes. Structural disease may give rise to short-lived headaches sometimes triggered by a Valsalva or postural change. Mass lesions, including those that interfere with cerebrospinal fluid egress, and pathology in the posterior fossa or base of the skull are particularly associated with short-lived Valsalva or cough-related headache. Even subarachnoid haemorrhage can give rise to brief headache. The secondary headaches are dealt with in Part III.

Chronic paroxysmal hemicrania

Chronic paroxysmal hemicrania (CPH), a relatively well characterized disorder[1-5], was first described in 1974.[6,7] The International Headache Society (IHS) defines it as frequent, short-lasting attacks of unilateral pain, usually in the orbital, supraorbital or temporal region, that last from 2 to 45 min. The characteristic frequency is five or more attacks a day, with a range of one to forty attacks a day. The pain is associated with at least one autonomic symptom, such as conjunctival injection, lacrimation, nasal congestion, rhinorrhoea, ptosis, or eyelid oedema.[8] The IHS criteria require that the attacks rapidly resolve following treatment with indomethacin. The dose is up to 150 mg/day orally and the response usually occurs within days of initiating an adequate dose. The IHS diagnostic criteria have proved to be very reliable in their practical application in CPH (Table 10.2).[9] Although the attack frequency may vary, by definition, the chronic form should not remit. The IHS classification noted that *the chronic stage may be precipitated by an episodic stage similar to the pattern seen in cluster headache, but this has not been sufficiently validated.*

The relationship between CPH and cluster headache is uncertain. The many clinical similarities argue that the disorders should be classified together. CPH is distinguished from cluster headache primarily by the shorter duration and higher frequency of headache attacks, by the female preponderance of the disorder and by the selective response to indomethacin. As cases have emerged[10-13], the clinical boundaries have become somewhat less distinct. It seems inappropriate at a biological level, and perhaps a clinical level, to insist on the absolute response to indomethacin being diagnostic. It may be better to reduce indomethacin responsiveness to a strong diagnostic indicator until the biological basis for that response is better understood.

Clinical features

CPH does not respect racial boundaries and is well described in black South Africans.[14,15] The sex distribution is a 3:1 female-to-male ratio. The age of onset is usually in the twenties[7], although there have been reports of the condition occurring in children at the age of three[16], nine[17], one[18] and eight[18], but these cases may be better characterized as cluster headache.[19] In paediatric cases, the syndrome may be characterized by daily attacks. The natural history will ultimately be determined by long-term observation. The pain is usually in the distribution of the ophthalmic division of the trigeminal nerve, but it has been reported in the occipital region. The syndrome is almost invariably unilateral, but one patient had bilateral pain that responded to indomethacin.[20] The pain is excruciating and may be throbbing as it builds up, although it is usually stabbing or boring. In contrast to patients with cluster

• **Table 10.1** *Primary short-lasting headaches*

Prominent autonomic features	Sparse or no autonomic features
Cluster headache*	Trigeminal neuralgia*
Chronic paroxysmal hemicrania*	Idiopathic stabbing headache*
	Cough headache*
Episodic paroxysmal hemicrania	Benign exertional headache*
SUNCT syndrome**	Headache associated with sexual activity*
Cluster–tic syndrome	Hypnic headache

*Denotes inclusion in current International Headache Society Criteria.[8]

**SUNCT = short-lasting, unilateral, neuralgiform headache with conjunctival injection and tearing.

● **Table 10.2** *IHS diagnostic criteria for paroxysmal hemicranias*

3.2 **Paroxysmal hemicrania** *(NOTE: This section replaces the previous section 3.2 by dividing paroxysmal hemicrania into an episodic and a chronic form.)*

3.2.1 Chronic paroxysmal hemicrania		3.2.2 Episodic paroxysmal hemicrania	
A	At least 30 attacks fulfilling B–E	A	At least 30 attacks fulfilling B–F
B	Attacks of severe unilateral orbital, supraorbital and/or temporal pain always on the same side lasting 2–45 mins	B	Attacks of severe unilateral orbital or temporal pain, or both, that is always unilateral and lasts 1–30 minutes
C	Attack frequency above five a day for more than half the time (periods with lower frequency may occur)	C	An attack frequency of 3 or more a day
		D	Clear intervals between bouts of attacks that may last from months to years
D	Pain is associated with at least one of the following signs/symptoms on the pain side: 1 Conjunctival injection 2 Lacrimation 3 Nasal congestion 4 Rhinorrhoea 5 Ptosis 6 Eyelid oedema	E	Pain is associated with at least one of the following signs or symptoms on the painful side: 1 Conjunctival injection 2 Lacrimation 3 Nasal congestion 4 Rhinorrhoea 5 Ptosis 6 Eyelid oedema
E	At least one of the following: 1 There is no suggestion of one of the disorders listed in groups 5–11 2 Such a disorder is suggested but excluded by appropriate investigations 3 Such a disorder is present, but the first headache attacks do not occur in close temporal relation to the disorder	F	At least one of the following: 1 There is no suggestion of one of the disorders listed in groups 5–11 2 Such a disorder is suggested but excluded by appropriate investigations 3 Such a disorder is present, but the first headache attacks do not occur in close temporal relation to the disorder

Note:
In most cases responds rapidly and absolutely to indomethacin (usually 150 mg/day or less)

headache, patients with CPH usually sit quietly and hold their heads or take to bed[21], behaviour that is rare in cluster headache. The attack frequency ranges from one to forty attacks a day, with a median frequency of about five to ten a day. Patients may have soreness or tenderness in the interval between attacks, especially if the attacks are frequent. This is not a special feature of CPH but is a generic feature of severe frequent headache, and may be expected with the significant nociceptive load being placed on the trigeminal pain system. The 2–45 min duration[3] is shorter than the 15–180 min typical duration for cluster headache.[8] The overlap creates diagnostic problems. The associated autonomic symptoms are almost completely accounted for by cranial parasympathetic activation (as in cluster headache; Figure 10.1)[22] except for the ptosis, which is likely to be a partial Horner's syndrome due to a functional sympathetic deficit.[23] Parasympathetic activation may cause oedema of the wall of the internal carotid artery and subsequent compression of the cervical sympathetic nerves as they pass through the base of the skull. Some patients with otherwise typical CPH, including indomethacin responsiveness, have no autonomic features.[24,25] Attacks may be precipitated by mechanical stimulation, particularly head movement[26–28] in some patients.

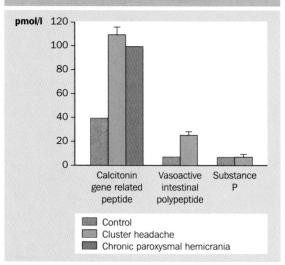

NEUROPEPTIDE CHANGES IN CLUSTER HEADACHE AND PAROXYSMAL HEMICRANIA

Control
Cluster headache
Chronic paroxysmal hemicrania

● **Figure 10.1** *This figure demonstrates the changes in calcitonin gene-related peptide (CGRP), vasoactive intestinal polypeptide (VIP) and substance P cluster headache and chronic paroxysmal hemicrania (CPH). The level of elevation of CGRP and VIP in the CPH patient is comparable with that seen in cluster headache patients.[30]*

Pathophysiology and investigations

The essential pathophysiology of CPH is unknown. The comparative rarity of the syndrome as well as the short-lasting nature of the individual attacks make CPH a difficult disorder to study. The available observations suggest similarities to cluster headache.

Blood and neuropeptide changes

Alterations in cylic release of catecholamines and β-endorphin occur in CPH[29], and are similar to those reported in cluster headache. We recently observed an increased level of calcitonin-gene related peptide (CGRP) and vasoactive intestinal polypeptide (VIP) in the cranial venous blood of a patient with CPH (Figure 10.1). The levels returned to normal with successful treatment with indomethacin.[30] These data are discussed below. Other observations in CPH include relative thrombocythemia[31] and increased phosphatidylserine labelling in neutrophils.[32] The relevance of these changes is not clear. Blood dyscrasias would not be a widespread experience of physicians treating primary headache syndromes and the neutrophil studies seem of doubtful significance.

Electrophysiological and autonomic studies

Patients with CPH are reported to have reduced pain thresholds, reduced corneal reflex thresholds, and normal blink reflexes.[33] Autonomic function studies, including salivation and nasal secretion, are normal.[34] Facial sweating is normal in CPH[35] in contrast to cluster headache.[36] The pupil ipsilateral to the pain (measured by pupillometry) is consistently smaller than its unaffected counterpart[37], most likely reflecting a partial Horner's syndrome. Similar findings were observed in studies of patients with cluster headache.[38] Bradycardia has been observed in CPH, and one of five patients studied developed a bundle branch block and atrial fibrillation during attacks.[39] Whether the bradycardia is a response to the severe pain or is part of an underlying autonomic problem requires further study.

Blood flow studies

Facial thermographic studies have shown either cold spots over the supraorbital margin or inner canthus interictally[40] or increased temperature over the affected area during the headache.[23] Mongini's thermographic results[40] were identical for patients with CPH and cluster headache. Cerebral blood flow studies of carbon dioxide reactivity, as measured by transcranial Doppler, were abnormal in three patients[41], while ocular blood flow was increased during attacks in a single patient.[42] The limited numbers of patients in these studies effectively mean that no judgment can usefully be made about the results. The modest changes that are seen are in line with what is reported in regional[43,44] or transcranial Doppler studies[45] in cluster headache in which the numbers of patients studied have been more convincing. The ocular blood flow changes observed in CPH are similar to those in cluster headache although, in comparison with normals, cluster headache patients had relatively reduced flow between attacks.[42]

Imaging

Magnetic resonance imaging (MRI) studies of patients with CPH have been normal[46], but segmental narrowing of ophthalmic veins on orbital phlebography has been reported[46], similar to the changes seen in cluster headache[47,48] and in the Tolosa–Hunt syndrome.[49,50] The findings on orbital phlebography are neither specific nor likely to be pathophysiologically relevant and the test has no practical place in patient management.

There are, therefore, no specific diagnostic investigations in CPH. The only clear conclusion from the pathophysiological and imaging studies is that attacks are associated with parasympathetic activation most likely mediated through the greater superficial petrosal outflow with an associated mild partial Horner's syndrome. There is little to suggest a fundamental neurobiological separation between CPH and cluster headache in regard to the final common pathways activated. The shorter attack duration, greater attack frequency, and different effect of indomethacin perhaps point to differences in the generation and thus central nervous system mechanisms, of these disorders.

Differential diagnosis

The differential diagnosis of CPH includes the other primary short-lasting headaches (Table 10.1) and the secondary causes of CPH (Table 10.3). Because secondary CPH, as

---

Table 10.3 *Secondary chronic paroxysmal hemicrania and clinical associations*

- Gangliocytoma of the sella turcica[52]
- Collagen vascular disease[51]
- Cerebrovascular disease[54]
- Pancoast tumour[57]
- Frontal lobe tumour[51]
- Cavernous sinus meningioma[55]
- Intracranial hypertension – increased cerebrospinal fluid pressure[56]
- Associations:
    Trigeminal neuralgia (CPH–tic syndrome)[114]
    Cluster headache[116]
    Migraine[117]

a proportion of all CPH, is relatively common, investigations are required to identify or exclude treatable underlying causes. A reasonably complete screen of a patient with CPH, considering the associated clinical problems reported, would include a blood count, looking for thrombo-cythemia[51], an erythrocyte sedimentation rate (ESR), vas-culitic investigations[51] and a brain imaging procedure, looking for an intracranial tumour such as a lesion in the region of the sella turcica[52,53] or elsewhere.[51] Other struc-tural mimics of CPH include an arteriovenous malforma-tion[54] or cavernous sinus meningioma. Secondary CPH is more likely if the patient requires high doses (>200 mg/day) of indomethacin.[55] Should the pain become bilateral, a lumbar puncture should be carried out to look for intracranial hypertension, even in the face of a response to indomethacin.[56] If bundle branch block or atrial fibrillation is suspected, an electrocardiogram and Holter monitor should be performed[39], and a chest X-ray should be considered to look for a Pancoast tumour.[57]

Treatment

The standard treatment of CPH is indomethacin 25 mg t.d.s., increasing to 50 mg t.d.s. after a week if there is no response. Occasional patients require higher doses or slow-release indomethacin preparations at night to treat breakthrough headaches. In some patients, gastrointesti-nal side effects require treatment with gastroprotective agents, such as H_2- or proton pump blockers. There seems to be no tachyphylaxis to the effects of indomethacin.[58] Although the IHS criteria require a response to indomethacin, this makes little absolute biological sense. CPH responds to other drugs, though less effectively. This includes other nonsteroidal antiinflammatory drugs (NSAID), such as naproxen[59] and calcium-channel block-ers, especially verapamil[60-62] (perhaps analogous to their use in cluster headache). One patient with an otherwise convincing clinical picture failed to respond to indomethacin 300 mg but responded to acetazolamide 250 mg t.d.s.[63] Sumatriptan was reported to be of benefit in a patient with bilateral CPH[56], although it was ineffective in a more typi-cal case.[64] In our experience, in contrast to its striking effects in cluster headache,[65] sumatriptan is not effective for CPH. This apparent contrast must be regarded as pre-liminary until there are sufficient reports of longer duration CPH that do not respond to sumatriptan. The lack of a response may be due to the very short duration of the headache. It takes sumatriptan 7–10 min to work.[66] It would be of great interest to see if a long attack of CPH responds to oxygen which is effective for cluster headache.[67] The only consistent preventive is verapamil, which is effective for both CPH and cluster headache.

Episodic paroxysmal hemicrania

Episodic paroxysmal hemicrania (EPH), named by Kudrow[68], is an extremely rare form of headache characterized by fre-quent, daily attacks of short-lived, unilateral, very severe headache with accompanying ipsilateral autonomic fea-tures.[69] Periods of frequent attacks are separated by rela-tively long remissions lasting weeks or months in a pattern similar to episodic cluster headache.[8] Some consider this headache an episodic variant of CPH[69], but definitive classi-fication will require more data. A case of one of the author's will serve to describe this condition.

Case report

A 35-year-old woman presented with an eight-year history of bouts of headache. She described stabbing, severe, left frontal and retro-orbital pains that would last 1–2 min and occur three to five times a day. The attacks were associated with marked watering of the left eye and left-sided ptosis. She had no nasal stuffiness or migrainous features. She would typically move rather than be still during an attack. The attacks came in bouts of six months with intervening breaks of 10–12 months. She had used numerous medications, including corticosteroids, methysergide, lithium, propranolol, pizotifen, amitriptyline and ergotamine, with no benefit. When first seen she was two months into a bout. She was commenced on indomethacin 25 mg t.d.s. and her headaches ceased completely after three days. The drug was stopped two weeks later and the attacks recurred within two days. Indomethacin was restarted and the attacks again settled rapidly.

Clinical features

There were 14 cases of EPH in the literature at the time of writ-ing.[68-75] The headache consists of bouts of short-lasting headache varying from 1 to 30 min that have been reported to occur 6–30 times per day. The pain is described as severe, throbbing, or stabbing and is localized to the orbital or tempo-ral region. There is no evidence for a sex-based predominance, and the age of onset varies from 12 to 51 years. All cases have demonstrated an absolute response to indomethacin. Calcium channel blockers have also been used.[76] Naproxen in a single patient produced an incomplete response. EPH may evolve from a disorder with distinct intervals into a chronic unremitting form that is identical to CPH. It is likely that the two conditions are ends of a spectrum, just as episodic and chronic cluster headache form ends of a spectrum. The clinical cases of transformation from the episodic phase to the chronic phase are perhaps the clearest evidence that EPH and CPH are closely biologically related. However, following the analogy of cluster headache, we prefer a nosology that distinguishes the two.

Short-lasting unilateral neuralgiform headache with conjunctival injection and tearing (SUNCT)

This form of short-lasting headache is also among the rarest of headache syndromes and again has curious autonomic associations.[77] Several clinical features differentiate SUNCT from other short-lasting headaches. A case seen by one of the authors will illustrate the clinical picture.

Case report

A 56-year-old woman presented with a five-year history of daily, episodic, short-lasting headaches. Attacks occurred up to five times a day and lasted 15–20 s each. The attacks were left-sided, moderately severe and retro-orbital. They were associated with marked tearing and redness of the ipsilateral eye and mild rhinorrhoea. There was no nausea, photophobia or phonophobia. There was no history of migraine nor family history of headache. There were no physical signs on examination of the nervous system and she was normotensive. MRI of the brain was normal. She had used amitriptyline, propranolol, pizotifen, methysergide, lithium, and verapamil without success. The latter lengthened the attacks and made the pain more severe. The patient had had a trial of steroids and used ergots and sumatriptan without success. She also had an unsuccessful trial of indomethacin, valproate and carbamazepine. She was refractory when lost to follow-up.

Clinical features

Patients who suffer from SUNCT are usually men[78], with a male:female gender ratio of 17:2.[79] The pain occurs in paroxysms that last 5–250 s [80], although longer, duller interictal pains have been reported, and two patients have had attacks that lasted up to 2 hours.[81] Although patients may have as many as 30 episodes an hour, five to six attacks an hour is the norm. The frequency may also vary in bouts. One man who suffered from as many as twenty attacks a day declined to a frequency of once or twice in one to four weeks[82], while another patient had almost continuous attacks for up to three hours.[83] Attacks over days

in an almost status-like pattern are reported.[84] A systematic study of attack frequency demonstrated a mean of twenty-eight attacks a day with a range of six to seventy - seven.[81] The conjunctival injection seen with SUNCT is often the most prominent autonomic feature, although tearing may also be very obvious. Other less prominent autonomic stigmata include sweating of the forehead or rhinorrhoea. The attacks may become bilateral, but the most severe pain remains unilateral. Most cases have some associated precipitating factors, which may be mechanical movements of the neck[85,86], a feature that is seen often in trigeminal autonomic cephalalgias (TACs) including cluster headache (Table 10.4).

Secondary SUNCT and associations

There have been three reported patients with secondary SUNCT syndromes. The first two patients had homolateral cerebellopontine angle arteriovenous malformations diagnosed on MRI.[87,88] The third patient had a cavernous haemangioma of the brainstem seen only on MRI.[89] A posterior fossa lesion causing otherwise typical SUNCT has also been noted in human immunodeficiency virus/acquired immunodeficiency syndrome (Graff-Radford, personal communication). These cases highlight the need for cranial MRI in investigating for secondary SUNCT.

● **Table 10.4** *IHS diagnostic criteria for SUNCT*

3.3 Short-lasting unilateral neuralgiform headache with conjunctival injection and tearing (SUNCT) *(Note: This section will replace the current unclassified section which then becomes section 3.5)*
A At least thirty attacks fulfilling B–E
B Attacks of unilateral moderately severe orbital or temporal stabbing or throbbing pain lasting 15 –120 s
C Attack frequency from three to one hundred per day
D Pain is associated with at least one of the following signs or symptoms of the affected side with feature (1) being most often present and very prominent: 1 Conjunctival injection 2 Lacrimation 3 Nasal congestion 4 Rhinorrhoea 5 Ptosis 6 Eyelid oedema
E At least one of the following: 1 There is no suggestion of one of the disorders listed in groups 5–11 2 Such a disorder is suggested but excluded by appropriate investigations 3 Such a disorder is present, but the first headache attacks do not occur in close temporal relation to the disorder

(Clinical note: The literature suggests that the most common secondary cause of SUNCT would be a lesion in the posterior fossa)

The connections between posterior structures and the trigeminal system proper are well documented in the laboratory[90] and in clinical practice.[91] Just as there is a reported associated case of CPH and trigeminal neuralgia, there is a single report of a patient with trigeminal neuralgia who developed a SUNCT syndrome.[92] These cases suggest that the trigeminal pathways may be involved in the entire range of short-lasting headache syndromes.

Investigations

Orbital phlebography is reported to be abnormal in patients with SUNCT, with a narrowed superior ophthalmic vein homolateral to the pain.[93] This finding led to the suggestion that SUNCT may be a form of orbital venous vasculitis[94], although there are similar reports in cluster headache, Tolosa–Hunt syndrome and CPH (see above). Forehead sweating, which is normal in CPH, is usually increased during bouts of SUNCT.[95] Pupillary studies using pupillometry and pharmacological approaches have revealed no abnormalities.[96] Since conjunctival injection occurs during SUNCT, it is not surprising that intraocular pressure and corneal temperatures are elevated during attacks.[97] This most likely reflects marked parasympathetic activation with local vasodilatation. Similarly, bradycardia in association with attacks of SUNCT may similarly indicate increased parasympathetic outflow.[98] Systolic blood pressure is sometimes elevated[99], although ventilatory function is normal.[100] The parasympathetic manifestations favour a central pathogenesis for SUNCT as a manifestation of the trigeminovascular reflex[101], rather than a peripheral vasculitic cause. Transcranial Doppler and SPECT studies have not demonstrated convincing change in the vasomotor activity[102] or cerebral blood flow[103] during attacks of pain.

Treatment

SUNCT is remarkably refractory to all treatments including indomethacin (Table 10.5). Most drugs used in the treatment of other short-lasting headaches are not useful in SUNCT.[104] Drugs and procedures reported to be either useful or without effect in SUNCT are recorded in Table 10.5 (drawn from the authors' personal experience and reference 105). Two patients with a provisional diagnosis of SUNCT that responded to sumatriptan most likely represent a spontaneous remission and are only described in a limited way.[105] Indomethacin is not useful in SUNCT.

Hemicrania continua

Hemicrania continua (HC) is characterized by a continuous, unilateral headache pain that is usually moderate in severity (Table 10.6).[106] Three-fifths of patients have superimposed attacks of more intense pains that are often short-lived but may last up to several days. The painful exacerbations are often associated with autonomic features, including ptosis, conjunctival injection, lacrimation and nasal congestion, hence the inclusion of this headache syndrome with the trigeminal-autonomic cephalgias. In general, these features are less prominent than the autonomic features of cluster headache or the paroxysmal hemicranias.

Classification

The nosology of these headaches is a difficult issue. They are clearly daily or near-daily by definition and have thus been sensibly listed with other headache syndromes that cause daily headache (see Chapter 8).[107] Medication overuse, a common aggravating factor in headache syndromes[108,109] may confuse the diagnosis of HC.[110] Whether or not medication overuse can produce HC is not settled. Given the overlap with the other TACs, HC could also be classified with those headaches. It is likely that the indomethacin response that is shared between the paroxysmal hemicra-

● **Table 10.5** *Treatment of SUNCT*

Treatment	Dosage (maximum /day)	Response	Number of reported patients
Pharmacological			
Aspirin	1800 mg	–	6
Paracetamol	4 g	–	6
Indomethacin	200 mg	–	3
Naproxen	1 g	–	3
Ibuprofen	1200 mg	–	7
Ergotamine (oral)	3 mg	–	1
Dihydroergotamine (i.v.i.)	3 mg	–	5
Sumatriptan (oral)	300 mg	–*	1
Sumatriptan (s.c.)	6 mg	–	7
Prednisone (oral)	100 mg	–	4
Methysergide	8 mg	–	5
Verapamil	480 mg	**	5
Valproate	1500 mg	–*	3
Lithium	900 mg	–	3
Propranolol	160 mg	–	2
Amitriptyline	100 mg	–	10
Carbamazepine	1200 mg	–	
Procedures or infusions			
Lignocaine (i.v.i.)	4 mg/min	–	2
Greater occipital nerve	block	–	4

* One patient with slight improvement.
** Treatment worsened condition.
– = Treatment had no effect.

nias and HC will have some clear linked pharmacological basis and further suggests that eventually we will have a convenient biological-based classification of these headaches.

Clinical features and differential diagnosis of TACs and related disorders

The TACs (Table 10.7) are characterized by short-lasting headaches with autonomic features. In CPH, EPH and SUNCT syndrome, autonomic features accompany attacks of severe pain. In HC, the autonomic features rarely present when the pain is mild and become more prominent during severe pain. Pain and autonomic features may be dissociated, as in CPH.[25] Hypnic headache attacks are short-lived, moderate in intensity, and not accompanied by autonomic features (Table 10.8). Thus, severe, short-lived pain is the usual concomitant of autonomic features. Despite their common elements, the TACs differ in the attack duration and frequency as well as their response to therapy (Table 10.9). Of the disorders discussed herein, the SUNCT syndrome has the shortest attack duration and the highest attack frequency. The paroxysmal hemicranias have

intermediate durations (1–45 min) and intermediate attack frequency. Cluster headache has longer attack durations (15–180 min) and relatively low attack frequency.

A point of diagnostic difficulty may arise with the cluster–tic syndrome which is characterized by the combination of idiopathic trigeminal neuralgia and cluster headache.[111,112] The pain of trigeminal neuralgia is lancinating, lasts for seconds, and is more common in the second and third divisions of the trigeminal nerve. It is often triggered by facial or buccal stimulation in the form of chewing, brushing the teeth, or touching the face. The cluster headache component spans the range of typical cluster headache, with attacks lasting 45 min and accompanied by autonomic features, such as lacrimation and nasal blocking, to shorter attacks of 30 s at a frequency of forty a day, more suggestive of a paroxysmal hemicrania.[113] As in trigeminal neuralgia occurring alone, carbamazepine may be useful in these patients. Given the report of CPH–tic syndrome[114] that responded to indomethacin, it

---

● **Table 10.6** *IHS diagnostic criteria for hemicrania continua*

3.4 Hemicrania continua

A	Headache present for at least 1 month
B	Unilateral headache
C	Pain has the following qualities **1** Continuous but fluctuating **2** Moderate severity **3** Lack of precipitating mechanisms
D	Headache must have either one of: **1** Complete response to indomethacin, or **2** One of the following autonomic features in association with exacerbations of pain: Conjunctival injection Lacrimation Nasal congestion Rhinorrhoea Ptosis Eyelid oedema
E	At least one of the following: **1** There is no suggestion of one of the disorders listed in groups 5–11 **2** Such a disorder is suggested but excluded by appropriate investigations **3** Such a disorder is present, but the first headache attacks do not occur in close temporal relation to the disorder

(Note: These headaches are usually non-remitting but rare cases of remission are reported. This clinical problem can be seen in the context of mediation overuse which may alter the clinical features and affect response to treatment. Whether this headache type can be further subdivided according to length and persistence of history is yet to be determined.[106])

● **Table 10.7** *Suggested reclassification for trigeminal autonomic cephalalgias (TACs)*

3	**Trigeminal autonomic cephalalgias (TACs)**
3.1	**Cluster headache**
	3.1.1 Episodic cluster headache
	3.1.2 Chronic cluster headache
3.2	Paroxysmal hemicranias (Table 10.4) **3.2.1** Episodic paroxysmal hemicrania **3.2.2** Chronic paroxysmal hemicrania
3.3	Short-lasting neuralgiform headache with conjunctival injection and tearing (Table 10.5)
3.4	Hemicrania continua (Table 10.6)

● **Table 10.8** *Suggested diagnostic criteria for hypnic headache.* *

4.7 Hypnic headache

A	Headaches occur at least 15 times per month for at least one month
B	Headaches awaken patient from sleep
C	Attack duration of 5–60 minutes
D	Pain is generalized or bilateral
E	Pain not associated with autonomic features
F	At least one of the following: **1** There is no suggestion of one of the disorders listed in groups 5–11 **2** Such a disorder is suggested but excluded by appropriate investigations **3** Such a disorder is present, but the first headache attacks do not occur in close temporal relation to the disorder

Note: A rapid clinical response to lithium at bedtime is usually expected.
**To be added as section to 4.7 to the current IHS classification of Miscellaneous Headaches Unassociated with a Structural Cause.*

● *Table 10.9* *Differential diagnosis of short-lasting headache.*

Feature		Cluster headache	Chronic paroxysmal hemicrania	Episodic paroxysmal hemicrania	SUNCT	Idiopathic stabbing headache	Trigeminal neuralgia
Gender (M:F)		9:1	1:3	1:1	8:1	F>M	F>M
Pain	Type	Boring	Throbbing/boring	Throbbing	Stabbing	Stabbing	Stabbing
	Severity	Very severe	Very severe	Very severe	More severe	Severe	Very severe
	Location	Orbital Temporal	Orbital Temporal	Orbital Temporal	Orbital Temporal	Any part	V2/V3
Attack duration		15–180 min	2–45 min	1–30 min	5–250 s	<1 s	<1 s
Attack frequency		1–8/day	1–40/day	3–30/day	1/day to 30/h	Few to many/day	Few to many/day
Autonomic features		+	+	+	+	–	–
Alcohol PPT		+	+	+	+	–	–
Indomethacin		±	+	+	–	+	–

Abbreviations: F = female; M = male; V1 = ophthalmic; V2 = maxillary; V3 = mandibular divisions of the trigeminal innervation;
+ = precipitates headaches; ± = effect not consistent; – = no effect on headache.

seems possible that various TACs may be associated with trigeminal neuralgia. Whether this is a distinct pathophysio-logical entity[113] or the coincidental overlap of two entities will require further study.[111,112] At this time, we suggest that the disorder be classified under the TACs in a miscellaneous sec-tion until more data are available. Lastly, one is sometimes left with patients who have pain that is short-lasting but longer than a conventional stab. Such a patient may have episodic pains lasting 2–3 min that are severe, triggerable

and responsive to carbamazepine.[115] We would consider these part of the spectrum of trigeminal neuralgia although recognize that without other data this is a somewhat arbitrary assignment.

While all of the TAC disorders may involve trigeminal–auto-nomic activation, the mechanisms that account for the differ-ences in clinical profile and treatment response are unknown. There are simply insufficient data to answer these questions at the moment, although it must be said, based on available data, that these headaches have more similarities than differences.

References

1. Antonaci F, Sjaastad O. Chronic paroxysmal hemicrania (CPH): a review of the clinical manifestations. *Headache* 1989; 29: 648–56.
2. Sjaastad O, Shen JM. Cluster headache. Our current concepts. *Acta Neurologica* 1991; 13: 500–5.
3. Russell D. Chronic paroxysmal hemicrania: severity, duration and time of occurrence of attacks. *Cephalalgia* 1984; 4: 53–6.
4. Spierings EL. Episodic and chronic paroxysmal hemicrania. *Clin. J. of Pain* 1992; 8: 44–8.
5. Sjaastad O. *Cluster Headache Syndrome.* London: Saunders, 1992.
6. Sjaastad O, Dale I. Evidence for a new (?) treatable headache entity. *Headache* 1974; 14: 105–8.
7. Sjaastad O. Chronic paroxysmal hemicrania. In: Vinken PJ, Bruyn GW, Klawans HL, Rose FC, eds. *Handbook of Clinical Neurology; vol. 48.* Amsterdam: Elsevier Science, 1986: 257–66.
8. Headache Classification Committee of The International Headache Society. Classification and diagnostic criteria for

headache disorders, cranial neuralgias and facial pain. *Cephalalgia* 1988; 8 (suppl 7): 1–96.
9. Leone M, Filippini G, D'Amico D, Farinotti M, Bussone G. Assessment of International Headache Society diagnostic criteria: a reliability study. *Cephalalgia* 1994; 14: 280–4.
10. Price RW, Posner JB. Chronic paroxysmal hemicrania: a disabling headache syndrome responding to indomethacin. *Ann. Neurol.* 1978; 3: 183–4.
11. Hochman MS. Chronic paroxysmal hemicrania: a new type of treatable headache. *Am. J. Med.* 1981; 71: 169–70.
12. Russell D, Christoffersen B, Hoerven I. Chronic paroxysmal hemicrania: case report. *Headache* 1978; 18: 99–100.
13. Rapoport AM, Sheftell FD, Baskin SM. Chronic paroxysmal hemicrania: case report of the second known definite occurrence in a male. *Cephalalgia* 1981; 1: 67–70.
14. Joubert J, Powell D, Djikowski J. Chronic paroxysmal hemicrania in a South African

Black. A case report. *Cephalalgia* 1987; 7: 193–6.
15. Joubert J. Cluster headache in black patients. A report of 7 cases. *S. African Med. J.* 1988; 73: 552–4.
16. Broeske D, Lenn NJ, Cantos E. Chronic paroxysmal hemicrania in a young child: possible relation to ipsilateral occipital infarction. *J. Child Neurol.* 1993; 8: 235–6.
17. Kudrow DB, Kudrow L. Successful aspirin prophylaxis in a child with chronic paroxysmal hemicrania. *Headache* 1989; 29: 280–1.
18. Gladstein J, Holden EW, Peralta L. Chronic paroxysmal hemicrania in a child. *Headache* 1994; 34: 519–20.
19. Solomon S, Newman LC. Chronic paroxysmal hemicrania in a child? *Headache* 1995; 35: 234.
20. Pollmann W, Pfaffenrath V. Chronic paroxysmal hemicrania: the first possible bilateral case. *Cephalalgia* 1986; 6: 55–7.
21. Stein HJ, Rogado AZ. Chronic paroxysmal hemicrania—two new patients. *Headache* 1980; 20: 72–6.

22. Goadsby PJ, Edvinsson L. Human *in vivo* evidence for trigeminovascular activation in cluster headache. *Brain* 1994; 117: 427–34.

23. Drummond PD. Thermographic and pupillary asymmetry in chronic paroxysmal hemicrania. A case study. *Cephalalgia* 1985; 5: 133–6.

24. Bogucki A, Szymanska R, Braciak W. Chronic paroxysmal hemicrania: lack of a pre-chronic stage. *Cephalalgia* 1984; 4: 187–9.

25. Pareja JA. Chronic paroxysmal hemicrania: dissociation of the pain and autonomic features. *Headache* 1995; 35: 111–13.

26. Sjaastad O, Egge K, Horven I, *et al*. Chronic paroxysmal hemicrania V. Mechanical precipitation of attacks. *Headache* 1979; 19: 31–6.

27. Sjaastad O, Russell D, Saunte C, Horven I. Chronic paroxysmal hemicrania VI. Precipitation of attacks. Further studies on the precipitation mechanism. *Cephalalgia* 1982; 2: 211–14.

28. Sjaastad O, Saunte C, Graham JR. Chronic paroxysmal hemicrania VII. Mechanical precipitation of attacks: new cases and localisation of trigger points. *Cephalalgia* 1984; 4: 113–18.

29. Micieli G, Cavallini A, Facchinetti F, Sanches G, Nappi G. Chronic paroxysmal hemicrania: a chronobiological study (case report). *Cephalalgia* 1989; 9: 281–6.

30. Goadsby PJ, Edvinsson L. Neuropeptide changes in a case of chronic paroxysmal hemicrania — evidence for trigemino-parasympathetic activation. *Cephalalgia* 1996; 16: 448–50.

31. MacMillan JC, Nukada H. Chronic paroxysmal hemicrania. *N.Z. Med. J.* 1989; 102: 251–2.

32. Fragoso YD, Seim S, Stovner LJ, Mack M, Bjerve KS, Sjaastad O. Arachidonic acid metabolism in polymorphonuclear cells in headaches. A methodological study. *Cephalalgia* 1988; 8: 149–55.

33. Antonaci F, Sandrini G, Danilov A, Sand T. Neurophysiological studies in chronic paroxysmal hemicrania and hemicrania continua. *Headache* 1994; 34: 479–83.

34. Saunte C. Chronic paroxysmal hemicrania: salivation, tearing and nasal secretion. *Cephalalgia* 1984; 4: 25–32.

35. Antonaci F. The sweating pattern in hemicrania continua. A comparison with chronic paroxysmal hemicrania. *Funct. Neurology* 1991; 6: 371–5.

36. Drummond PD, Lance JW. Pathological sweating and flushing accompanying the trigeminal lacrimation reflex in patients with cluster headache and in patients with a confirmed site of cervical sympathetic deficit. Evidence for parasympathetic cross-innervation. *Brain* 1992; 115: 1429–45.

37. de Souza Carvalho D, Salvesen R, Sand T, Smith SE, Sjaastad O. Chronic paroxysmal hemicrania. XIII. The pupillometric pattern. *Cephalalgia* 1988; 8: 219–26.

38. Drummond PD. Autonomic disturbance in cluster headache. *Brain* 1988; 111: 1199–1209.

39. Russell D, Storstein L. Chronic paroxysmal hemicrania: heart rate changes and ECG rhythm disturbances. A computerized analysis of 24h ambulatory ECG recordings. *Cephalalgia* 1984; 4: 135–44.

40. Mongini F, Caselli C, Macri V, Tetti C. Thermsographic findings in cranio-facial pain. *Headache* 1990; 30: 497–504.

41. Shen JM. Transcranial Doppler sonography in chronic paroxysmal hemicrania. *Headache* 1993; 33: 493–6.

42. Horven I, Russell D, Sjaastad O. Ocular blood flow changes in cluster headache and chronic paroxysmal hemicrania. *Headache* 1989; 29: 373–6.

43. Krabbe AA, Henriksen L, Olesen J. Tomographic determination of cerebral blood flow during attacks of cluster headache. *Cephalalgia* 1984; 4: 17–23.

44. Meyer JS, Kawamura J, Terayama Y. CT-CBF and ^{133}Xe inhalation cerebral blood flow studies in cluster headache. In: Olesen J, ed. *Migraine and Other Headaches. The Vascular Mechanisms*. New York: Raven Press, 1991: 305–10.

45. Dahl A, Russell D, Nyberg-Hansen R, Rootwelt K. Cluster headache: transcranial Doppler ultrasound and rCBF studies. *Cephalalgia* 1990; 10: 87–94.

46. Antonaci F. Chronic paroxysmal hemicrania and hemicrania continua: orbital phlebography and MRI studies. *Headache* 1994; 34: 32–4.

47. Hannerz J. Pathoanatomic studies in a case of Tolosa–Hunt syndrome. *Cephalalgia* 1988; 8: 25–30.

48. Hoes MJAJM, Bruyn GW, Vielvoye GJ. The Tolosa–Hunt syndrome- literature review: seven new cases and a hypothesis. *Cephalalgia* 1981; 1: 181–94.

49. Tolosa E. Periarteritic lesions of the carotid siphon with the clincial features of a carotid infraclinoidal aneurysm. *J. Neurol. Neurosurg. Psychiatry* 1954; 17: 300–2.

50. Hunt WE, Meagher JN, LeFever HE, Zeman W. Painful ophthalmoplegia. Its relation to indolent inflammation of the cavernous sinus. *Neurology (Minneap.)* 1961; 11: 56–62.

51. Medina JL. Organic headaches mimicking chronic paroxysmal hemicrania. *Headache* 1992; 32: 73–4.

52. Vijayan N. Symptomatic paroxysmal hemicrania. *Cephalalgia* 1992; 12: 111–13.

53. Gawel MJ, Rothbart P. Chronic paroxysmal hemicrania which appears to arise from either third ventricle pathology or internal carotid artery pathology. *Cephalalgia* 1992; 12: 327.

54. Newman LC, Herskovitz S, Lipton R, Solomon S. Chronic paroxysmal headache: two cases with cerebrovascular disease. *Headache* 1992; 32: 75–6.

55. Sjaastad O, Stovner LJ, Stolt-Nielsen A, Antonaci F, Fredriksen TA. CPH and hemicrania continua: requirements of high dose indomethacin dosages — an ominous sign? *Headache* 1995; 35: 363–7.

56. Hannerz J, Jogestrand T. Intracranial hypertension and sumatriptan efficacy in a case of chronic paroxysmal hemicrania which became bilateral. (The mechanism of indomethacin in CPH). *Headache* 1993; 33: 320–3.

57. Delreux V, Kevers L, Callewaert A. Hemicranie paroxystique inaugurant un syndrome de Pancoast. *Rev. Neurolog.* 1989; 145: 151–2.

58. Sjaastad O, Antonaci F. Chronic paroxysmal hemicrania: a case report. Long-lasting remission in the chronic stage. *Cephalalgia* 1987; 7: 203–5.

59. Hannerz J, Ericson K, Bergstrand G. Chronic paroxysmal hemicrania: orbital phlebography and steroid treatment. A case report. *Cephalalgia* 1987; 7: 189–92.

60. Schlake HP, Bottger IG, Grotemeyer KH, Husstedt IW, Schober O. Single photon emission tomography (SPECT) with 99mTc-HMPAO (hexamethyl propylenamino oxime) in chronic paroxysmal hemicrania – a case report. *Cephalalgia* 1990; 10: 311–15.

61. Shabbir N, McAbee G. Adolescent chronic paroxysmal hemicrania responsive to verapamil monotherapy. *Headache* 1994; 34: 209–10.

62. Evers S, Husstedt I-W. Alternatives in drug treatment of chronic paroxysmal hemicrania. *Headache* 1996; 36: 429–32.

63. Warner JS, Wamil AW, McLean MJ. Acetazolamide for the treatment of chronic paroxysmal hemicrania. *Headache* 1994; 34: 597–9.

64. Dahlof C. Subcutaneous sumatriptan does not abort attacks of chronic paroxysmal hemicrania (CPH). *Headache* 1993; 33: 201–2.

65. Goadsby PJ. Cluster headache and the clinical profile of sumatriptan. *Eur. Neurol.* 1994; 34 (Suppl): 35–9.

66. Ekbom K. Treatment of acute cluster headache with sumatriptan. *N. Eng. J. Med.* 1991; 325: 322–6.

67. Kudrow L. Response of cluster headache attacks to oxygen inhalation. *Headache* 1981; 21: 1–4.

68. Kudrow L, Esperanca P, Vijayan N. Episodic paroxysmal hemicrania? *Cephalalgia* 1987; 7: 197–201.

69. Newman LC, Gordon ML, Lipton RB, Kanner R, Solomon S. Epsidoic paroxysmal hemicrania: two new cases and a literature review. *Neurology* 1992; 42: 964–6.

70. Blau JN, Engel H. Episodic paroxysmal hemicrania: a further case and review of the literature. *J. Neurol. Neurosurg. Psychiatry* 1990; 53: 343–4.

71. Spierings EL. The chronic paroxysmal hemicrania concept expanded. *Headache* 1988; 28: 597–8.

72. Geaney DP. Indomethacin-responsive episodic cluster headache. *J. Neurol. Neurosurg. Psychiatry* 1983; 46: 860–1.

73. Bogucki A, Niewodniczy A. Case report: chronic cluster headache with unusual high frequency of attacks: differential diagnosis with CPH. *Headache* 1984; 24: 150–1.

74. Alberca R, Sureda B, Marquez C, Navarro A. Episodic paroxysmal hemicrania or chronic paroxysmal hemicrania in a pre-chronic state? *Neurologia* 1991; 6: 219–21.

75. Goadsby PJ, Lipton RB. A review of paroxysmal hemicranias, SUNCT syndrome and other short-lasting headaches with autonomic features, including new cases. *Brain* 1997; 120: 193–209.

76. Coria F, Claveria LE, Jimenez-Jimenez FJ, Seijas EV. Episodic paroxysmal hemicrania responsive to calcium channel blockers. *J. Neurol. Neurosurg. Psychiatry* 1992; 55: 166.

77. Sjaastad O, Saunte C, Salvesen R, et al. Shortlasting unilateral neuralgiform headache attacks with conjunctival injection, tearing, sweating, and rhinorrhea. *Cephalalgia* 1989; 9: 147–56.

78. Pareja JA, Sjaastad O. SUNCT syndrome. A clinical review. *Headache* 1997; 37: 195–202.

79. Pareja JA, Sjaastad O. SUNCT syndrome in the female. *Headache* 1994; 34: 217–220.

80. Pareja JA, Ming JM, Kruszewski P, Caballero V, Pamo M, Sjaastad O. SUNCT syndrome: duration, frequency and temporal distribution of attacks. *Headache* 1996; 36: 161–5.

81. Pareja JA, Joubert J, Sjaastad O. SUNCT syndrome. Atypical temporal patterns. *Headache* 1996; 36: 108–10.

82. Sjaastad O, Zhao JM, Kruszewski P, Stovner LJ. Short-lasting unilateral neuralgiform headache attacks with conjunctival injection, tearing, etc. (SUNCT): III. Another Norwegian case. *Headache* 1991; 31: 175–7.

83. Pareja JA, Pareja J, Palomo T, Caballero V, Pamo M. SUNCT syndrome: repetitive and overlapping attacks. *Headache* 1994; 34: 114–16.

84. Pareja JA, Caballero V, Sjaastad O. SUNCT syndrome. Status-like pattern. *Headache* 1996; 36: 622–4.

85. Becser N, Berky M. SUNCT syndrome: a Hungarian case. *Headache* 1995; 35: 158–60.

86. Calvo JF, Tinetti N, Leston J. SUNCT. The first Argentinian case. *J. Neurol. Sci.* 1997; 150(Suppl): S34.

87. Bussone G, Leone M, Volta GD, Strada L, Gasparotti R. Short-lasting unilateral neuralgiform headache attacks with tearing and conjunctival injection: the first symptomatic case. *Cephalalgia* 1991; 11: 123–7.

88. De Benedittis G. SUNCT syndrome associated with cavernous angioma of the brain stem. *Cephalalgia* 1996; 16: 503-6.

89. Morales F, Mostacero E, Marta J, Sanchez S. Vascular malformation of the cerebellopontine angle associated with SUNCT syndrome. *Cephalalgia* 1994; 14: 301–2.

90. Goadsby PJ, Hoskin KL. The distribution of trigeminovascular afferents in the non-human primate brain *macaca nemestrina*: a c-fos immunocytochemical study. *J. of Anatomy* 1997; 190: 367–75.

91. Martins IP, Baeta E, Paiva T, Campo T, Gomes L. Headaches during intracranial endovascular procedures: a possible model of vascular headache. *Headache* 1993; 33: 227–33.

92. Bouhassira D, Attal N, Esteve M, Chauvin M. SUNCT syndrome. A case of transformation from trigeminal neuralgia. *Cephalalgia* 1994; 14: 168–70.

93. Kruszewski P. Short-lasting, unilateral, neuralgiform headache attacks with conjunctival injection and tearing (SUNCT syndrome): V. Orbital phlebography. *Cephalagia* 1992; 12: 387–9.

94. Hannerz J, Greitz D, Hansson P, Ericson K. SUNCT may be another manifestation of orbital venous vasculitis. *Headache* 1992; 32: 384–9.

95. Kruszewski P, Zhao JM, Shen JM, Sjaastad O. SUNCT syndrome: forehead sweating pattern. *Cephalalgia* 1993; 13: 108–13.

96. Zhao JM, Sjaastad O. SUNCT syndrome: VIII. Pupillary reaction and corneal sensitivity. *Funct. Neurology* 1993; 8: 409–14.

97. Sjaastad O, Kruszewski P, Fostad K, Elsas T, Qvigstad G. SUNCT syndrome: VII. Ocular and related variables. *Headache* 1992; 32: 489–95.

98. Kruszewski P, Sand T, Shen JM, Sjaastad O. Short-lasting, unilateral, neuralgiform headache attacks with conjunctival injection and tearing (SUNCT) syndrome: IV. Respiratory sinus arrhythmia during and outside paroxysms. *Headache* 1992; 32: 377–83.

99. Kruszewski P, Fasano ML, Brubakk AO, Shen JM, Sand T, Sjaastad O. Short-lasting, unilateral, neuralgiform headache attacks with conjunctival injection, tearing, and subclinical forehead sweating (SUNCT syndrome): II. Changes in heart rate and arterial blood pressure during pain paroxysms. *Headache* 1991; 31: 399–405.

100. Kruszewski P, White LR, Shen JM, et al. Respiratory studies in SUNCT syndrome. *Headache* 1995; 35: 344–8.

101. Goadsby PJ, Zagami AS, Lambert GA. Neural processing of craniovascular pain: a synthesis of the central structures involved in migraine. *Headache* 1991; 31: 365–71.

102. Shen JM, Johnsen HJ. SUNCT syndrome: estimation of cerebral blood flow velocity with transcranial Doppler ultrasonography. *Headache* 1994; 34: 25–31.

103. Poughias L, Aasly J. SUNCT syndrome: cerebral SPECT images during attacks. *Headache* 1995; 35: 143–5.

104. Pareja JA, Kruszewski P, Sjaastad O. SUNCT syndrome: trials of drugs and anesthetic blockades. *Headache* 1995; 35: 138–42.

105. Ghose RR. SUNCT syndrome. *Med. J. Aust.* 1995; 162: 667–8.

106. Sjaastad O, Spierings EL. Hemicrania continua: another headache absolutely responsive to indmethacin. *Cephalalgia* 1984; 4: 65–70.

107. Silberstein SD, Lipton RB, Solomon S, Mathew NT. Classification of daily or near-daily headaches: proposed revisions to the IHS criteria. *Headache* 1994; 34: 1–7.

108. Mathew NT. Transformed or evolutional migraine. *Headache* 1987; 27: 305–6.

109. Sheftell FD. Chronic daily headache. *Neurology* 1992; 42 (suppl 2): 32–6.

110. Young WB, Silberstein SD. Hemicrania continua and symptomatic mediation overuse. *Headache* 1993; 33: 485–7.

111. Solomon S, Apfelbaum RI, Guglielmo KM. The cluster-tic syndrome and its surgical therapy. *Cephalalgia* 1985; 5: 83–9.

112. Watson P, Evans R. Cluster-tic syndrome. *Headache* 1985; 25: 123–6.

113. Alberca R, Ochoa JJ. Cluster-tic syndrome. *Neurology* 1994; 44: 996–9.

114. Hannerz J. Trigeminal neuralgia with chronic paroxysmal hemicrania: the CPH-tic syndrome. *Cephalalgia* 1993; 13: 361–4.

115. Mulleners WM, Verhagen WIM. Cluster–tic syndrome. *Neurology* 1996; 47: 302.

116. Tehindrazanarivelo AD, Visy JM, Bousser MG. Ipsilateral cluster headache and chronic paroxysmal hemicrania: two case reports. *Cephalalgia* 1992; 12: 318–20.

117. Pareja J, Pareja J. Chronic paroxysmal hemicrania coexisting with migraine. Differential response to pharmacological treatment. *Headache* 1992; 32: 77–8.

118. Newman LC, Lipton RB, Solomon S. The hypnic headache syndrome: a benign headache disorder of the elderly. *Neurology* 1990; 40: 1904–5.

119. Raskin NH. The hypnic headache syndrome. *Headache* 1988; 28: 534–36.

Secondary headache disorders

chapter 11

Post-traumatic headache

Introduction

Post-traumatic headache is a form of secondary headache that arises after head injury and is often a part of the post-traumatic syndrome. It can follow a mild-to-moderate closed head injury, even when there has been no loss of consciousness. In addition to headache, symptoms include depression, irritability, memory impairment, loss of libido, dizziness or vertigo, alcohol intolerance, and attention and concentration difficulties.[1]

Most physicians agree that some patients have headache as a sequela to cranial trauma, but this relationship is hotly debated. Unfortunately, this debate has, to some extent, lost its intellectual way, or at least had it confused, by arguments that cross medicolegal barriers. The concept that cranial trauma can induce headache that persists long after the trauma occurs is not restricted to motor vehicle accidents; it may be invoked as a mechanism for head pain after blunt trauma, such as falling from a horse, or even iatrogenic trauma, such as from a craniotomy. Moreover, the discussion is rendered more complex as one attempts to classify the various clinical presentations that may be seen after cranial trauma. We take the view that the problem exists and should be managed as the patient's presenting headache syndrome dictates.

Epidemiology

Motor vehicle accidents account for 45% of head injury, falls for 30%, and occupational and recreational accidents for 20%.[2] Patients with mild head injury, defined as a Glasgow coma scale of 13–15 (Table 11.1), are hospitalized at a rate of approximately 200/100,000 per year.[3] Post-traumatic headache develops in many of these patients.[4–10]

● **Table 11.1** Glasgow coma scale

Eye opening (E)		Best motor response (M)	
Spontaneous	4	Obeys	6
To sound	3	Localizes	5
To pain	2	Withdraws	4
None	1	Abnormal flexion	3
Verbal response (V)		Extends	2
		None	1
Oriented	5		
Confused	4		
Inappropriate	3	Score equals sum (of)	
Incomprehensible	2	E+M+V and ranges between 3–15	
None	1		

Whiplash refers to the sequence of extension, flexion and lateral motions of the neck that follows impact, with or without direct trauma to the head. Its symptomatology is similar to post-traumatic syndrome and post-traumatic headache and includes neck pain, headaches, dizziness and paraesthesias. Cognitive and psychological sequelae are extremely common.

Clinical features

The International Headache Society (IHS) criteria for post-traumatic headache[11] (Table 11.2) are not primarily concerned with the headache's clinical features, but with the pathogenetic and temporal relationship of the headache to the trauma. The IHS criteria for post-traumatic headache require the onset of headache within two weeks of either the head injury or regaining consciousness. However, in clinical practice it is often difficult to determine when the headache actually started, since head pain may be mild and other pains (particularly neck pain) more prominent.

Migraine with or without aura may be triggered by impact.[12] Alternatively, a pattern of recurring migraine-like headaches may begin some time after a head injury.[4,13–16] In one study,[14] 35 patients had newly-acquired migraine with or without aura, beginning within a few days of mild head injury or whiplash injury.

Since trauma can trigger typical primary headaches, such as migraine, tension-type headache, or cluster headache, the IHS advised a fourth digit code to account for such a situation. It is difficult to discuss a clinically *typical* post-traumatic headache. The essence of the diagnosis is that the cranial trauma triggered the headache from which the patient suffers. The headache is often mixed with symptoms of the post-traumatic syndrome, a symptom complex that also includes vertigo, blurred vision and cognitive complaints. Post-traumatic syndrome symptoms (Table 11.3) may be delayed or develop immediately following trauma. Local occipital tenderness occurs immediately, while head, neck and shoulder pain usually begins within 24–48 hours of the injury. Neuralgic pain in the frontal or occipitocervical region may occur and may be associated with the other headache types.

Orthostatic headache can occur secondary to intracranial hypotension, with features similar to those of a post-lumbar puncture headache. Intracranial hypotension could result from a cerebrospinal fluid (CSF) leak through a dural root sleeve tear or a cribriform plate fracture. Idiopathic

● **Table 11.2** *IHS criteria for post-traumatic headache*[11]

5.1 Acute post-traumatic headache

5.1.1 With significant head trauma and/or confirmatory signs

Diagnostic criteria:

A Significance of head trauma documented by at least one of the following:

  1 Loss of consciousness

  2 Post-traumatic amnesia lasting more than 10 minutes

  3 At least two of the following exhibit relevant abnormality: clinical neurological examination, X-ray of skull, neuroimaging, evoked potentials, spinal fluid examination, vestibular function test, neuropsychological testing

B Headache occurs less than 14 days after regaining consciousness (or after the trauma, if there has been no loss of consciousness)

C Headache disappears within 8 weeks after regaining consciousness (or after trauma, if there has been no loss of consciousness)

5.1.2 With minor head trauma and no confirmatory signs

Diagnostic criteria:

A Head trauma that does not satisfy 5.1.1 A

B Headache occurs less than 14 days after injury

C Headache disappears within 8 weeks after injury

5.2 Chronic post-traumatic headache

A Significance of head trauma documented by at least one of the following:

  1 Loss of consciousness

  2 Post-traumatic amnesia lasting more than 10 minutes

  3 At least two of the following exhibit relevant abnormality: clinical neurological examination, X-ray of skull, neuroimaging, evoked potentials, spinal fluid examination, vestibular function test, neuropsychological testing

B Headache occurs less than 14 days after regaining consciousness (or after the trauma, if there has been no loss of consciousness)

C Headache continues for more than 8 weeks after regaining consciousness (or after trauma, if there has been no loss of consciousness)

5.2.2 With minor head trauma and no confirmatory signs

Diagnostic criteria

A Head trauma that does not satisfy 5.1.1 A

B Headache occurs less than 14 days after injury

C Headache continues for more than 8 weeks after injury

● **Table 11.3** *Sequelae of mild head injury*

Headaches	Psychological and somatic complaints
Tension-type	Irritability
Migraine	Anxiety
Cluster	Depression
Low cerebrospinal pressure	Personality change
Occipital neuralgia	Fatigue
Idiopathic intracranial hypotension	Sleep disturbance
Supraorbital and infraorbital neuralgia	Decreased libido
Cervicogenic	Decreased appetite
Temporomandibular joint syndrome or dysfunction	**Rare sequelae**
Local neuroma	Subdural and epidural haematomas
Mixed	Seizures
Cranial nerve symptoms and signs	Transient global amnesia
Dizziness	Tremor
Vertigo	Dystonia
Tinnitus	
Hearing loss	
Blurred vision	
Diplopia	
Convergence insufficiency	
Light and noise sensitivity	
Diminished taste and smell	

intracranial hypertension (pseudotumour) with and without papilloedema has also been reported as a consequence of head injury.[17]

Dysautonomic cephalalgia can follow injury to the carotid sheath. This rare, severe, unilateral headache is localized to the frontotemporal area and is associated with ipsilateral increased facial sweating and pupillary dilation.[1,18]

Temporomandibular joint injury may occur. Symptoms include incomplete jaw opening, clicking on lateral movements, jaw pain with mastication or prolonged talking, and pain on palpation of the jaw joint or the muscles of mastication. Temporomandibular joint dysfunction may be a headache trigger.

Impaired memory and difficulty concentrating are common in the post-traumatic syndrome.[10] Some patients have neurocognitive deficits and a documented inability to process information.[19] Many have difficulty processing different stimuli simultaneously and appear absent-minded because they must devote their full concentration to the task at hand. Other frequently reported symptoms include anger, depression, irritability and personality changes.

Non-specific dizziness and episodic and positional vertigo are commonly associated with post-traumatic headache.[20] Sleep disturbances, including insomnia and daytime drowsiness, are frequent. Non-specific staring episodes, non-vestibular dizziness and periodic loss of consciousness are rare.

Risk factors

Age, gender and certain mechanical factors are risks for a poor outcome after head injury or whiplash injury. Women have a 1.9-fold increased risk of post-traumatic headache compared to men.[21] Increased age is associated with a less rapid and less complete recovery.[22–24] Post-traumatic headache is more likely if the head is inclined or rotated prior to impact or if there is a rear-end collision or an unprepared occupant.[25]

The relationship between the severity of the injury and the severity or incidence of the post-traumatic headache is uncertain. The persistence of the headache does not correlate with the duration of unconsciousness, post-traumatic amnesia, skull fracture, electroencephalogram (EEG) abnormalities, or bloody CSF.[20,26]

Pathophysiology

Post-traumatic headache is a group of traumatically-induced disorders with overlapping symptoms. Peripheral nerve injury may result in neuralgic pain; soft tissue or skeletal injuries may initiate or trigger chronic daily headache; and injury to the neck, jaw and tissues of the scalp cause pain that is referred into the head.

Head injury causes shear forces to the brain that can produce diffuse axonal injury. Direct impact is not necessary.[27] Diffuse axonal injury is most common in the corpus callosum, internal capsule, fornices, dorsolateral midbrain and pons.[28]

Head injury usually involves a combination of translational and rotational forces. Restricted rotation makes it more difficult to produce a concussion in animals.[29] Unsynchronized rotations often develop between the cerebral hemispheres and the cerebellum,[29] making axons in the upper brainstem particularly vulnerable to diffuse axonal injury. Midbrain haemorrhage can result. Ischaemic brain injury, abnormal cerebrovascular autoregulation and vasospasm may follow severe headache (Figure 11.1).

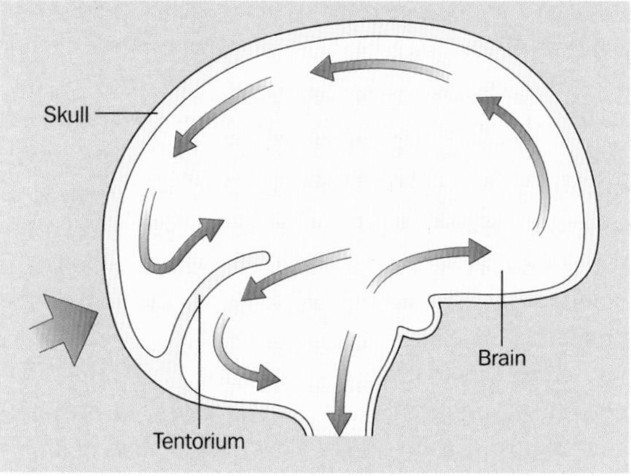

● **Figure 11.1** *Brain motion. (From Ward C. Status of head injury modeling. Head and Neck injury Criteria, Washington D.C., USA, Department of Transportation, 1981.)*

Testing

Neuroimaging

Most hospitalized patients with mild or moderate head injury have magnetic resonance imaging (MRI) abnormalities. These abnormalities eventually decrease, with many resolving within one month.[30] Because of the risk of subsequent deterioration, all patients with mild behavioural abnormalities, equivocal findings on examination, or a Glasgow coma scale of <15 should be neuroimaged. With subacute or chronic post-traumatic syndrome, however, guidelines are less clear. If neuroimaging was not done, brain computed tomography or MRI should be performed to exclude chronic subdural haematoma, hydrocephalus or a structural lesion unrelated to the trauma. If neck pain is prominent and persistent, a cervical MRI may be indicated, but if the neurological examination is normal or severe radicular symptoms are absent, an abnormal MRI usually does not change therapy. Of concern is a possible fracture or dislocation of the cervical spine, and the patient should have cervical spine films to rule out this problem.

Single photon emission computed tomography (SPECT)

Single photon emission computed tomography observes the physiological behaviour of the brain. In the acute phase of head injury, technetium-99m hexamethylpropyleneamineoxine (Tc-HMPAO) SPECT is more sensitive than computed tomography and is helpful in predicting outcome.[31–33] In 20 patients with head injury, Tc-HMPAO SPECT showed abnormalities in 60%, whereas only 25% had abnormalities on computed tomography.[34] In 12 patients with mild-to-moderate head injury one to nine years after injury, Tc-HMPAO SPECT was abnormal in 10 patients, while computed tomography was abnormal in 6 patients.[35]

Electroencephalography (EEG)

The EEG is usually of little value in evaluating post-traumatic headache. While often abnormal immediately after injury, it normalizes within minutes to weeks. Persistent findings that were once considered abnormal are now considered normal variants with the same incidence as is found in the general population.[36]

Evoked potentials

Short latency somatosensory evoked potentials have not been shown to be of value in head injury.[37] On the other hand, brainstem auditory evoked potentials have been found to be abnormal in 10–20% of patients with head injury and postconcussion syndrome. While the brainstem auditory evoked potential separates groups of patients with post-traumatic headache from groups of controls, it does not differentiate an individual with post-traumatic headache from one without post-traumatic headache.

Neuropsychological testing

Neuropsychological testing in patients with head injury is often markedly abnormal early on and improves or resolves with time. Abnormalities are found in information processing, auditory vigilance, reaction time, sustained divided and distributed attention, visual and verbal memory, design fluency imagination and analytic capacity.

Neuropsychological tests were performed on 30 patients with post-traumatic syndrome after whiplash injury. Deficits in attention and concentration resolved within six weeks. Visual memory, imagination and analytic capacity were recovered within the next six weeks. Verbal memory abstraction, cognitive selectivity and information processing speed took more than 12 weeks to recover.[38] This suggests that there is a hierarchy of functional recovery following mild head injury.

Relationship between cranial trauma and headache

Migraine,[14] cluster headache or chronic daily headache can occur after even trivial head injury.[39] Post-traumatic headache is more common in patients with a history of headache.[40,41] Post-traumatic headache usually lasts for three to five years and then abates[42] independent of financial compensation.[43,44,45] Since 10% of most populations studied have migraine, and many more suffer from other headache types (see Chapter 3), the association between trauma and headache could at times be one of chance. We think not, but the question is difficult to resolve. It has been suggested that post-traumatic headache may be seen up to 24 months after the injury and that as many as 12% of patients acquire their headaches more than six months after the trauma.[24] The problem with such assertions is that we do not know how many people would acquire a headache in a suitable control group. The IHS thus set a somewhat arbitrary limit that the headache should come on within two weeks of the head injury. While this criterion is *ad hoc*, it is useful in practice. If cranial trauma induces a headache process, it seems likely that it would have a relatively short latency from a physiological point of view; certainly the concept that a headache starting years after cranial trauma has a causative relationship to the trauma seems difficult to accept.

Diagnosis

The diagnosis of post-traumatic headache and post-traumatic syndrome, therefore, is established by symptoms that are consistent with the syndrome and onset that is related to trauma.

The differential diagnoses include subdural or epidural haematoma, CSF hypotension, cerebral vein thrombosis, cavernous sinus thrombosis, cervical or carotid artery dissection, cerebral haemorrhage, epilepsy and hydrocephalus.

Management

Management of post-traumatic headache is dictated by the clinical syndrome. Structural problems, such as low cerebrospinal fluid pressure syndromes, must be excluded by neuroimaging and a careful history and physical examination. Patients with post-traumatic headache are often misunderstood. They may be distressed and require support and an objective, comprehensive approach to treatment. An explanation of the existence and recognition of the syndrome can be very therapeutic.

A recognizable primary headache syndrome (e.g. migraine or cluster headache) that has been triggered by cranial trauma is managed in the usual manner. Cervical and soft-tissue injuries should be identified and treated, as should anxiety, depression and cognitive dysfunction. Post-traumatic chronic daily headache is very difficult to treat, but again the management principles are as outlined in Chapter 8.

Few studies have evaluated specific drug treatments for post-traumatic headache. Most have involved the use of the antidepressant, amitriptyline. We have found tricyclics, such as amitriptyline and imipramine, as well as valproate, to be extremely useful in these patients. Like many patients with chronic daily headache syndromes, medication overuse can be a complicating variable that must be addressed if treatment is to be successful. Perhaps the most effective tool is a careful and straightforward explanation of the syndrome. The fact that the pain-producing structures of the brain, when disturbed, can effectively 'wind themselves up' to produce the pain that was triggered by, but persists independent of, the original trauma can help patients cope with what must be to them a bizarre situation.

Sumatriptan and zolmitriptan are effective for the migrainous exacerbation of post-traumatic headache, but not for the baseline headache.[46] Repetitive intravenous dihydroergotamine is effective for post-traumatic headache that meets the criteria of chronic daily headache[47,48] and appeared to improve cognitive function in one study.[48] Intravenous chlorpromazine has been effective in acute post-traumatic headache. One must be on the lookout for analgesic and ergotamine overuse[49] in patients with daily or near-daily headache; preventive medications should be used preferentially and abortive medications limited.

Physical modalities, such as physical therapy and exercise, chiropractic treatment and massage, have been beneficial for some patients, particularly when the headache is related to, or occurs in association with, cervical trauma. Cervical orthoses, electrotherapy, heat and cold have been used successfully, particularly in the acute stage, to improve functioning. These methods have not been rigorously tested and such data will be of great value in planning treatment regimens. In one open study, manual therapy was more successful than cold packs in relieving chronic post-traumatic headache.[50] After the initial, acute phase, exercise programmes are important to prevent deconditioning and a decrease in the overall level of functioning.

Since prognostic studies have used different study designs, varying subject characteristics, and various definitions of head injury, it has been difficult to accurately ascertain the prognosis of post-traumatic headache. One month after mild head injury, 31%[51] to 90%[52] of patients had headache. Two to three months post-injury, 32%[53] to 78%[10] of patients had headache. One year after injury, the range was 8%[54] to 35%.[55] Two to four years after injury, three studies show that 20–24% of patients have persistent headache.

Approximately one-third of patients are unable to return to work after head injury.[56] In one study, 34% of previously employed patients admitted to a hospital had not returned to work three months after injury. Older patients with higher levels of education and employment, greater income, and higher socioeconomic status are, however, likely to return to work.[10]

In the post-traumatic headache patient, two processes may occur simultaneously. The first process is diffuse axonal injury, which is due to acceleration/deceleration forces. When diffuse axonal injury is more severe, it is associated with abnormalities on MRI, positron emission tomography, SPECT and certain neuropsychological tests. Clinical improvement may occur over several months, with these tests normalizing or improving. A second process, separate from diffuse axonal injury, may be responsible for the persistent headache, psychopathology and neurocognitive deficits that occur after head injury. This process is often heralded by more severe early headache. A pre-existing factor or vulnerability may be a necessary precondition for this process to present itself fully in a given individual.

References

1. Young WB, Packard RC. Post-traumatic headache. In: Silberstein SD, Goadsby P (eds.). *Headache*. Newton MA: Butterworth Heinemann, 1997.
2. Jennett B, Frankowski RF. The epidemiology of head injury. In: Braakman R (ed). *Handbook of Clinical Neurology*. New York: Elsevier, 1990: 116.
3. Kraus JF, McArthur DL, Silberman TA. Epidemiology of mild brain injury. *Seminars in Neurol* 1994; 14(1): 17.
4. Evans RW. The postconcussion syndrome and the sequelae of mild head injury. *Neurol Clin* 1992; 10: 815–47.
5. Raskin NH. Post-traumatic headache: the postconcussion syndrome. In: Rashkin NH (ed). *Headache*. New York: Churchill Livingstone, 1988.
6. Brenner C, Friedman AP, Merritt HH *et al*. Post-traumatic headache. *J Neurosurg* 1944; 1: 379–91.
7. Elkind AH. Posttraumatic headache. In: Diamond S, Dalessio DJ (eds). *The Practising Physician's Approach to Headache*. 5th edition. Baltimore: Williams and Wilkins, 1992: 146–61.
8. Speed WG. Psychiatric aspects of post-traumatic headaches. In: Adler C, Adler S, Packard R (eds). *Psychiatric Aspects of Headache*. Baltimore: Williams and Wilkins, 1987: 210–17.
9. Gfeller JD, Chibnall JT, Duckro PN. Postconcussion symptoms and cognitive functioning in posttraumatic headache patients. *Headache* 1994; 34: 503–7.
10. Rimel RW, Giordani B, Barth JT, Boll TJ, Jane JA. Disability caused by minor head injury. *Neurosurgery* 1981; 9(3): 221–8.
11. Headache Classification Committee of the International Headache Society. Classification and diagnostic criteria for headache disorders, cranial neuralgias and facial pain. *Cephalalgia* 1988; 88(7): S1–96.
12. Haas DC, Lourie T. Trauma-triggered migraine: an explanation for common neurologic attacks after mild head injury. *J Neurosurg* 1988; 68: 181–8.
13. Mandel S. Minor head injury may not be 'minor'. *Postgrad Med* 1989;85: 213–15.
14. Weiss HD, Stern BJ, Goldbert J. Post-traumatic migraine: chronic migraine precipitated by minor head or neck trauma. *Headache* 1991; 31: 451–6.
15. Binder LM. Persisting symptoms after mild head injury: a review of the postconcussive syndrome. *J Clin Exp Neuropsychol* 1986; 8(4): 323–46.
16. Winston KR. Whiplash and its relationship to migraine. *Headache* 1987; 27: 452–7.
17. Silberstein S, Marcelis J. Pseudotumor cerebri without papilledema. *Headache* 1990; 30: 304.

18. Vijayan N. A new post-traumatic headache syndrome. *Headache* 1977; 17: 19–22.

19. Gronwall D, Wrightson P. Delayed recovery of intellectual function after minor head injury. *Lancet* 1974;2:605–9.

20. Lidvall HF, Linderoth B, Norlin B. Causes of the postconcussional syndrome. *Acta Neurol Scand* 1974; 50(56): 1143.

21. Jensen OK, Nielsen FF. The influence of sex and pretraumatic headache on the incidence and severity of headache after head injury. *Cephalalgia* 1990; 10: 285–93.

22. Bohnen N, Twijnstra A, Jolles J. Posttraumatic and emotional symptoms in different subgroups of patients with mild head injury. *Brain injury* 1992; 6(6): 481–7.

23. McClelland RJ, Fenton GW, Rutherford W. The postconcussional syndrome revisited. *J Royal Soc Med* 1994; 87: 508–10.

24. Cartlidge N, Shaw D. *Head Injury.* Philadelphia: WB Saunders, 1981: 951–54.

25. Mendelson G. Not 'cured by a verdict'. *Med J Aust* 1982; 2: 132–4.

26. DeBenedittis G, DeSantis A. Chronic post-traumatic headache: clinical, psychopathologic features and outcome determinants. *J Neurosurg Sci* 1983; 27: 177–86.

27. Gennarelli TA. Mechanisms of brain injury. *J Emerg Med* 1993; 1: 511.

28. Blumbergs PC, Jones NR, North JB. Diffuse axonal injury in head trauma. *J Neurol Neurosurg Psychiatr* 1989; 52: 838–41.

29. Elson LM, Ward CC. Mechanisms and pathophysiology of mild head injury. *Semin Neurol* 1994; 14: 818.

30. Levin HS, Amparo E, Eisenberg HM *et al.* Magnetic resonance imaging and computerized tomography in relation to the neurobehavioral sequelae of mild and moderate head injuries. *J Neurosurg* 1987; 66: 706–13.

31. Abdel-Dayem HM, Sadek SA, Kouris K *et al.* Changes in cerebral perfusion after acute head injury: comparison of CT with Tc-99m-PAO SPECT. *Radiology* 1987; 165: 221–6.

32. Reid RH. Gulenchyn K, Ballinger JR *et al.* Cerebral perfusion imaging with Tc-HM PAO following cerebral trauma. *Clin Nucl Med* 1990; 15: 383–8.

33. Abdel-Dayem H, Masdeu J, O'Connel R *et al.* Brain perfusion abnormalities following minor/moderate closed head injury: comparison between early and late imaging in two groups of patients. *Eur J Nucl Med* 1994; 21: 750.

34. Gray BG, Ichise M, Chung D *et al.* Technetium-99m-HMPAO SPECT in the evaluation of patients with a remote history of traumatic brain injury: a comparison with X-ray computed tomography. *J Nucl Med* 1992; 33: 52–8.

35. Krelina M, Reid R, Ballinger J. Regional cerebral blood flow in patients with remote close-head injuries. *Can J Neurol Sci* 1989; 2: 279.

36. Schoenhuber R, Gentilini M. Neurophysiologic assessment of mild head injury. In: Levin HS, Eisenberg HM, Benton AL (eds). *Mild Head Injury.* New York: Oxford University Press 1989: 142–50.

37. Bricolo AP, Turella GS. Electrophysiology of head injury. In: Braakman R (ed). *Handbook of Clinical Neurology, Volume 13(57): Head injury.* New York: Elsevier 1990: 181–206.

38. Keidel M, Yaguez L, Wilhelm H, Diener HC. Prospective follow-up of neuropsychologic deficits after cervicocephalic acceleration trauma. Neurologische Klinik and Poliklinik, Universitat Essen. *Nervenarzt* 1992; 63(12): 731–40.

39. Haas DC, Lourie H. Trauma-triggered migraine: an explanation for common neurologic attacks after mild head injury. *J Neurosurg* 1988; 68: 181–8.

40. Jensen OK, Nielsen FF. The influence of sex and pretraumatic headache on the incidence and severity of headache after head injury. *Cephalalgia* 1990; 10: 285–93.

41. Russell MB, Olesen J. Migraine associated with head trauma and its relation to migraine. *Eur J Neurol* 1996; 3: 424–8.

42. Medina JL. Efficacy of an individualized outpatient program in the treatment of chronic post-traumatic headache. *Headache* 1992; 32: 180–3.

43. Packard RC, Ham LP. Post-traumatic headache: determining chronicity. *Headache* 1993; 33: 133–4.

44. De Benedittis G, De Santis A. Chronic post-traumatic headache: clinical, psychopathological features and outcome determinants. *J Neurosurg Sci* 1983; 27: 177–86.

45. Packard RC. Post-traumatic headache: permanency and relationship to legal settlement. *Headache* 1992; 32: 496–500.

46. Gawel MJ, Rothbart P, Jacobs H. Subcutaneous sumatriptan in the treatment of acute episodes of post-traumatic headache. *Headache* 1993; 33(2): 96–7.

47. McBeath JG, Nanda A. Use of dihydroergotamine in patients with postconcussion syndrome. *Headache* 1994; 34: 148–51.

48. Young WB, Hopkins MM, Janyszek B, Primavera JP. Repetitive intravenous DHE in the treatment of refractory posttraumatic headache. *Headache* 1994; 34(5): 297 (abstr.).

49. Herd A, Ludwig L. Relief of post-traumatic headache by intravenous chlorpromazine. *J Emerg Med* 1994; 12(6): 849–51.

50. Jensen OK, Nielsen FF, Vosmar L. An open study comparing manual therapy with the use of cold packs in the treatment of post-traumatic headache. *Cephalalgia* 1990; 10: 241–50.

51. Munderhoud JM, Boclens ME, Huizenga J *et al.* Treatment of minor head injuries. *Clin Neurol Neurosurg* 1980; 82: 127–40.

52. Denker PG. The postconcussion syndrome: prognosis and evaluation of the organic factors. *N.Y. State J Med* 1944; 44: 379–84.

53. Denny-Brown D. Disability arising from closed head injury. *JAMA* 1945; 127: 429–36.

54. Rutherford WH, Merrett JD, McDonald JR. Symptoms of one year following concussion from minor head injuries. *Injury* 1978; 10: 225–30.

55. Dencker SJ, Lofving BA. A psychometric study of identical twins discordant for closed head injury. *Acta Psychiatr Neurol Scand* 1958; (Suppl.33): 1958.

56. Rutherford WH, Merrett JD, McDonald JR. Sequelae of concussion caused by minor head injuries. *Lancet* 1977; 1: 14.

chapter 12

Headache associated with non-vascular intracranial disease

Introduction

Headache is one of the most common clinical manifestations of altered intracranial pressure. Any disruption of cerebrospinal fluid (CSF) production, flow or absorption may lead to alterations in intracranial pressure and headache. Clinical syndromes include post-lumbar puncture headache, spontaneous intracranial hypotension, brain tumour, idiopathic intracranial hypertension, hydrocephalus, intracranial haemorrhage and subdural haematoma. Mass lesions can produce traction on pain-sensitive intracranial structures, impede CSF flow, or directly increase pressure by mass effect, all of which can produce headache. Some disorders produce unique symptoms that aid in their diagnosis, for example, the orthostatic headache, characteristic of intracranial hypotension, or the cough headache associated with hindbrain abnormalities.

The International Headache Society (IHS)[1] classifies these disorders as 'headache associated with non-vascular intracranial disorder [7.0]' (Table 12.1). Patients may have worsening of a pre-existing headache or may develop a new form of headache (including migraine, tension-type headache, or cluster headache) in close temporal relationship to a non-vascular intracranial disorder. Causality is *not* necessarily implied.

Cerebrospinal fluid (CSF)

History

The ventricular cavities were first described by Galen, in the 2nd century, but it was left to Contugno, in 1764, to describe the CSF. Earlier anatomists never encountered the CSF, since decapitation, performed before dissection, allowed it to escape. In 1825, Magendie tapped the cisterna magna in animals. He named the CSF and discovered,

between the IVth ventricle and the subarachnoid space, the foramen that bears his name.[2]

Dandy's work supported the view that the CSF originated from the choroid plexus and the perivascular spaces of the brain. Key and Retzius demonstrated that the CSF passes from the subarachnoid space through the Pacchionian bodies into the cerebral venous sinuses (Figure 12.1).[2]

Lumbar puncture was introduced by Quinke in 1891. Using a percutaneous needle with a stylet, he measured the components of CSF and its pressure in normal and disease states. Bier first described post-lumbar puncture headache in 1898, when he injected cocaine into his own subarachnoid space and developed a violent post-dural headache.[3] Schaltenbrand, in 1938, was the first to describe spontaneous intracranial hypotension using the term 'spontaneous aliquorhea'.[4]

Production, flow, absorption and pressure

The major source of CSF is the choroid plexus; however, some CSF is formed in extrachoroidal sites. The choroid plexus of the lateral ventricle is continuous with that of the IIIrd ventricle, but separate from that of the IVth ventricle. Both active transport and serum dialysis are involved in CSF production (Figure 12.2).[5]

The estimated rate of CSF formation in humans is 0.37 ± 0.1 ml/min, which represents a formation rate of 500 ml/day. This rate is unaffected by intracranial pressures

● **Table 12.1** *Headache associated with non-vascular intracranial disorder: Diagnostic criteria*

- Symptoms and/or signs of intracranial disorder
- Confirmation by appropriate investigation
- Headache as a new symptom or of a new type occurs temporally related to intracranial disorder

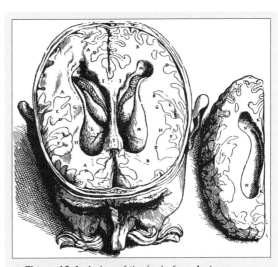

● **Figure 12.1** *A view of the brain from Andreas Vesalius' Fabrica, showing the ventricles.*

CSF PATHWAYS

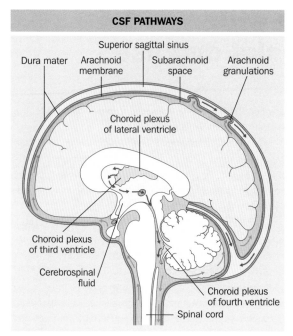

Superior sagittal sinus

Dura mater Arachnoid Subarachnoid Arachnoid
membrane space granulations

Choroid plexus
of lateral ventricle

Choroid plexus
of third ventricle

Cerebrospinal
fluid

Choroid plexus
of fourth ventricle

Spinal cord

● *Figure 12.2* CSF pathways.

● *Table 12.2* Factors determining CSF pressure

- CSF secretion pressure
- CSF absorption rate
- Intracranial arterial pressure
- Intracranial venous pressure
- Brain bulk
- Hydrostatic pressure
- Presence of intact/surrounding coverings

● *Table 12.3* Mechanisms for elevated intracranial pressure

- Increased CSF production or secretion pressure
- Decreased CSF absorption
- Increased venous pressure
- Obstruction of normal CSF flow
- Increase in brain bulk: mass lesion/cerebral oedema
- Increased bulk or pressure in dura
- Combination of above

of −10 to 240 mmH$_2$O.[5] The total CSF volume is renewed every 6–8 hours.

The zero reference level of lumbar CSF pressure is the right atrial pressure level. In normal subjects, minor CSF pressure pulsations are seen, with pulsations between 2 and

CSF PRESSURES IN THE FOUR GROUPS

	Acute pseudo-tumor (N=116)	Chronic pseudo-tumor (N=18)	Normal obese (N=41)	Normal non-obese (N=15)
CSF pressure (mmH2O) 550 500 450 400 350 300 250 200 150 100 50				

* Papilledema   ■ Same patient, two LP

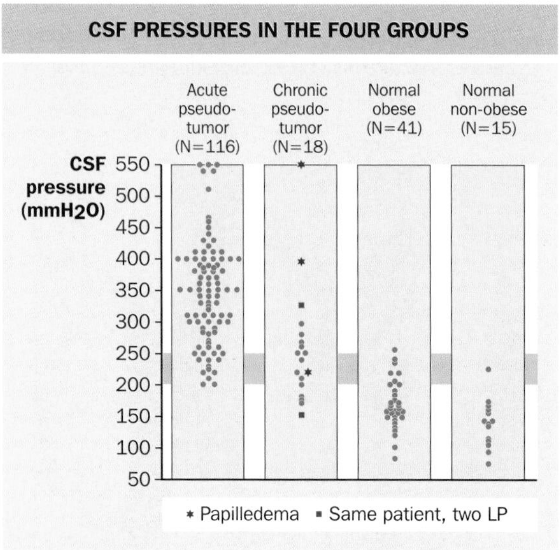

● *Figure 12.3* CSF pressures in the four groups. Three patients in the chronic group still had papilledema (asterisks). One patient in the chronic group had two lumbar punctures (squares). One lumbar puncture was normal and the other showed elevated pressure.[6]

5 mmH$_2$O being synchronous with respiration and pulsations between 1 and 2 mmH$_2$O with systole. In humans, in the lateral recumbent position, the average CSF pressure is 150 mmH$_2$O, with a range of 70–200 mmH$_2$O.[2,5] Corbett and Mehta[6] recorded CSF pressures between 200 and 250 mmH$_2$O in normal non-obese controls, suggesting that the upper limit of normal may be 250 mmH$_2$O.(Figure 12.3) When CSF pressure falls below 50–90 mmH$_2$O, symptoms of intracranial hypotension occur. At times the CSF pressure is not measurable and CSF can only be obtained by aspiration.[2,5,7] If simultaneous pressures are taken from the cerebral ventricles, the cisterna magna, and the lumbar sac during a change from the recumbent to the erect posture, there is a significant change in pressure throughout the system. The pressure rises to 375–565 mmH$_2$O in the lumbar sac, becomes 0 mmH$_2$O at the level of the cisterna magna, and can fall to −85 mmH$_2$O in the ventricles.[5,8–11]

The factors that determine CSF pressure are listed in Table 12.2. Of these, transmitted venous pressure is the most important determinant.[5] Intracranial pressure can be elevated by any of the mechanisms in Table 12.3. A mass lesion can produce elevated intracranial pressure when it:

- reaches a critical size;
- obstructs the intracranial venous system producing increased venous pressure; or
- obstructs the CSF pathways.

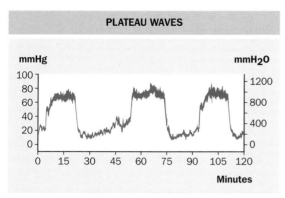

PLATEAU WAVES

● *Figure 12.4* Plateau waves as visualized with an intracranial pressure transducer in a patient with a malignant brain tumour. During the waves a rapid increase in signs of cerebral dysfunction was noted.[2]

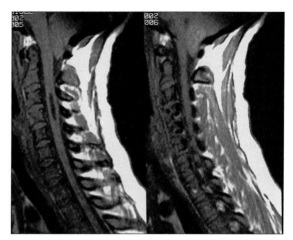

● *Figure 12.5* Chiari malformation.

According to the Monro–Kellie doctrine, any increase in intracranial volume leads to increased intracranial pressure; since an adult's skull has rigid walls, it forms a closed chamber, with a small exit, the foramen magnum, providing the only outlet for CSF into the vertebral canal.

Patients with intracranial hypertension who are monitored continuously with isovolumetric pressure transducers show frequent rapid pressure fluctuations. Two fluctuations are related to respiration and systole. The third, now called plateau waves (Figure 12.4), is an acute elevation of pressure, lasting 5–20 minutes, that can reach levels as high as 600–1300 mmH$_2$O.

When intracranial hypotension is present, intracranial CSF pressure falls more when the upright posture is assumed. This produces increased traction on the supporting structures of the brain (the blood vessels and dural sinuses), which may cause headache in the upright position. Secondary compensatory venous dilation may contribute to the headache as well.[12,13] Intracranial CSF volume loss, measured by magnetic resonance imaging (MRI), occurs mainly in the cortical sulci and has been correlated to post-lumbar puncture low CSF pressure headache. Venous dilation compensates for the volume loss.[14] Jugular compression, which causes more venous dilation but increases intracranial pressure, aggravates low pressure headache. Grant found no change in the position of the intracranial structures in patients with intracranial hypotension on MRI.[14] However, other workers have found downward displacement of the brain with incisural or cerebellar tonsillar herniation which could be mistaken for a Chiari malformation (Figure 12.5)[15,16] descent of the brainstem, flattening of the basis pontis and bowing of the optic chiasm over the pituitary gland. The downward displacement might have been worse if an upright scan had been performed. These MRI abnormalities often resolve with headache improvement.[17–20] Thus, headache may result from either painful venous dilation or displacement of and traction on pain-sensitive intracranial structures.

Intracranial hypotension

Headache is the most common clinical symptom of intracranial hypotension (Table 12.4). Unlike intracranial hypertension, where headache occurs in 30–80% of symptomatic patients, headache is present in almost all patients with symptomatic intracranial hypotension.[21] The headache may be frontal, occipital or diffuse. It is accentuated by the erect position and relieved with recumbency (orthostatic headache). The pain is severe, dull or throbbing in nature, and usually not relieved with analgesics. It is aggravated by head-shaking, coughing, straining or sneezing and jugular compression. The more severe the headache, the more frequently it is associated with dizziness, nausea, vomiting and tinnitus, and the longer the patient is upright, the longer it takes the headache to subside with recumbency.[22] Physical

● *Table 12.4* Features of low CSF pressure headache

- Pain: aggravated by upright position; relieved with recumbency. Aggravated by head shaking and jugular compression.
- Associated symptoms: nausea, vomiting, dizziness, tinnitus, photophobia, anorexia, and generalized malaise.
- Physical exam: within normal limits (rare neck stiffness, slow pulse rate 'vagus pulse').
- Lumbar puncture: opening pressure from 0–70 mmH$_2$O CSF in the lateral decubitus position.

examination is usually normal; however, there may be mild neck stiffness and a slow pulse rate ('vagus pulse'). Spinal fluid pressure usually ranges from 0–70 mmH$_2$O. The CSF composition is usually normal, but there may be a slight protein elevation and a few red blood cells.[21]

Intracranial hypotension can be divided into two categories (Table 12.5):

- spontaneous, in which there is no evidence of CSF leak or systemic illness, and
- symptomatic, which may be associated with a CSF leak.[23]

The IHS[1] classifies low CSF pressure headache as one that 'occurs or worsens less than 15 minutes after assuming the upright position and disappears or improves less than 30 minutes after resuming the recumbent position'.

The most common cause of intracranial hypotension is lumbar pressure. Head or back trauma, craniotomy, and spinal surgery can produce CSF hypotension as a result of a dural tear or a traumatic avulsion of a nerve root, resulting in a CSF leak.[24–26] In addition, craniotomy and trauma can produce intracranial hypotension not associated with a CSF leak. This may be a result of decreased CSF formation, decreased cerebral blood flow, or both.[27] Low pressure syndromes can occur secondary to CSF rhinorrhoea, either spontaneous, post-traumatic or because of a pituitary tumour. Spontaneous dural tears must be ruled out in all cases of spontaneous intracranial hypotension. A systemic medical illness, including severe dehydration, hyperpnoea, meningoencephalitis, uraemia, severe systemic infection and infusion of hypertonic solution, can cause CSF hypotension. Postural headache can also occur in patients who have had

CSF shunts. This is one of the complications of treating idiopathic intracranial hypertension.[28,40] Other causes of spontaneous positional headache, such as a colloid cyst of the IIIrd ventricle, need to be ruled out.[29]

It is believed that post-lumbar puncture headache is caused by low CSF pressure secondary to CSF leakage. In fact, dural holes and subdural collections of CSF have been observed at laminectomy or autopsy performed post-lumbar puncture.[2,52] Kunkle induced post-lumbar puncture headache in normal subjects by draining CSF.[30] Headache appeared when pressure was reduced by removing 20 ml of CSF. The estimated intracranial pressure fell to between –220 and –290 mmH$_2$O from a normal –100 mmH$_2$O in the sitting position. Performing spinal drainage on a patient who had a prior section of the Vth and IXth cranial nerves and upper cervical nerves on the left side did not produce left-sided headache.[2] No direct correlation exists between the level of pressure on a subsequent lumbar puncture and the presence of low- (as well as high-) pressure headache, but a correlation exists between CSF volume loss and headache.[14,31] Jugular compression increases severity despite increasing intracranial pressure, suggesting that headache is not caused solely by intracranial hypotension.[31]

As the low-pressure headache improves, the associated tinnitus and feeling of ear blockage disappear. An anatomical connection between the subarachnoid space and the cochlea would allow development of labyrinthine hypotension and cochlear symptoms.[2]

The clinical syndrome of spontaneous intracranial hypotension is similar to that of post-lumbar puncture headache. Schaltenbrand described three possible mechanisms to explain the pathophysiology of spontaneous intracranial hypotension:

- decreased CSF production,
- increased CSF absorption, and
- CSF leakage from cryptic small dural tears.

By definition, there is no evidence of central nervous system (CNS) trauma or prior lumbar puncture. Cases of spontaneous intracranial hypotension have been reported in which the radionucleide cisternogram showed rapid uptake in the bladder and kidneys and rapid transport of isotope with no evidence of CSF leak.[23,32–34] DiChiro believes this is abnormal and consistent with CSF hyperabsorption. Rando and Fishman reported rapid uptake in the bladder and kidney in two cases of spontaneous intracranial hypotension secondary to CSF spinal leaks.[35] They believe that hyperabsorption is due to an occult CSF leak and that increased CSF absorption only occurs with elevated intracranial pressure.

● **Table 12.5** *Causes of low pressure headache syndrome*

- **Spontaneous intracranial hypotension**
- **Symptomatic**

    Lumbar puncture: diagnostic, myelographic and spinal anaesthesia

    Traumatic: head or back trauma
       With CSF leak (dural tear, traumatic nerve root avulsion)
       Without CSF leak

    Postoperative: craniotomy, spinal surgery, post pneumonectomy (thoracoarachnoid fistula)
       With CSF leak
       Without CSF leak

    Spontaneous CSF leak: CSF rhinorrhoea, occult pituitary tumour, dural tear.

    Systemic illnesses: dehydration, diabetic coma, hyperpnoea, meningoencephalitis, uraemia, severe systemic infection.

Slowing of isotope flow, which is evidence for decreased CSF production, has also been reported.[36–39] This could lead to brain sagging with compression of the pituitary–hypothalamic axis and further reduction in CSF production.[38] Slit-like ventricles and tight basilar cisterns have been reported on computed tomographic (CT) scan in spontaneous intracranial hypotension, leading to speculation that this contributed to decreased CSF production.[40] However, small ventricles due to a compensatory increase in brain volume is most likely a result, rather than a cause, of decreased CSF production.

Many believe that occult CSF leakage is the major cause of idiopathic intracranial hypertension.[41] A history of minor trauma is often elicited.[42] In 39 Mayo Clinic cases, 52% had a history of minor trauma or an inciting event.[20] These included falling onto the buttocks,[43,44] a sudden twist or stretch,[41,45] sexual intercourse or orgasm,[46] a sudden sneeze or paroxysmal coughing,[47] vigorous exercise[48] or strenuous effort during racket sports.[49] Traumatic rupture of spinal epidural cysts (formed during development), perineural cysts, or a nerve sheath tear[16,35,41,42,44,49,50] could then produce a cryptic CSF leak. CSF can also leak into the petrous or ethmoidal regions[51] or through the cribriform, and the patient may swallow the fluid and be unaware of the leak.

The Mayo Clinic[20] series had an equal representation of men and women. The true incidence of spontaneous low CSF pressure headache is unknown. This syndrome is often under-recognized since the neurological examination is normal and headache is such a common complaint.

Headache is the most common complication of lumbar puncture, occurring in 15–30% of patients. Onset varies from 15 minutes to 4 days following lumbar puncture, but it can take as long as 12 days to manifest itself. If untreated, the headache can last 2–14 days (most commonly 4–8 days) or even months.[52]

The volume of CSF leakage after lumbar puncture, measured by MRI, does not correlate to the occurrence of post-lumbar puncture headache.[53] Post-lumbar puncture headache is more common in younger patients and in women, who are affected twice as often as men.[22,31,52,54,55,56] This sex difference is most marked in younger women in most, but not all, studies.[22] A lower incidence of post-lumbar puncture headache in patients with higher opening pressures has been reported but not confirmed.[55,56] Patients reporting headache before lumbar puncture were more likely to report post-lumbar puncture headache.[56] Race, quantity of CSF removed, a blood tap, multiple perforations of the dura, or the qualifications of the operator do not influence the incidence of post-lumbar puncture headache.[52,56] The incidence is dependent upon the type of procedure: surgical lumbar puncture, 13%; obstetrical, 18%, and diagnostic, 32%.[57] Torrey observed that post-lumbar puncture headache was rare among schizophrenic

• **Table 12.6** *Post-LP headache*

Contributing factors
Prior headache
Female sex
Type of procedure

Non-contributing factors
Race
Quantity of CSF removed
Bloody tap
Multiple perforations of the dura?
Qualifications of the operation?

patients, perhaps due to their insensitivity to pain.[58] This finding was not confirmed in another study.[59] A low frequency of post-lumbar puncture headache has been reported in demented patients (Table 12.6).[60]

Vilming has reported a 7% incidence of short duration, non-postural, post-lumbar puncture headache. This has not been included in past series of post-lumbar puncture headache, and it is uncertain whether this is a low-grade post-lumbar puncture headache or is totally unrelated.[55] Rare neurological sequelae include IIIrd, IVth, VIth and VIIIth nerve palsies causing diplopia, tinnitus and bilateral deafness.[61] Most patients with post-lumbar puncture headache improve spontaneously.

There is no evidence that post-lumbar puncture headache is prevented by keeping the patient supine after the lumbar puncture, keeping the patient prone after the lumbar puncture, removing the needle with the patient prone and head down, or maintaining adequate hydration.[2,22,52] In fact, prolonged recumbency may increase the risk of post-lumbar puncture headache.[56] Evidence suggests that using a small gauge needle (smaller than 22 gauge) may decrease the incidence of post-lumbar puncture headache in most[31,62,63,64] but not all[65] studies. However, it is very difficult to use this size needle for a diagnostic lumbar puncture. Recently a non-traumatic lumbar puncture needle has been used, which reportedly is associated with a low incidence of post-lumbar puncture headache.[66,67]

A distinction must be made between a patient with an orthostatic headache that is relieved by recumbency and a patient with a headache that is aggravated by movement or assuming the upright posture. If the headache is orthostatic and the patient does not have orthostatic hypotension, then the diagnosis is intracranial hypotension, the causes of which are listed in Table 12.5.

The diagnosis of low CSF pressure headache is easily made in the presence of orthostatic headache, particularly if there is an obvious aetiology, such as a recent lumbar puncture, head or back trauma, a recent craniotomy, or one of the associated medical illnesses (Table 12.5). If no obvious cause is apparent or the diagnosis is uncertain, lumbar puncture (perhaps at the time of cisternography) is indicated, following a neuroimaging procedure (CT or MRI). Lumbar punctures in these patients can be difficult with either traumatic or 'dry taps'. Some patients require cisternal taps for fluid collection. When the CSF pressure is below atmospheric pressure, a 'sucking noise' may be heard when the stylet is removed from the lumbar puncture needle, and air within the lateral ventricles may be visible on X-ray.[20] The opening pressure usually ranges from 0–70 mmH$_2$O. However, in the Mayo Clinic series in spontaneous intracranial hypotension, the opening pressure was at times in the normal range especially if the measurement was made after a period of recumbency.[20]

CSF analysis is benign in low-pressure headache. Common abnormalities include a moderate pleocytosis, the presence of red blood cells and elevated protein. The elevated protein may be due to disruption of normal hydrostatic and oncotic pressure across the venous sinus and arachnoid villi, resulting in the passage of serum protein into the CSF.[12,35,68]

If the cause of the low pressure is known, one should proceed with the appropriate treatment modalities. If, however, the aetiology is uncertain, one should proceed with radioisotope cisternography or ionic myelography to identify CSF leaks, which can be caused by a dural tear or nerve avulsion.[69] One should also search for occult CSF rhinorrhoea by examining the collection of radioisotope in the nose, through the use of numbered cotton pledgets. A radioactive tracer is instilled into the lumbar subarachnoid space. Its pattern of distribution is followed by scanning the entire neuraxis with a gamma camera at 4, 8 and 24 hours. CSF normally flows upward to the cerebral convexities and the sylvian fissures.[23] Early isotope accumulation in the bladder and kidneys or leakage outside the subarachnoid space is abnormal and should be looked for (Figure 12.6).

CSF hyperabsorption is one explanation for intracranial hypotension.[32,34,70] However, the early appearance of tracer in the bladder may be secondary to an occult CSF leak and not necessarily due to hyperabsorption.[35] Water-soluble myelography and CT-myelography have been used to help localize site(s) of CSF leakage, and still some leaks may be missed. Although CT-myelography has a somewhat higher yield, the yield of both of these studies may be suboptimal.[51] Non-ionic (pantopaque) myelography, which is no longer available, revealed dural tears even when cisternography and ionic myelography were normal. If no secondary cause is present and no dural leak can be demonstrated, spontaneous intracranial hypotension should be considered.[4,23,39,41,71] However, the inability to detect a leak despite early filling of the bladder does not necessarily mean the mechanism is hyperabsorption.

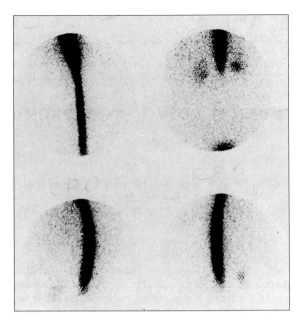

● **Figure 12.6.** *Scintigraph at 45 minutes showing early bladder and kidney uptake. No evidence of CSF leak. (Reproduced from ref. 23, with permission.)*

Neuroimaging

Both CT and MRI are useful in evaluating patients with low-pressure headache. Subdural haematomas due to tears in bridging veins have been associated with intracranial hypotension.[17,68]

Diffuse meningeal enhancement (DME) on enhanced gadolinium MRI has been reported by Mokri *et al.*[72] and others (Figure 12.7, Table 12.7).[18] Meningeal enhancement occurs with severe post-traumatic[73] positional,[16,17,74,75] spontaneous and post-lumbar puncture headache. One spontaneous case had a negative meningeal biopsy.[17] After the patient recovered, the meningeal enhancement disappeared.

Before DME was a recognized feature of spontaneous intracranial hypotension, patients often had extensive testing to rule out other causes of meningeal enhancement, such as meningeal carcinomatosis, meningitis, subarachnoid haemorrhage, neuroborreliosis and neurosarcoidosis.[72,74]

● **Table 12.7** *Diffuse meningeal enhancement*

- Both supra- and infratentorial
- Pachymeningeal
- No enhancement of depths or cortical sulci
- No brainstem enhancement

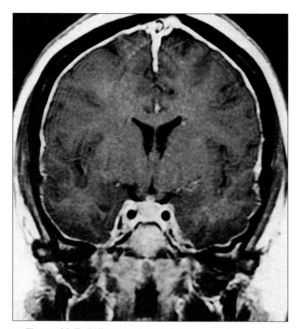

● *Figure 12.7* Diffuse meningeal enhancement.
(Reproduced from ref. 163, with permission.)

Meningeal enhancement could account for the low CSF pressure by enhancing arachnoid villi CSF transport. Meningeal inflammation could, in addition, produce pain in dilated venous sinuses. Meningeal (dural) enhancement may be secondary to venous dilatation as a consequence of reduced CSF volume. Venous engorgement would result in a greater concentration of gadolinium in the dural vasculature since dural microvessels lack tight junctions, unlike the arachnoid membranes that are part of the blood–brain barrier.

Based upon results of meningeal biopsy, some believe DME is due to inflammation of the pachymeninges,[15,73,74] while others have found normal results on meningeal biopsy.[17,18] Good and Ghobrial reported a case of intracranial hypotension with meningeal enhancement on gadolinium MRI.[15] A biopsy showed involvement of fibrocollagenous proliferation of the arachnoid, not the dura. Meningeal biopsies in nine Mayo Clinic patients did not show inflammatory changes.[20] Fishman and Dillon[16] believe that the meningeal fibrosis is a late manifestation of chronic venous congestion. DME may improve or resolve headache with resolution of the headache.[16,18,72,74,76]

Treatment

Many treatment modalities exist for intracranial hypotension, including bedrest, peripheral intravascular volume expansion, steroids, caffeine, blood patch, abdominal binder, and continuous intrathecal saline infusion (Table 12.8).[33,47,40,77,78,79,80] Treatment should be based on aetiology (Table 12.5). Any

associated illness should be treated and if a CSF leak exists, it should be treated appropriately and repaired if it is accessible and can be identified. The treatment of post-lumbar puncture headache and spontaneous intracranial hypotension are similar. Post-craniotomy hypotension will not be discussed.

Treatment of low CSF pressure headache begins with non-invasive therapeutic modalities (Table 12.8) of bedrest and an abdominal binder. If these modalities are prolonged, however, they are not cost-effective; therefore, if there is no improvement, intravenous or oral caffeine can be used and may produce significant relief.

Caffeine produces intracerebral arterial constriction, probably through blockade of brain adenosine receptors.[22] Caffeine sodium benzoate 500 mg intravenously was dramatically effective in 75% of patients with low CSF pressure who had undergone previous lumbar puncture.[77] A second dose 2 hours later raised the success rate to 85%. In an open study, 2 litres of intravenous Ringer's lactate solution containing 500 mg of caffeine sodium benzoate was given at a rate of 1 litre for the first hour and then 1 litre over 2 hours. Both could be repeated after 4 hours. The total response rate in 18 patients was 75%.[81]

In a placebo-controlled double-blind study, 40 postpartum patients were given oral caffeine (300 mg): 120% the dose of caffeine in caffeine sodium benzoate (250 mg caffeine, 250 mg sodium benzoate). Beneficial effects were rapid, with 70% of patients experiencing relief within 4 hours and no symptom recurrence.[82]

A brief trial of steroids and caffeine, bedrest or an abdominal binder, may be beneficial. If relief is not obtained within 24 hours, a quick steroid taper is recommended because of potential side effects. If the patient continues to be symptomatic after a non-invasive medical approach, a blood patch is indicated.

With a 90% success rate, the blood patch, originally described by Gormley in 1960, is the most successful treatment for low CSF pressure headache.[83–86] It is performed by infusing 10–20 ml of autologous blood in the epidural space under sterile conditions. A prospective study conducted to evaluate the efficacy of different volumes of blood found no difference between 10 ml and 10–15 ml of blood

● *Table 12.8* Treatment of low CSF headache

- Bedrest
- Abdominal binder
- Caffeine
- Steroids
- Epidural blood patch
- Continuous epidural saline infusion

(determined by patient height). The blood patch was initially successful in 91% of patients 2 hours after the procedure. Long-term, 87% were satisfied, but only 61% had both immediate and permanent relief. There was no difference depending on volume injected.[87] Many investigators have performed blood patches for spontaneous intracranial hypotension and have described similar results.

The presumed mechanism of action of the blood patch is an immediate gelatinous tamponade of a dural leak followed by fibrin deposition and fibroblastic activity. The blood patch can tolerate a pressure as high as 40 mmHg soon after coagulation.[87] Collagen deposition and scar formation are complete within three weeks. However, this mechanism has recently been challenged by several investigators who have noted a recurrence of orthostatic headache four to six months after a successful blood patch.[22] They propose that compression of the dural sac with an increment in CSF pressure may serve as a signal that de-activates the low CSF pressure headache, possibly by antagonizing adenosine receptors.[22]

MRI at 30 minutes and 3 hours has shown the extradural blood patch to have a mass effect, compressing the dural sac and displacing the conus medullaris and cauda equina(Figure 2.8). The main bulk of the clot occupied four or five vertebral levels, with a thinner spread cephalad and caudad. Initially some blood entered the CSF and changed the MRI signal, but this concentrated to a focal dural clot by 3 hours. After 7 hours, the mass effect had disappeared.[88]

If the headache of intracranial hypotension recurs, a repeat blood patch should be performed or a continuous intrathecal saline infusion attempted.[80,84] In the latter procedure, an epidural catheter is placed at the L2–3 level and a saline infusion begun at a rate of 20 ml/hour and continued for as long as 72 hours.

A retrospective study of 196 patients treated with the epidural blood patch revealed no major complications. Thirty-seven percent had pain at the injection site, 12% had leg pain, 10% had sensory disturbances in the lower extremities, 8% had gait disturbances and 8% had leg weakness. These symptoms were mild and transient.[89]

Increased intracrania pressure

Many disorders are associated with the syndrome of increased intracranial pressure (Table 12.9). It may be difficult to correlate the clinical features with the underlying pathological process, since increased intracranial pressure is not always associated with either headache or papilloedema, and no direct correlation exists between the degree of pressure elevation and the presence of headache. Headache does not usually occur with mild-to-moderate elevations of intracranial pressure when there is no associated traction or distortion of pain-sensitive structures; however, in at least two conditions (acute hydrocephalus and idiopathic intracranial hypertension) this is not the case.

Postulated mechanisms for headache are listed in Table 12.10. A convexity meningioma may distort the adjacent middle meningeal artery and cause pain, which may be referred to the ipsilateral frontotemporal region (Figure 12.9). A posterior fossa tumour may impinge upon the VIIth cranial nerve, producing a headache that is referred to the ipsilateral ear.

Although increased CSF pressure is not necessary for headache development, it clearly plays a role in some patients with CNS neoplasms, acute obstructive hydrocephalus, and idiopathic intracranial hypertension. The rate of the change in pressure may be critical. Sudden increases in intracranial pressure by tumours obstructing the foramen

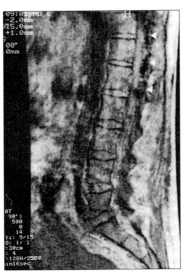

● **Figure 12.8** *Midline T1 weighted sagittal section (GE 500/14/90) after blood patch showing extensive blood clot displacing the conus medullaris and cauda equina anteriorly (Reproduced from ref. 164, with permission.)*

● **Table 12.9** *Syndromes of increased intracranial pressure*

Primary
Idiopathic intracranial hypertension with papilloedema
Idiopathic intracranial hypertension without papilloedema
Secondary
Hydrocephalus

Mass lesion
  neoplasm
    stroke – haematoma

Meningitis/encephalitis
Trauma
Major intracranial and extracranial venous obstruction
Drugs: vitamin A, nalidixic acid, anabolic steroids, steroid withdrawal
Systemic disease: renal disease, hypoparathyroidism, systemic lupus erythematosus

● **Table 12.10** *Mechanisms for headache with increased intracranial pressure*

- Traction on pain-sensitive intracerebral vessels (venous sinuses and arteries at the base of the brain)
- Transient herniation of hippocampal gyri
- Traction on cranial or cervical nerves, or elevation of intracranial pressure

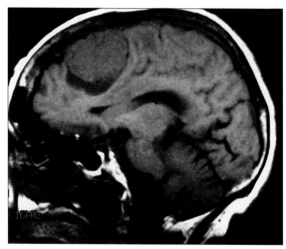

● **Figure 12.9** *Meningioma.*

of Monro or the cerebral aqueduct may cause abrupt, severe headache associated with gait disturbance, syncope, incontinence or visual obscurations.

Intracranial neoplasms

Headache occurs at presentation in up to half of patients with brain tumours and develops in the course of the disease in 60%. Headache is a rare initial symptom in patients with pituitary tumours, craniopharyngiomas or cerebellopontine angle tumours.[90,91] It is a very common initial symptom with infratentorial tumours (other than cerebellopontine angle tumours), occurring in 80–85% of patients.[92,93] Elevation of intracranial pressure is not necessary for its production. In one older, pre-CT series of 72 brain-tumour patients, headache occurred in those patients without elevated intracranial pressure as often as it did in those with increased intracranial pressure.[91] The headache is usually bilateral, but it can be on the side of the tumour.[90,91] Supratentorial tumours that impinge on structures innervated by the ophthalmic division of the Vth cranial nerve may produce frontotemporal headache, while posterior fossa tumours may compress the IXth and Xth cranial nerves and

produce occipitonuchal pain. Metastatic brain tumours may invade the meninges (meningeal carcinomatosis) and produce generalized headache and other signs of meningeal irritation. Occasionally, brain tumours produce a migraine-like headache, even with a visual aura.

One pre-CT/MRI series looked at the characteristic headache features of 221 patients who had brain tumours, only 60% of whom had headache. Tumour location had no significant bearing on the presence or absence of headache. Pain intensity was mild to moderate in 63% of patients and severe in 37%. The headaches were intermittent in 85%, throbbing in 15%, aggravated by changing position in 20%, by coughing or exertion in 25% and on the side of the tumour in 30%. Five patients had exertional headache. Half of the patients had nausea or vomiting. Twenty-five percent had headache during sleep, on arising, or both. Increased intracranial pressure was observed in 42% of patients with headache and in 6% of patients without headache.[94]

In a survey of 778 patients with cerebral tumour, headache was the earliest or principal symptom in 54%. No difference in headache frequency was noted between rapidly-growing and slow-growing tumours. The headache could occur intermittently and mimic migraine.[95]

In a modern series of 111 consecutive patients with primary (34%) or metastatic (66%) brain tumour, diagnosis was based on neuroimaging. Increased intracranial pressure was defined by the presence of papilloedema, obstructive hydrocephalus, communicating hydrocephalus from leptomeningeal metastasis or a lumbar puncture opening pressure >250 mm of CSF. Headache was present in 48% of both primary and metastatic tumours. It was similar to tension-type headache (TTH) in 77%, to migraine in 9% and to other headache types in 14%. Unlike true TTH, brain-tumour headaches were worsened by bending in 32%, and nausea or vomiting was present in 40%.[96]

Patients with increased intracranial pressure usually had headaches (86%) that were typically frontal in location and pressure-like or aching in character. Only 1% of patients had a unilateral headache. The headache was constant in 61%. The pain was severe in intensity, associated with nausea and vomiting, and resistant to common analgesics. Ataxia was present in 61%. In contrast, only 36% of patients with a supratentorial tumour without increased intracranial pressure had headaches. These headaches were milder and more likely to be intermittent (however, they were constant in 20% of patients). Nausea, vomiting, and ataxia were much less common.[96]

Patients with a history of prior headache were more likely to have brain tumour headache. In many cases this headache was similar in character to the prior headache, but it was more severe, more frequent, or associated with neurologic signs or symptoms.

In another modern prospective study of patients with brain tumour, only 8% had headache as their first and isolated clinical manifestation at the time of diagnosis. Thirty-one percent had headache, but only one of the original patients continued to have headache as an isolated symptom.[97] The prevalence of headache as an initial symptom of brain tumour has decreased in many series due to earlier detection by neuroimaging.

Headaches are a more common symptom of brain tumour in children (over 90%) than in adults (ca. 60%), due in part, perhaps, to the greater prevalence of posterior fossa tumours.[98] The following characteristics occur frequently: headache awakening the child from sleep or present on awakening, severe or prolonged headache, increased severity or frequency of headache and increased frequency of vomiting. Most children (94%) with headache had neurological signs. In 96%, diagnostic clues appeared within four months of the onset of headache.[99]

Rossi and Vassella[100] compared 600 children with migraine to 67 children with brain tumours. Characteristic features in the brain-tumour group were nocturnal headache or headache present on arising, both associated with vomiting and increased headache frequency. These symptoms were present in 32% of the brain-tumour group and 10% of the childhood migraine group. Nocturnal headache or headache present on arising associated with vomiting or progressive neurological symptoms or signs occurred in 65/67 children with brain tumour within two months of the onset of their headaches.

Zammarano[101] found 5 of 2416 tumour patients who presented with migraine-like headache without other signs of tumour. As changes in cognition may be the first sign of tumour, children with headache must be observed long enough to establish that they have normal growth and intellectual and motor development.

In Kennedy and Nathwanil's[102] brain-tumour series, headache was the presenting symptom in 53% of children, but most had other symptoms and signs as well, and 46% had papilloedema. The median duration of headache before tumour diagnosis in these children was five months.[103] In this series, brain-tumour headache could mimic migraine or tension-type headaches, sometimes for years.

In 1991, the Childhood Brain Tumor Consortium published their retrospective record review on the incidence of headache in children with CNS tumours. The overall incidence of headache was 62%, ranging from 70% with infratentorial lesions, to 58% with supratentorial tumours, to 35% in patients with spinal canal tumours, approximately the incidence of benign headache in elementary school children. Headache was typically associated with other signs or symptoms and was rarely an isolated symptom (<1%). Symptoms of intracranial tumour included abnormal academic performance, difficulty walking, back or abdominal pain, bladder symptoms, increasing head circumference and failure to thrive. Headache frequency increased through age seven and leveled off regardless of tumour location. The low percentage of headache in the very young may be due to the expansile nature of the infant skull or may be an artifact of the inability of young children to communicate the source of their discomfort.[104]

Following successful combined whole brain radiotherapy and chemotherapy of their posterior fossa or pineal tumours (actually 14–32 months after termination of therapy), four children developed episodic, severe hemicranial headaches associated with nausea and transient visual loss, hemisensory deficit, dysphasia or hemiparesis.[105] These children had no prior history of similar headaches, no family history of migraine and no evidence of tumour recurrence. It is unclear what produces these migrainous manifestations. The occurrence of headaches in treated brain-tumour patients does not necessarily mean tumour recurrence.

There is a significant overlap between the headache of brain tumour and that of migraine or TTH. A headache of recent onset, a headache that has changed in character or a headache accompanied by a neurological sign or symptom that cannot be easily explained by the aura of migraine requires a thorough evaluation, particularly if the headache is severe or occurs with nausea or vomiting. Morning or nocturnal headache associated with vomiting and increased headache frequency can be seen with both migraine and brain tumour. Brain tumour headache is more common in patients with a history of prior headache, increased intracranial pressure and large tumours with a midline shift (Figure 12.10).

In other space-occupying lesions such as subdural haematomas and brain abscesses, headache is an earlier and more frequent symptom. Eighty-one percent of McKissock's[106] 216 patients with chronic subdural haematoma had headache; only 11% of acute, and 53% of subacute, subdural haematoma patients had headache. The difference in headache prevalence between tumour and subdural haematoma is believed to be due to the more rapid evolution and greater extent of the haematomas. The lesser occurrence of headache in acute and subacute subdural haematomas compared with chronic subdural haematoma may be due to the underlying traumatic cerebral changes in the former, obtunding consciousness early and making it difficult to elicit a history of headache (Figure 12.11).

In brain abscesses, a progressively severe, intractable headache is common. In published clinical series, headache was present in 70–90% of patients (Figure 12.12).[107] The higher headache prevalence in patients with abscesses, compared to tumours, may be due to the faster evolution, the associated meningeal reaction, and the occasional low-grade fever that may accompany abscess (see Chapter 14).

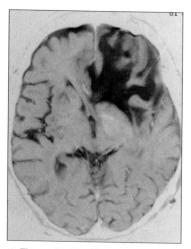

● *Figure 12.10* Glioma.

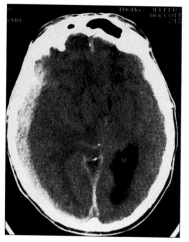

● *Figure 12.11* Subdural haematoma.

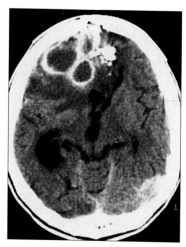

● *Figure 12.12* Brain abscess.

Intracranial hypertension

Intracranial hypertension may be either *idiopathic*, with no clear identifiable cause, or *symptomatic*, a result of venous sinus occlusion, radical neck dissection, hypoparathyroidism, vitamin A intoxication, systemic lupus, renal disease or drug side effects (nalidixic acid, danocrine, steroid withdrawal) (Table 12.9).[128]

The syndrome of idiopathic intracranial hypertension, also known as 'pseudotumour cerebri' or 'benign intracranial hypertension', is a condition of increased intracranial pressure of unknown cause that occurs predominantly in obese women of childbearing age (Table 12.11). Definitive diagnosis cannot be made without excluding brain tumours and other intracranial mass lesions, infections, hypertensive encephalopathy, pulmonary encephalopathy (related to chronic carbon dioxide toxicity), and obstruction of the cerebral ventricles. The adjective 'benign' is no longer employed because, although spontaneous recovery usually occurs, this is not invariable and, indeed, permanent visual loss may occur. In fact, visual loss occurs in 80% of patients and blindness occurs in 10%.[108,109] The symptoms of idiopathic intracranial hypertension are those of generalized increased intracranial pressure, with headache occurring in most, but not all, patients. Idiopathic intracranial hypertension can cause unilateral, bilateral, frontal or occipital headache, although bifrontotemporal headache is the most common.[110] Unilateral headache with increased CSF pressure due to idiopathic intracranial hypertension may be an exacerbation of a migraine diathesis or a new local phenomenon. Transient visual obscuration (TVO),[111] an episode of visual clouding in one or both eyes, usually lasting seconds, occurs with all forms of increased intracranial pressure with papilloedema but is not a specific symptom. TVO can occur in patients without increased intracranial pressure who have elevated optic discs from other causes, such as disc oedema, nerve sheath tumour, drusen or coloboma. Other common symptoms include pulsatile tinnitus, diplopia and visual loss. Some patients report shoulder and arm pain (perhaps secondary to nerve root dilatation) and retroorbital pain.[108] Signs include papilloedema and VIth nerve palsy.

Idiopathic intracranial hypertension occurs with a frequency of about 1 case per 100 000 per year in the general population and 19.3 cases per 100 000 per year in obese women aged 20–44 years.[112] The patient with idiopathic intracranial hypertension is commonly a young, obese woman with chronic daily headaches, normal laboratory studies, a normal neurological examination (except for papilloedema) and an empty sella (Table 12.11, Figures 12.13 and 12.14).

● *Table 12.11* Features of idiopathic intracranial hypertension

- Headache: chronic tension type headache with migrainous features, may be present upon awakening. Can be intermittent or absent.

- Associated features: pulsatile tinnitus, transient visual obscurations, diplopia, visual loss, shoulder and arm pain.

- Patients: predominantly obese women aged 20–50 years.

- Physical and neurological exam: within normal limits, except for papilloedema, visual loss, obesity, and a VIth nerve palsy.

- Neuroradiology: CT or MRI show no evidence of intracranial mass, hydrocephalus, or venous sinus thrombosis. (Empty sella may be present.)

- Lumbar puncture: demonstrates increased CSF pressure with a normal composition. (May show decreased protein.)

- No other causes of increased CSF pressure present

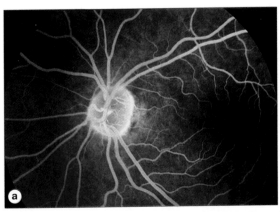
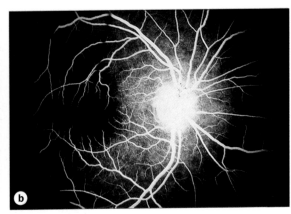

● **Figure 12.13** *Fluoroscein angiography of fundi. (a) Normal. (b) Papilloedema.*

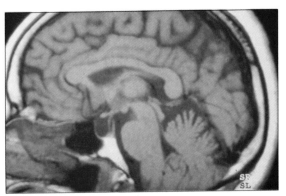

● **Figure 12.14** *Empty sella.*

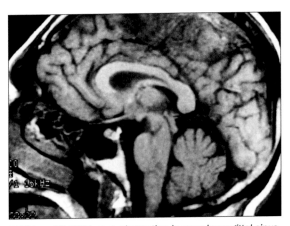

● **Figure 12.15** *Venous obstruction in superior sagittal sinus.*

There is no evidence to associate idiopathic intracranial hypertension with pregnancy, hypertension, diabetes, thyroid disease, iron-deficiency anaemia or the use of tetracyclines or oral contraceptives. Arterial hypertension may be overreported in patients with idiopathic intracranial hypertension if a large blood pressure cuff is not used for obese patients.[108]

Symptomatic intracranial hypertension can be secondary to changes in cranial venous outflow, which may influence intracranial pressure by:

- increasing cerebral blood volume,
- producing brain oedema, and
- impairing CSF absorption.

Intracranial venous outflow obstruction can be caused by chronic otitis, head trauma, tumours, hypercoaguable states and cerebral oedema.[113] Extracranial venous outflow obstruction occurs with surgical ligation and further compression of venous outflow. Cranial venous outflow hypertension can also occur without obstruction in patients with arteriovenous malformations, cardiac failure and pulmonary failure.

The pathophysiology of idiopathic intracranial hypertension is unknown. Postulated mechanisms are listed in Table 12.12. Some studies suggest that interstitial brain oedema and a decreased rate of absorption at the arachnoid villi are the major contributors.[114–122] The disturbances of CSF hydrodynamics in idiopathic intracranial hypertension persist for years.[123]

Malm et al.[123] believe that increased CSF pressure in idiopathic intracranial hypertension is a result of either a rise in venous sagittal sinus pressure secondary to extracellular oedema causing venous obstruction or a low conductance for CSF reabsorption producing a compensatory increase in CSF pressure. King et al.[124] evaluated nine idiopathic intracranial hypertension patients with cerebral venography and manometry. Elevated venous pressure was found in the superior sagittal and proximal transverse sinuses, which dropped at the level of the lateral third of the transverse sinus. The abnormality, not as well demonstrated on venography, resembled mural thrombosis. Two patients with intracranial hypertension due to minocycline did not have venous hypertension. The authors suggested that most patients with idiopathic intracranial hypertension may have partial venous outflow obstructions,[124] blurring the distinction between idiopathic and symptomatic causes (Figure 12.15).

Karakalios *et al.*[125] studied ten patients with idiopathic intracranial hypertension using angiography and manometry. Five patients had dural venous outflow obstruction on venography while five had normal anatomy. Pressure was elevated in the superior sagittal sinus in all patients. In those with obstruction, there was a high-pressure gradient across the stenosis. In those without obstruction, the right atrial pressure was elevated. Angioplasty or infusion of thrombolytic agents improved outlet obstruction but not the clinical picture. The authors suggested that elevated intracranial venous pressure may be the universal mechanism of idiopathic intracranial hypertension, and that all cases are symptomatic. Our major concern with this observation is the absence of any sign of right heart failure in the patients with elevated right atrial pressure.

Headache due to idiopathic intracranial hypertension occurs in about 75% of idiopathic cases. It is more common in patients who present to neurologists (in Weisberg's series 100% had headache) than in those who present to ophthalmologists with visual loss or to otolaryngologists with tinnitus.[126] Patients with idiopathic intracranial hypertension are, on the whole, not particularly ill although their headaches may be very severe. Somnolence, fever, or other systemic symptoms should suggest venous sinus occlusion or some other cause of increased pressure. If the patient has been headache prone in the past, the headaches of idiopathic intracranial hypertension may be qualitatively similar but more constant and more severe than the prior headache. In patients with idiopathic intracranial hypertension, the headaches are usually daily and continuous and qualify for the designation of chronic daily headache.

Wall *et al.* described the headache of idiopathic intracranial hypertension. Ninety-three percent of patients described their headache as the most severe ever.[110] Chronic daily headache present upon awakening and pulsating in character, retro-ocular pain with eye movement, and associated symptoms of nausea, vomiting and pulsatile tinnitus were common features.

Most of the patients were women (93%) and obese (93%). The mean age was 31 years. Headache was reported by 92%. Of those, 73% had chronic daily headache, 93%

said it was the most severe ever, and 83% said it was pulsatile. Nausea occurred in 57%, vomiting in 38%, and orbital pain in 43%. TVO was present in 71%, diplopia in 38% and visual loss in 31%.[110]

Pain on eye movement, while not a common feature of migraine, occurs in up to 20% of patients with idiopathic intracranial hypertension.[108,110] The typical ocular pain is retrobulbar and bilateral, in contrast to the unilateral pain on eye movement associated with visual loss that occurs with optic neuritis.

Another feature of idiopathic intracranial hypertension is a cranial bruit that may be audible to observers. This pulse-synchronous, pulsatile noise stops with carotid compression and is a common reason for otolaryngologic consultation. The bruit is caused by turbulence in the major venous sinuses. It may be soft-or high-pitched and is best auscultated with the bell over the mastoid or the temporalis with the mouth held open.[127]

Occasionally while being examined for another purpose patients with idiopathic intracranial hypertension are incidentally found to have papilloedema. Five to 10% of patients are essentially asymptomatic.[128] Loss of visual field and visual acuity are the only significant complications of idiopathic intracranial hypertension with papilloedema. Ophthalmological examination should include intraocular pressure, visual fields (Goldmann or Humphrey), optic disc photos, visual acuity and a search for a relative afferent pupil.[128]

Idiopathic intracranial hypertension without papilloedema

Intracranial hypertension can occur without papilloedema.[129,130,131,132] The clinical, historical, radiographic and demographic characteristics are identical to patients with papilloedema except for:

- possible association with prior head trauma or meningitis,
- extended delay in diagnosis, which requires lumbar puncture in the absence of papilloedema, and
- no evidence of visual loss as seen in patients with idiopathic intracranial hypertension with papilloedema.

Patients, particularly obese women, with chronic daily headache and symptoms of increased intracranial pressure, i.e. pulsatile tinnitus, a history of head trauma or meningitis, an empty sella on neuroimaging studies, or a headache that is unrelieved by standard therapy, should have a diagnostic lumbar puncture.

● **Table 12.12** *Pathophysiology of idiopathic intracranial hypertension*

- Increased rate of CSF formation
- Increased intracranial venous pressure
- Decreased rate of CSF absorption
- Increase in brain interstitial fluid (oedema)

Why there is no papilloedema in these cases of intracranial hypertension is not known. Congenital or acquired optic nerve sheath defects, 'chronic idiopathic intracranial hypertension' with resolution of papilloedema, or early idiopathic intracranial hypertension are alternative explanations.

In a spinal fluid examination study of 85 patients with refractory transformed migraine, 12 patients had elevated CSF pressures ranging from 230–450 mmH$_2$O.[133] Ten of the twelve were women and half were obese. This observation supports our position that a subset of patients with chronic daily headache, who fit the stereotype of the obese female of childbearing age, may have idiopathic intracranial hypertension without papilloedema. These patients may respond to CDH treatment, but often, although not always, respond better if the elevated CSF pressure is treated. These patients would not have been identified without a lumbar puncture.[134]

Treatment

The treatment of elevated intracranial pressure depends on the underlying cause. In many cases, the history, clinical examination and neuroradiographical studies may define the syndrome, with distinctive therapy preceding any further diagnostic studies. Thus, AVM, abscess, cerebral neoplasm, cerebral infarct, acute meningitis, subarachnoid haemorrhage, subdural haematoma, and acute obstructive hydrocephalus may be treated with appropriate surgical (drainage, shunt) or medical (antibiotics, hyperventilation, steroids, hypertonic osmotic diuretics) intervention.

In patients with idiopathic intracranial hypertension (with or without papilloedema), chronic meningitis, and some cases of subarachnoid haemorrhage, diagnosis is based on lumbar puncture following neuroimaging (paying attention to empty sella and sinus thrombosis). If lumbar puncture is unremarkable and intracranial pressure is elevated to greater than 200 mmH$_2$O (in nonobese subjects), then idiopathic intracranial hypertension is the likely diagnosis. Routine blood chemistries (PT, PTT, ANA, VDRL,chemistry profile, thyroxine, and thyroid-stimulating hormone) are helpful.

Once the diagnosis of idiopathic intracranial hypertension is made, secondary causes should be sought and eliminated. Over fifty diseases, conditions, toxins or pharmaceuticals have been associated with idiopathic intracranial hypertension. Obese patients should be encouraged to lose weight. If the patient is asymptomatic and has no visual loss, then no treatment is indicated, but careful ophthalmologic follow-up is needed. If there is no papilloedema, or papilloedema with no visual loss, and the only complaint is headache, then it should be treated aggressively.

Headache associated with idiopathic intracranial hypertension and papilloedema frequently responds to standard headache treatment (Table 12.13). Surgical treatment of idiopathic intracranial hypertension has been directed towards preventing visual loss secondary to papilloedema. Improvement in headache occurs in many patients with optic nerve sheath fenestration.

If rigorous headache therapy is unsuccessful, or if there is visual loss, then a four to six week trial of furosemide or a potent carbonic anhydrase inhibitor (acetazolamide) should be given. The starting dose is 500 mg twice daily, which can even be increased to ≥ 2 g daily. Side effects include nausea, depression, acral and perioral numbness and tingling, and renal stones. Rare cases of hepatic failure have been reported. Patients thus treated develop a compensated metabolic acidosis, which serves as a marker of compliance. Furosemide (40–160 mg/day) with potassium supplementation may also reduce the headache.[128] These drugs decrease elevated intracranial pressure. The use of high dose steroids (prednisone or dexamethasone) is controversial but may be effective in idiopathic intracranial hypertension. Rebound headache is common when steroids are withdrawn.

Lumbar puncture typically relieves headache in idiopathic intracranial hypertension. Occasionally a post-lumbar puncture headache will occur. The failure of headache to improve following the first or subsequent lumbar puncture may be because the headache is generated by a mechanism other than elevated CSF pressure or a venous sinus occlusion. In some of our intractable headache patient's there is a dissociation between the CSF pressure and the headache. At times, lumbar puncture reduces the pressure and relieves the headache, and at other times there is no improvement. Since CSF is rapidly replaced, prolonged symptomatic relief may reflect a persistent CSF leak. Alternatively, transient reduction of CSF pressure may allow decompression of the arachnoid villi, allowing for prolonged enhanced CSF absorption. Patients with idiopathic intracranial hypertension who have visual loss or a severe incapacitating headache that does not respond to medical therapy or repeated lumbar puncture may need surgical management.

● **Table 12.13** Treatment of idiopathic intracranial hypertension

- Eliminate symptomatic causes
- Weight loss if obese
- Standard headache treatment
- Carbonic anhydrase inhibitors and loop diuretics
- Short course of high dose corticosteroids
- Serial lumbar punctures
- Lumboperitoneal or ventriculoperitoneal shunt
- Optic nerve sheath fenestration

Some suggest treating idiopathic intracranial hypertension with a lumboperitoneal shunt, but this has a high re-operation rate and the potential for development of hindbrain herniation and a new headache. Others believe ventriculoperitoneal shunt is the preferred shunting procedure. Eggenberger *et al.*[135] retrospectively reviewed the efficacy of lumboperitoneal shunt in 27 patients with idiopathic intracranial hypertension. A functioning shunt always alleviated symptoms. None of the patients had low pressure headache or abdominal pain for the first two months. However, 56% required shunt revision. There were no major complications other than shunt failure. In the series, 67% of the patients were shunted for intractable headache; all had headache improvement or relief postoperatively. Shunt revision was performed for obstruction (in 65% of patients) or secondary intracranial hypotension (in 15.1%). Two patients had asymptomatic tonsillar herniation, neither of whom were re-operated.

Optic nerve sheath fenestration (ONSF) entails surgical incision of the dura covering the intraorbital optic nerve. The proposed mechanism is improved optic nerve axoplasmic flow and continuous intraorbital CSF drainage; 65–76% get relief of medically-uncontrolled headache with ONSF. Although ONSF has been performed on patients with unilateral papilloedema, to our knowledge it is untried in patients with idiopathic intracranial hypertension without papilloedema. Without threatened vision loss, the small risk of visual loss due to the surgery probably outweighs the potential benefits.

Exertional and cough headaches

Although coughing and exertion rarely provoke headache, these manoeuvres can aggravate any type of headache. However, transient, severe head pain upon coughing, sneezing, weight-lifting, bending, straining at stool or stooping, defines cough headache. Originally described by Tinel[136] in 1932 as '*la céphalée à l'effort*' and later by Symond,[137] cough headache mainly affects middle-aged men. It runs its course over a few years, and is uncommon in the clinic: only 93 diagnoses were made at the Mayo Clinic over a 14-year period by Rooke.[138] He proposed the broader term 'benign exertional headache' for any headache that is precipitated by exertion, has an acute onset, and is unassociated with structural central nervous system disease, thus combining cough and exertional headache. In a population-based study,[139] benign cough headache and benign exertional headache each had a prevalence of about 1%.

The most recent classification of these disorders was done by the International Headache Society (IHS)[1] (Tables 12.14 and 12.15). The IHS separates 'benign cough headache' and 'benign exertional headache', since these entities have different clinical features, diagnostic evaluations, and treatment responses.[140,141]

Headache associated with sexual activity describes bilateral headaches precipitated by masturbation or coitus, also in the absence of any intracranial disorder. Benign sexual headache is now a well-defined entity with three types recognized in the IHS classification (Table 12.16).[1] They are described according to the presumed clinical pathophysiological mechanism. The most frequent, type 2, begins suddenly at the time of orgasm and is thought to be related to haemodynamic changes. It is often associated with exertional headache.

● **Table 12.14** *Benign cough headache*

- Benign cough headache is a bilateral headache of sudden onset, lasting less than one minute, precipitated by coughing.
- It may be prevented by avoiding coughing.
- It may be diagnosed only after structural lesions such as posterior fossa tumour have been excluded by neuroimaging.

● **Table 12.15** *Benign exertional headache*

- Benign exertional headache is specifically brought on by physical exercise.
- It is bilateral, throbbing in nature at onset, and may develop migrainous features in patients susceptible to migraine.
- It lasts from 5 minutes to 24 hours.
- It is prevented by avoiding excessive exertion, particularly in hot weather or at high altitude.
- It is not associated with any systemic or intracranial disorder.

● **Table 12.16** *Headache associated with sexual activity*

Headache is:
- precipitated by sexual excitement
- bilateral at onset
- prevented or eased by ceasing sexual activity before orgasm
- not associated with any intracranial disorder such as aneurysm.

Dull type
  A dull ache in the head and neck that intensifies as sexual excitement increases.

Explosive type
  A sudden severe ('explosive') headache occurring at orgasm.

Postural type
  Postural headache resembling that of low CSF pressure developing after coitus.

Benign cough headache

This is infrequent. The mean age of onset is 55 years, with a range of 19 to 73 years. It is twice as common in patients over 40 years of age and is four times more common in men than in women.[138] The pain begins immediately[137,142] or within seconds after coughing, sneezing or a Valsava manoeuvre (lifting, straining at stool, blowing, crying or singing).[136,143,144] The pain is severe in intensity, with a bursting, explosive or splitting quality that lasts a few seconds or minutes. The headache is usually bilateral, with maximal pain at the vertex or in the occipital, frontal or temporal region. Bending the head or lying down may be impossible.[145] The headache is not generally associated with nausea or vomiting and the neurological examination is usually normal. Vomiting suggests an organic basis for the headache.[141] As many as 25% of cases have an antecedent respiratory infection.[137,138,146] Most patients are pain-free between attacks of head pain, but in some cases the paroxysms are followed by dull, aching pain that may persist for hours; 5 of the 21 patients reported by Symonds had such additional headaches.[137] As these patients often express their complaint as a continuous headache, they should be asked directly about the role of exertion as a trigger factor.

Symptomatic cough headache

Age at onset is significantly lower for symptomatic cough headache than for benign cough headache (Table 12.17) Pascual *et al.* found that symptomatic cough headache could be precipitated by laughing, weight-lifting or acute body or head postural changes in addition to coughing. Symptomatic cough headache can be caused by hindbrain abnormalities, posterior fossa meningioma, midbrain cysts, basilar impression, acoustic neurinoma and brain tumour such as Arnold–Chiari malformation.[147,148,149] In the Pascual *et al.* series, headache was the only symptom, at first, of Arnold–Chiari type I malformation in three patients; however, all patients had or eventually developed posterior fossa signs or syringomyelia. Besides beginning earlier in life than benign cough headache, symptomatic cough headache does not respond to indomethacin. If a patient does not respond to indomethacin, has posterior fossa signs, or is younger than 50 years, MRI must be done.

Cough headache can be confused with other disorders, such as exertional headache, effort migraine and coital headache.[146,150] In fact, 40% of patients with coital headache of the vascular type had exertional headache, suggesting a relationship between these entities.[151]

Benign exertional headache

This begins significantly earlier than benign cough headache ($P < 0.005$), by almost 40 years. It is typically throbbing, lasts from 5 minutes to 24 hours and is provoked by physical exercise. The pain usually begins during exertion, is non-explosive, and can be either bilateral or unilateral.

Symptomatic exertional headache

Symptomatic exertional headache is usually explosive in onset, severe, and bilateral. Twelve of the Pascual *et al.* patients presented because of acute headache that coincided with physical exercise. Aetiologies included SAH, sinusitis and brain mass.

● **Table 12.17 Cough, exertional and sexual headache**

Parameter	Cough headache		Exertional headache		Sexual headache	
	Benign	Symptomatic	Benign	Symptomatic	Benign	Symptomatic
Patients (n)	13	17	16	12	13	1
Age, range (years)	67 ± 11, 44–81	39 ± 14, 15–63	24 ± 11, 10–48	42 ± 14, 18–61	41 ± 9, 24–57	60
Sex (% men)	77	59	88	43	85	100
Duration	Secs to 30 min	Seconds to days	Min to 2 days	1 day to 1 month	1 min to 3 hours	10 days
Bilateral localization	92%	94%	56%	100%	77%	Yes
Quality	Sharp, stabbing	Bursting, stabbing	Pulsating	Explosive, pulsating	Explosive + pulsating	Explosive + pulsating
Other manifestations	No	Posterior fossa signs	Nausea, photophobia	Nausea, vomiting, double vision, neck rigidity	None	Vomiting, neck rigidity
Diagnosis	Idiopathic	Chiari Type I malformation	Idiopathic	SAH, sinusitis, brain metastases	Idiopathic	SAH

Modified from Pascual et al.[140]

Benign sexual headache

Benign sexual headache (type 2) begins later than benign exertional headache and earlier than benign cough headache. The headache is usually bilateral, but it can be unilateral. It is usually severe and explosive with occasional throbbing and stabbing. Its duration varies, lasting from <1 minute to 3 hours (average 30 minutes). The frequency of the episodes was directly related to that of sexual intercourse or masturbation. Up to one-third of patients have similar episodes with physical exertion.

Symptomatic sexual headache

Explosive headache that occurs during coitus, is usually symptomatic of a subarachnoid haemorrhage (SAH).

Rooke[138] followed 103 patients who had exertional headache but no detectable intracranial disease on initial examination. After three or more years of follow-up, 10 patients subsequently developed organic intracranial lesions; 30 of the remaining 93 had complete headache relief within five years. The remainder improved or were headache-free after 10 years. This pre-CT era study emphasizes the importance of careful evaluation for organic disease.

Apart from that of Rooke,[138] the largest series of headaches of sudden onset provoked by cough, physical exercise or sexual excitement was performed by Pascual et al.[140] Benign and symptomatic cases differed in several clinical aspects. Symptomatic cough headache began earlier in life, tended to last longer, and was more frequent than benign cough headache. Chiari type I malformation was the only cause. SAH, sinusitis and brain metastases were the causes of symptomatic exertional headache.

Of the 219 cases of exertional and cough headache reviewed by Sands et al.,[141] 48 had an identifiable organic aetiology. Table 12.18 (adapted from Sands et al.) summarizes cases of cough and exertional headache, grouping together aetiologically-related cases from several selected series. The group with posterior fossa space-occupying lesions includes cases with Arnold–Chiari deformity and hindbrain herniation. Post-traumatic and postcraniotomy cases were also grouped together. From his review one cannot accurately estimate how many patients with exertional headache have structural disease.[136–138,142,144,145,150,147,152–154]

Symptomatic exertional and sexual headaches began later in life and lasted longer than benign exertional and sexual headaches. Male predominance was not present in the symptomatic exertional headache group. Furthermore, all patients with symptomatic headaches had manifestations of meningeal irritation or intracranial hypertension. Patients with subarachnoid bleeding had only had one headache episode. Although neuroradiological studies could be avoided in cases with clinically typical benign sexual or exertional headaches (men around the third decade of life, with a normal examination and short-duration, multiple episodes of pulsating pain that responded to ergotamine or to preventive beta-blockers), the remaining patients must have a brain CT (and a CSF examination if the CT scan is normal).

Benign cough headache and benign exertional headache are separate conditions. Besides the different precipitants (sudden Valsalva manoeuvres and sustained physical exercise respectively), benign cough headache begins later than benign exertional headache. Cough headache starts 43 years later, on average, than exertional headache, and while the youngest patient with benign cough headache in the Pascual series was 44 years old, the oldest patient with benign exertional headache was 48 years. Benign cough headache tended to be shorter than benign exertional headache and the pain quality and response to treatment were different. Benign cough headache was described as sharp or stabbing and responsive to indomethacin, whereas benign exertional headache was pulsating, tending to last longer and improving with ergotamine or propranolol. It is not uncommon for patients to experience both benign sexual headache and benign exertional headache; this occurred in 31% of patients in the Pascual et al. series.

Other types of headache may be exacerbated by exertion. Severe migraine, post-lumbar puncture headache, and, rarely, idiopathic intracranial hypertension may be aggravated by coughing.[155] Paroxysmal headache may also occur in patients with IIIrd ventricular colloid cysts, which may produce intermittent obstruction of cerebrospinal fluid (CSF) flow through the foramen of Monroe resulting in abrupt increases of intracranial pressure. Similar headache has also been experienced by patients who have lateral ventricular tumours, craniopharyngiomas, pinealomas and tumours of the cerebellum and cerebrum. Phaeochromocytomas[155,156] may also cause paroxysmal headache, especially during exercise. In Rooke's series of 303 patients with intracranial lesions, however, none

Table 12.18 Aetiologies for cough and exertional headache in literature[141]

Condition	Patients, n (%)
Structural (organic)	48
Posterior fossa space-occupying lesions	18 (37.5)
After trauma or after craniotomy	13 (27.0)
Supratentorial space-occupying lesions	9 (18.7)
Basilar impression/platybasia	6 (12.5)
Syrinx	2 (4.2)
Benign exertional headache	171
Total	**219**

of the 27 patients with an unruptured cerebral aneurysm or vascular anomaly complained of exertional headache.

Van den Bergh[157] reported two patients with Arnold–Chiari malformation who had headache paroxysms brought on by coughing, sneezing and laughing. In Arnold–Chiari malformation, a ball-valve mechanism may be responsible for CSF passing more easily from the spine to the cranium than vice versa. Lumbar CSF pressure waves following a cough occur sooner and rise higher than cisternal pressure waves; the lumbar pressure waves also fall sooner and lower. Therefore, there is a phase during which the lumbar pressure exceeds the cisternal pressure, followed by a phase in which the cisternal pressure is greater than the lumbar pressure; this is aggravated by the ball-valve effect and can produce cough headache.[159,160]

Stevens et al.[161] retrospectively studied 141 patients with adult Arnold–Chiari malformation (defined as descent of the hindbrain into the cervical canal, with meningomyelocele absent and hydrocephalus rare). Headache was present in 41 patients and was considered a symptom only if it was exacerbated by head movement, exercise or coughing.

Outcomes of pre-operative cough and posture-related headache showed no relationship to tonsillar descent or any other imaging parameter, including the size of the cisterna magna, yet the latter feature was significantly improved in 62.6% of cases. Posture- and cough-related headache, like drop attacks, are thought to result from intermittent tonsillar impaction in the foramen magnum. Therefore, the lack of association of such features with small or obliterated cisterna magna or low-lying tonsils both pre- and postoperatively suggests that the origin of these symptoms is more complex.[161]

The long-term outlook for these patients is favourable. If the headaches are frequent or severe, prophylactic therapy is required, as the short duration of the headaches renders abortive therapy impractical. Some patients respond dramatically to indomethacin in doses of 25–150 mg daily.[145] If there is gastrointestinal intolerance to indomethacin, concomitant treatment with misoprostol, sulcralfate or antacids may be helpful. When indomethacin fails, Raskin[146] reports that naproxen, ergonovine and phenelzine are useful, but propranolol is not.

Symonds[137] performed four lumbar punctures or pneumoencephalograms on each of 21 patients with benign cough headache syndrome. One patient developed a typical post-lumbar puncture headache following the lumbar puncture, but her cough headache syndrome remitted for three weeks, and then recurred. Some patients with benign cough headache respond to lumbar puncture to treat the disorder.[162]

References

1. International Headache Society. Classification and diagnostic criteria for headache disorders, cranial neuralgias, and facial pain. *Cephalalgia* 1988; 8(Suppl. 7): 1–96.
2. Fishman RA. *Cerebrospinal fluid in diseases of the nervous system*. 2nd edition. Philadelphia: W.B. Saunders Company, 1992.
3. Morewood GH. A rational approach to the cause, prevention and treatment of postdural puncture headache. *Can Med Assoc J* 1993; 148: 1087–93.
4. Schaltenbrand G. Neure Anschauen zor Pathophysiologie der Liquorzirkulation. *Zentralb Nforchir* 1938; 3: 290–300.
5. Milhorat TH. *Hydrocephalus and the cerebrospinal fluid*. Baltimore: Williams and Wilkins, 1972.
6. Corbett JJ, Mehta MP. Cerebrospinal fluid pressure in normal obese subjects and patients with pseudotumor cerebri. *Neurology* 1983; 33: 1386–8.
7. Gamache FW, Patterson RH, Alksne JF. Headache associated with changes in intracranial pressure. In: Dalessio DJ (ed). *Wolff's Headache and Other Head Pain*. 5th edition. New York: Oxford University Press, 1987: 352–5.
8. Von Storch T, Carmichael A, Banks T. Factors producing lumbar cerebrospinal fluid pressure in man in the erect position. *Arch Neurol Psychiat* 1987; 38: 1158.
9. Loman J, Myerson A, Goldman D. Effects of alteration of posture on cerebrospinal fluid pressure. *Arch Neurol Psychiat* 1935; 33: 1279–84.
10. Loman J. Component of cerebrospinal fluid pressure as affected by changes in posture. *Arch Neurol Psychiat* 1934; 31: 679–81.
11. Freemont-Smith F, Kubie L. Relation of vascular hydrostatic pressure and osmotic pressure to cerebrospinal fluid pressure. *Assoc Res Nerv Dis Proc* 1929; 8: 154.
12. Cass W, Edelist G. Post spinal headache. *JAMA* 1974; 227: 786–7.
13. Dalessio D (ed.). *Wolff's Headache and Other Head Pain*. 3rd edition. New York: Oxford University Press, 1972.
14. Grant R, Condon B, Hart I, Teasdale GM. Changes in intracranial CSF volume after lumbar puncture and their relationship to post-LP headache. *J Neurol Neurosurg Psychiatry* 1991; 54: 440–2.
15. Good DC, Ghobrial M. Pathologic changes associated with intracranial hypotension and meningeal enhancement on MRI. *Neurology* 1993; 43: 2698–2700.
16. Fishman RA, Dillon WP. Dural enhancement and cerebral displacement secondary to intracranial hypotension. *Neurology* 1993; 43: 609–11.
17. Pannullo S, Reich J, Posner J. Meningeal enhancement associated with low intracranial pressure. *Neurology* 1992; 42(suppl. 3): 430.
18. Pannullo S, Reich JB, Krol G *et al*. MRI changes in intracranial hypotension. *Neurology* 1993; 43: 919–26.
19. Kasner SE, Rosenfeld J, Farber RE. Spontaneous intracranial hypotension: headache with a reversible Arnold-Chiari malformation. *Headache* 1995; 35: 557–9.
20. Lay CL, Campbell JK, Mokri B. Low cerebrospinal fluid pressure headache. In: Goadsby P, Silberstein SD (eds). *Blue Books of Practical Neurology: Headache*. Boston: Butterworth Heinemann, 1997: 355–68.
21. Silberstein SD, Marcelis J. Headache associated with abnormalities in intracranial structures or pressure including brain tumor and post-LP headache. In: Dalessio D, Silberstein SD (eds). *Wolff's Headache and Other Head Pain*. 6th edition. New York: Oxford University Press, 1993: 438–61.
22. Raskin NH. Headaches caused by alterations of structure or homeostasis. In: *Headache*. New York: Churchill-Livingstone, 1988: 283–316.
23. Marcelis J, Silberstein SD. Spontaneous low cerebrospinal fluid pressure headache. *Headache* 1990; 30: 192–6.
24. Sharrock NE. Postural headache following thoracic somatic paravertebral nerve block. *Anaesthesiology* 1980; 52: 360–2.
25. Kieffer SA, Wolff JM, Prentice WB, Loken MK. Scinticesternography in individuals without known neurological disease. *Am J Roentgenology* 1971; 112: 225–36.
26. Front D, Penning L. Subcutaneous extravasation of CSF demonstration by scinticisternography. *J Nuc Med* 1973; 15:200–201.
27. Bell WB, Joynt RJ, Sahs AL. Low spinal fluid pressure syndrome. *Neurology* 1960; 10: 512–21.
28. Major O, Fedorcsak I, Sipos L *et al*. Slit-ventricle syndrome in shunt operated children. *Acta Neurchirurgica* 1994; 127: 69–72.
29. Young WB, Silberstein SD. Paroxysmal headache caused by colloid cyst of the third ventricle: case report and review of the literature. *Headache* 1997; 37: 15–20.
30. Kunkle EL, Ray BS, Wolff HG. Experimental studies on headache: analysis of the headache associated with changes in intracranial pressure. *Arch Neurol Psychiatry* 1943; 49: 323–59.
31. Raskın NH. Lumbar puncture headache: a review. *Headache* 1990; 30: 197–200.
32. Labadie EL, Antwerp JV, Bamford CR. Abnormal lumbar isotope cisternography in an unusual case of spontaneous hypoliquorrheic headache. *Neurology* 1976; 26: 135–9.
33. Kraemer G, Hanns HC, Eissner D. CSF hyperabsorption: a cause of spontaneous low CSF pressure headache. *Neurology* 1987; (suppl. 1): 238A.
34. Molins A, Alvarez J, Somalla J, Titus F, Codina A. Cisternographic pattern of spontaneous liquoral hypotension. *Cephalalgia* 1990; 10: 59–65.
35. Rando TA, Fishman RA. Spontaneous intracranial hypotension: report of two cases and review of the literature. *Neurology* 1992; 42: 481–7.
36. Bell WE, Joynt RJ, Sahs AL. Low spinal fluid pressure syndromes. *Neurology* 1958; 8: 157–63.
37. Teng P, Papatheodorou C. Primary cerebrospinal fluid hypotension. *Los Angeles Neurol Soc.* 1968; 33(3): 121–8.
38. Yamamoto M, Suehiro T, Nakata H *et al*. Primary low cerebrospinal fluid pressure syndrome associated with galactorrhea. *Internal Medicine* 1993; 32(3): 228–31.
39. Huber M. Spontaneous hypoliquorrhea: seven observations. *Schweiz Arch Neurol Neurochir Psychiatry* 1970; 106: 923.
40. Murros K, Fogelholm R. Spontaneous intracranial hypotension with slit ventricles. *J Neurol Neurosurg Psychiatry* 1983; 46: 1149–51.
41. Lasater GM. Primary intracranial hypotension. *Headache* 1970; 10: 63–6.
42. Lake AP, Minckler J, Scanlan RL. Spinal epidural cyst: theories of pathogenesis. *J Neurosurg* 1974; 40: 774–8.
43. Bell WE, Joynt RJ, Sahs AL. Low spinal fluid pressure syndromes. *Neurology* 1958; 8: 157–63.
44. Nosik WA. Intracranial hypotension secondary to lumbar nerve sleeve tear. *JAMA* 1955; 157: 1110–11.
45. Horton JC, Fishman RA. Neurovisual findings in the syndrome of spontaneous intracranial hypotension from aural cerebrospinal fluid leak. *Ophthalmology* 1994; 101(2): 244–51.
46. Paulson GW, Klawans HL. Benign orgasmic cephalalgia. *Headache* 1974; 13: 181–7.
47. Baker CC. Headache due to spontaneous low spinal fluid pressure. *Minn Med* 1983; 66: 325–8.
48. Capobianco DJ, Kuczler FJ. Case report: primary intracranial hypotension. *Nilit Med* 1990; 155: 64–6.

49. Garcia-Albea E, Cabrera F, Tejeiro J et al. Delayed postexertional headache, intracranial hypotension and racket sports (letter). *J Neurol, Neurosurg, Psychiatry* 1992; 55(10): 975.

50. Farraraccio BE. Positional headache due to spontaneous intracranial hypotension (letter). *Southern Medical Journal* 1992; 85(1): 57.

51. Fernandez E. Headaches associated with low spinal fluid pressure. *Headache* 1990; 30: 122–8.

52. Tourtellote WW, Haerer AF, Heller GL et al. *Post-lumbar puncture headaches.* Springfield, IL: Charles C. Thomas, 1964.

53. Iqbal J, Davis LE, Orrison WW. An MRI study of lumbar puncture headaches. *Headache* 1995; 35: 420–2.

54. Dripps RD, Vandam LD. Longterm follow-up of patients who received 10,098 spinal anesthetics. *JAMA* 1954; 156: 1486–91.

55. Vilming ST, Schrader H, Monstad I. The significance of age, sex, and cerebrospinal fluid pressure in post lumbar puncture headache. *Cephalalgia* 1989; 9: 99–106.

56. Kuntz KM, Kokmen E, Stevens JC et al. Post-lumbar puncture headaches: experience in 501 consecutive procedures. *Neurology* 1992; 42: 1884–7.

57. DiGiovanni AJ, Dunbar BS. Epidural injections of autologous blood for postlumbar puncture headache. *Anesth Analg* 1970; 49(2): 268–71.

58. Torrey EF. Headaches after lumbar puncture and insensitivity to pain in psychiatric patients. *N Engl J Med* 1979; 301: 111.

59. Daniels AM, Sallie R. Headache, lumbar puncture, and expectation. *Lancet* 1981; I: 1003.

60. Blennow K, Wallin A, Häger O. Low frequency of post-lumbar puncture headache in demented patients. *Acta Neurol Scand* 1993; 88: 221–3.

61. Reid JA, Thorburn J. Headache ofter spinal anesthesia. *Br J Anaesth* 1991; 67: 674.

62. Lynch J, Krings-Ernst I, Stick K et al. Use of a 25-guage Whitacre needle to reduce the incidence of postdural puncture headache. *Br J Anaesth* 1991; 67: 690–3.

63. Rasmussen BS, Blom L, Hansen P, Mikkelsen SJ. Postspinal headache in young and elderly patients. *Anesthesia* 1989; 44: 571–3.

64. Geurts JW, Haanschoten MC, Van Wijk RM, Kraak K, Besse TC. Post-dural headache in young patients. *Acta Anaesthesiol Scand* 1990; 34: 350–3.

65. McGann GM, Gleeson FV, Kelly I et al. The influence of needle size on postmyelography headache: a controlled trial. *Br J Radiol* 1992; 65: 1102–04.

66. Engelhardt A, Oheim S, Neundorrfer B. Post lumbar puncture headache: experiences with an 'atraumatic' needle. *Cephalalgia* 1991; 11(Suppl 11): 356–7.

67. Braune H-J, Huffman G. A prospective double-blind clinical trail, comparing the sharp Quincke needle (22G) with an 'atraumatic' needle (22G) in the induction of post-lumbar puncture headache. *Acta Neurol Scand* 1992; 86: 50–54.

68. Sipe JC, Zyroff J, Waltz TA. Primary intracranial hypotension and bilateral isodense subdural hematomas. *Neurology* 1981; 31: 334–7.

69. Vilming ST, Titus F. Low cerebrospinal fluid pressure. In: Olesen J, Tfeldt-Hansen P, Welch MA (eds). *The Headaches.* New York: Raven Press, 1993: 687–95.

70. Weber WE, Heidendal GA, de Krom MC. Primary intracranial hypotension and abnormal radionuclide cisternography. Report of a case and review of the literature. *Clin Neurol Neurosurg* 1991; 93: 55–60.

71. Lindquist T, Moberg E. Spontaneous hypoliquorrhea. *Acta Med Scand* 1949; 132: 556–61.

72. Mokri B, Krueger BR, Miller GM, Piepgras DG. Meningeal gadolinium enhancement in low-pressure headaches. *J Neuroimag* 1993; 3: 11–15.

73. Sable SG, Ramadan NM. Meningeal enhancement and low CSF pressure headache. An MRI study. *Cephalalgia* 1991; 11: 275–6.

74. Hockman MS, Naidich TP, Kobetz SA, Fernandez-Maitin A. Spontaneous intracranial hypotension with pachymeningeal enhancement on MRI. *Neurology* 1992; 42: 1628–30.

75. Bourekas EC, Jonathan SL, Lanzieri CF. Postcontrast meningeal MR enhancement secondary to intracranial hypotension caused by lumbar puncture. *J Comput Assist Tomogr* 1995; 19(2): 299–301.

76. Berlit P, Berg-Dammer E, Kuehne D. Abducens nerve palsy in spontaneous intracranial hypotension (scientific note). *Neurology* 1994; 44: 1552.

77. Sechzer PH, Abel L. Post-spinal anesthesia headache treated with caffeine. Evaluation with demand method. Part 1. *Current Therapeutic Research* 1978; 24: 307–12.

78. Gaukroger PB, Brownridge P. Epidural blood patch in treatment of spontaneous low CSF pressure headache. *Pain* 1987; 29: 119–22.

79. Parris WCV. Use of epidural blood patch in treating chronic headache: report of six cases. *Can J Anaesth* 1987; 34: (4): 403–6.

80. Peterson RC, Freeman DP, Knox CA, Gibson BE. Successful treatment of spontaneous low cerebrospinal fluid pressure headache. *Ann Neurol* 1987; 22:148A.

81. Jarvis AP, Greenawalt JW, Fagraeus L. *Anesth Analg* 1986; 65: 313–21.

82. Camann WR, Murray RS, Mushlin PS, Lambert DH. Effects of oral caffeine on postdural puncture headache. A double-blind, placebo-controlled trial. *Anesth Analg* 1990; 70: 181–4.

83. Gormley JB. Treatment of post-spinal headache. *Anesthesiology* 1960; 21: 565–6.

84. Bart AJ, Wheeler AS. Comparison of epidural saline infusion and epidural blood placement in the treatment of post lumbar puncture headache. *Anesthesiology* 1978; 48: 221–3.

85. Millette PC, Paqacz A, Charest C. Epidural blood patch for the treatment of chronic headache after myelography. *Journal de l'Association Canadienne des Radiologistes* 1982; 33: 236–8.

86. Ostheimer GW, Palahniuk RJ, Shnider SM. Epidural blood patch for post-lumbar puncture headache. *Anesthesiology* 1974; 41: 307–8.

87. Taivainen T, Pitkänen M, Tuominen M, Rosenberg PH. Efficacy of epidural blood patch for postdural puncture headache. *Acta Anaesthesiol Scand* 1993; 37:702–5.

88. Beards SC, Jackson A, Griffiths AG, Horsman EL. Magnetic resonance imaging of extradural blood patches: appearances from 30 min to 18 h. *Br J Anaesth* 1993; 71:182–8.

89. Tarkkila PJ, Miralles JA, Palomaki EA. The subjective complications and efficiency of the epidural blood patch in the treatment of postdural puncture headache. *Reg Anaesth* 1989; 14: 247–50.

90. Jaeckle KA. Clinical presentation and therapy of nervous system tumors. In: WG Bradley, RB Daroff, GM Fenichel, and CD Marsden (eds). *Neurology in Clinical Practice.* Boston: Butterworth-Heinemann, 1991: 1008–30.

91. Lavyne MH, Patterson RH. Headache and brain tumor. In: DJ Dalessio (ed.). *Wolff's Headache and Other Head Pain.* 5th edition. New York: Oxford University Press, 1987: 343–9.

92. Kunkle EC, Pfeiffer JB, Wilholt WM, Hamrick LD Jr. Recurrent brief headache in 'cluster' pattern. *Trans Am Neurol Assoc* 1942; 77: 240–3.

93. Northfield DWC. Some observations on headache. *Brain* 1938; 61: 133.

94. Rushton JG, Rooke ED. Brain tumor headache. *Headache* 1962; 2: 147–52.

95. Heyck H. Examination and differential diagnosis of headache. In: *Handbook of Clinical Neurology, Volume 5.* 1968: 25–36.

96. Forsyth PA, Posner JB. Headaches in patients with brain tumors. A study of 111 patients. *Neurology* 1993; 43: 1678–83.

97. Vazquez-Barquero A, Ibanez FJ, Herrara S *et al*. Isolated headache as the presenting clinical manifestation of intracranial tumor: A prospective study. *Cephalalgia* 1994; 14: 270–2.

98. Zulch KJ, Mennel HD, Zimmerman V. Intracranial hypertension. In: *Handbook of Clinical Neurology, Volume 16*. 1974: 89–149.

99. Honig PJ, Charney EB. Children with brain tumor headaches. *Am J Dis Child* 1982; 136: 121–4.

100. Rossi LN, Vassella F. Headache in children with brain tumour. *Childs Nerv Syst* 1989; 5: 307–9.

101. Zammarano CB, D'Ancona ML, Miceli MC. Headache and cerebral neoplasm in childhood. In: Lanzi G, Balottin U, Cernibori A (eds). *Headache in Children and Adolescents*. The Netherlands: Elsevier, 1989: 177–8.

102. Kennedy CR, Nathwani A. Headache as a presenting feature of brain tumours in children. *Cephalalgia* 1995; 15(suppl. 16): 15.

103. Galicich JH, Sundaresan N. Metastatic brain tumors. In: Wilkins RH, Rengachary SS (eds). *Neurosurgery*. New York: McGraw-Hill, 1985: 600.

104. Childhood Brain Tumor Consortium. The epidemiology of headache among children with brain tumor: headache in children with brain tumors. *J Neurooncol* 1991; 10: 31–46.

105. Shuper A, Packer RJ, Vezina LG *et al*. Complicated migrainelike episodes in children following cranial irradiation and chemotherapy. *Neurology* 1995; 45: 1837–40.

106. McKissock W. Subdural hematoma. A review of 389 cases. *Lancet* 1960; 1: 1365–70.

107. Britt RH. Brain abscess. In: Wilkins RH, Rengachary SS (eds). *Neurosurgery*. New York: McGraw-Hill, 1985: 1928–56.

108. Giuseffi V, Wall M, Siegal PZ, Rojas PB. Symptoms and disease associations in *Neurology* 1991; 41: 239–44.

109. Wall M, George D. Idiopathic intracranial hypertension: a prospective study of 50 patients. *Brain* 1991; 114: 155–80.

110. Wall M. The headache profile of idiopathic intracranial hypertension. *Cephalalgia* 1990; 10: 331–5.

111. Sadun AA, Currie JN, Lessell S. Transient visual obscurations with elevated optic discs. *Ann Neurol* 1984; 16: 489–94.

112. Durcan FJ, Corbett JJ, Wall M. The incidence of pseudotumor cerebri: population studies in Iowa and Louisiana. *Arch Neurol* 1988; 45: 875–7.

113. Johnston I, Hawke S, Kalmagyi M, Antyeo C. The pseudotumor syndrome. *Arch Neurol* 1991; 48: 740–7.

114. Borgesen SE, Gjerris F. Relationships between intracranial pressure, ventricular size, and resistance to CSF outflow. *J Neurosurg* 1987; 67: 535–9.

115. VanAlphen HAM. Migraine, a result of increased CSF pressure: a new pathophysiologic concept (preliminary report). *Neurosurg Rev* 1986; 9: 121–4.

116. Gjerris F, Sorenson S, Vorstrup S, Paulson OB. Intracranial pressure, conductance to cerebrospinal fluid outflow, and cerebral blood flow in patients with benign intracranial hypertension (pseudotumor cerebri). *Ann Neurol* 1985; 17: 158–62.

117. Fishman RA. The pathophysiology of pseudotumor cerebri. An unsolved puzzle. Editorial. *Neurology* 1984; 41: 257–8.

118. Bjerre P, Lindholm J, Gyldensted C. Pseudotumor cerebri: a theory on etiology and pathogenesis. *Acta Neurol Scand* 1982; 66:472 –81.

119. Donaldson JO, Binstock ML. Pseudotumor cerebri in an obese woman with Turner syndrome. *Neurology* 1981; 31: 758–60.

120. Janny P, Chazal J, Colnet G, Irthorn B, Georget AM. Benign intracranial hypertension and disorders of CSF absorption. *Surg Neurol* 1981; 15: 168–74.

121. Fishman RA. Pathophysiology of pseudotumor. *Ann Neurol* 1979; 5: 496.

122. Johnston I. Reduced CSF absorption syndrome. Reappraisal of benign intracranial hypertension and related conditions. *Lancet* 1973; 8: 2418–21.

123. Malm J, Kristensen B, Markgren P, Ekstedt J. CSF hydrodynamics in idiopathic intracranial hypertension: a long-term study. *Neurology* 1992; 42: 851–8.

124. King JO, Mitchell PJ, Thomson KR, Tress BM. Cerebral venography and manometry in idiopathic intracranial hypertension. *Neurology* 1995; 45: 2224–8.

125. Karahalios DG, Rekate HL, Khayata MH, Apostolides PJ. Elevated intracranial venous pressure as a universal mechanism in pseudotumor cerebri of varying etiologies. *Neurology* 1996; 46: 198–202.

126. Weisberg LA. Benign intracranial hypertension. *Medicine* 1975; 54: 197–207.

127. Corbett JJ. Headache due to idiopathic intracranial hypertension. In: Goadsby P, Silberstein SD (eds). *Blue Books of Practical Neurology: Headache*. Boston: Butterworth Heinemann, 1997: 279–83.

128. Corbett JJ, Thompson HS. The rational management of idiopathic intracranial hypertension. *Arch Neurol* 1991; 48: 1049–51.

129. Marcelis J, Silberstein SD. Idiopathic intracranial hypertension without papilledema. *Arch Neurol* 1991; 48: 392–9.

130. Spence JD, Amacher AL, Willis NR. Benign intracranial hypertension without papilledema: role of 24 hour cerebrospinal fluid pressure monitoring in diagnosis and management. *Neurosurgery* 1980; 7: 326–36.

131. Scanari M, Mingrino S, d'Avella D, DellaCort V. Benign Intracranial hypertension without papilledema: a case report. *Neurosurgery* 1979; 5: 376–7.

132. Lipton HL, Michelson PE. Pseudotumor cerebri syndrome without papilledema. *JAMA* 1972; 220: 1591–2.

133. Mathew NT, Ravishankar K, Sanin LC. Coexistence of migraine and idiopathic intracranial hypertension without papilledema. *Neurology* 1996; 46: 1226–30.

134. Silberstein SD, Corbett JJ. The forgotten lumbar puncture. *Cephalalgia* 1993; 13: 212–13.

135. Eggenberger ER, Miller NR, Vitale S. Lumboperitoneal shunt for the treatment of pseudotumor cerebri. *Neurology* 1996; 46: 1524–30.

136. Tinel J. Un syndrome d'algie veineuse intracranienne. La cephalee a l'effort. *Prat Med Fr* 1932;13:113–19.

137. Symonds C. Cough headache. *Brain* 1956; 79: 557–68.

138. Rooke ED. Benign exertional headache. *Med Clin North Am* 1968; 52: 801–8.

139. Rassmussen BK, Jensen R, Schroll M, Olesen J. Epidemiology of headache in a general population — a prevalence study. *J Clin Epidemiol* 1991; 44: 1147–57.

140. Pascual J, Igelsias F, Oterino A, Vazquez-Barquero A, Berciano J. Cough, exertional, and sexual headaches: an analysis of 72 benign and symptomatic cases. *Neurology* 1996; 46: 1520–4.

141. Sands GH, Newman L, Lipton R. Cough, exertional, and other miscellaneous headaches. *Med Clin N Amer* 1991; 75: 733–43.

142. Nick J. La céphalée d'effort. A propos d'une série de 43 cas. *Sem Hop Paris* 1980; 56: 621–8.

143. Tinel J. La cephalee d'effort. Syndrome de distension douloureuse des veines intracraniennes. *Medicine (Paris)* 1932; 13: 113–18.

144. Nightingale S, Williams B. Hindbrain hernia headache. *Lancet* 1987; 1: 731–2.

145. Mathew NT. Indomethacin responsive headache syndromes. *Headaches* 1981; 21: 147–50.

146. Raskin NH. The indomethacin-responsive syndromes. In: *Headache*. New York: Churchill Livingstone 1988: 255–68.

147. Williams B. Cough headache due to craniospinal pressure dissociation. *Arch Neurol* 1980; 37: 226–30.

148. Rushton JG, Rooke ED. Brain tumor headache. *Headache* 1962; 2: 147–52.

149. Raskin N. Headaches associated with organic diseases of the nervous system. *Med Clin North Am* 1978; 62: 459–66.

150. Ekbom K. Cough headache. In: Vinken PJ, Bruyn GW, Klawans HL *et al* (eds). *Headache (Handbook of Clinical Neurology, Vol 48)* New York: Elsevier Science Publishing, 1986: 67–371.

151. Silbert PL, Edis RH, Stewart-Wynne EG, Gubbay SS. Benign vascular sexual headache and exertional headache: interrelationships and long term prognosis. *J Neurol Neurosurg Psychiatry* 1991; 54: 417–21.

152. Ibbotson S. Weightlifter's headache. *Br J Sports Med* 1987; 3: 138.

153. Paulson GW. Weightlifter's headache. *Headache* 1983; 23: 193–4.

154. Powell B. Weightlifter's cephalalgia. *Ann Emerg Med* 1982; 11: 449–51.

155. Silberstein SD, Marcelis J. Headache associated with abnormalities in intracranial structures or pressure including brain tumor and post-LP headache. In: Dalessio D, Silberstein SD (eds). *Wolff's Headache and Other Head Pain, (6th Edition).* New York: Oxford University Press, 1993: 438–61.

156. Lance JW, Hinterberger H. Symptoms of pheochromocytoma with particular reference to headache correlated with catecholamine production. *Arch Neurol* 1976; 33: 281–8.

157. Paulson GW, Zipf RE, Beekman JF. Pheochromocytoma causing exercise-related headache and pulmonary edema. *Ann Neurol* 1979; 5: 96–9.

158. Thomas JE, Rooke ED, Kvale WF. The neurologist's experience with pheochromocytoma: A review of 100 cases. *JAMA* 1966; 10: 100–4.

159. Van den Bergh V, Amery WK, Waelkens J. Trigger factors in migraine: a study conducted by the Belgian migrain society. *Headache* 1987; 27: 191–6.

160. Williams B. Cerebrospinal fluid pressure changes in response to coughing. *Brain* 1976; 99: 331–46.

161. Stevens JM, Serva WAD, Kendall BE, Valentine AR, Ponsford JR. Chiari malformation in adults: relation of morphological aspects to clinical features and operative outcome. *J Neurol Neurosurg Psychiatry* 1993; 56: 1072–7.

162. Raskin NH. The cough headache syndrome: treatment. *Neurology* 1995; 45: 1784.

163. Ramadan NM. Headache caused by raised intracranial pressure and intracranial hypotension. *Curr Opin Neurol* 1996; 9: 214–18.

164. Griffiths AG, Beards SC, Jackson A *et al*. Visualization of extradural blood patch for post lumbar puncture headache by magnetic resonance imaging. *Br J Anaesth* 1993; 70: 223–5.

chapter 13

Headache associated with vascular disease: migraine and stroke

Introduction

Migraine and stroke each produce various combinations of headache, focal neurological deficits and alterations of cerebral blood flow (CBF). Charcot[1,2] noted that migraine's transient neurological deficits could persist and suggested that the disorders may be associated. Ever since, the relationships between these disorders have challenged clinicians and scientists. The migraine aura can mimic transient ischaemic attacks (TIA). Conversely, in stroke, headache may occur as a preictal, ictal or postictal feature.[3,4,5] In addition to the problem of differential diagnosis, there are causal relationships between migraine and stroke on several levels.

In this chapter we will review the clinical and epidemiological evidence that suggests that migraine and stroke are comorbid. We will then consider a classification for migraine-related stroke prepared by Welch. We will address migraine-related stroke. We will then consider, in detail, carotid dissection and subarachnoid haemorrhage (SAH), and finally, examine the treatment complications of comorbidity.

Are migraine and stroke associated?

Hospital series suggest that 1–17% of strokes are attributed to migraine in patients under 50 years of age.[6,7] In general, the relationship between migraine and stroke is stronger for migraine with aura[8,9] than for migraine without aura. Strokes related to migraine are commonly found in the distribution of the posterior cerebral artery.[10,11] Efforts have been made to determine the mechanism of migraine-associated stroke. Bougousslavsky et al. (1988) reported that patients who had a stroke during an attack of migraine with aura had arterial lesions, compared to 91% of migraine with aura patients who experienced a stroke remote from a migrainous event and 82% of patients with a stroke and no history of migraine.[12] The low prevalence of arterial lesions suggests that mechanisms other than focal arterial pathology may underlie migrainous infarction.

In an attempt to identify factors associated with migrainous infarction, Rothrock et al.[9] compared the clinical features of 310 patients with migraine and 30 patients with acute migrainous stroke. They found no significant differences in gender, mean age of migraine onset, mitral valve prolapse, hypertension, active smoking or active oestrogen use. Migraine with aura was substantially overrepresented in patients with migrainous stroke (80%) compared to migraine patients without stroke. In this study, migrainous infarction carried a poor prognosis. Six recurrent ischaemic infarcts (all migraine-associated) were diagnosed in 28 of these patients who were followed for a mean of 25.3 months. No strokes occurred in 173 of the control migraine patients followed for at least one year. As the two groups were similar in this vascular risk profile, migraine with aura may be an independent risk factor for stroke.

The case-control design has been used to examine migraine as a risk factor for stroke. The Collaborative Group for the Study of Stroke in Young Women compared hospitalized stroke patients with both community- and hospital-based controls.[13] There was a twofold increase in the risk of stroke for women with migraine when compared with community controls but not relative to hospital controls; thus, the study was inconclusive. A hospital-based, case-controlled study of 89 patients found an association between migraine and stroke; after adjusting for vascular risk factors, however, this was no longer statistically significant.[14] Tzourio et al.[15,16] reported that migraine was associated with a fourfold increased risk of stroke in women under the age of 45 years. A strong association between stroke and migraine occurs in women under 45 years of age for migraine without aura (odds ratio, OR = 3.0) and migraine with aura (OR = 6.2). The risk is significantly increased in migrainous women who smoke more than one pack a day (OR = 10.2) or use oral contraceptives (OR = 13.9).

Carolei et al.[17] conducted a case-control study of 308 patients aged 15–44 years with either TIA or stroke, and 591 prospectively recruited age- and sex-matched controls to evaluate the relationship of migraine and stroke. For each case, a hospital control and population control were randomly selected. A history of migraine was more frequent in patients than in controls (14.9% vs. 9.1%; adjusted OR = 1.9, 95% confidence interval CI = 1.1–3.1). In the prospectively designed subgroup analyses, a history of migraine reached the highest odds ratio (3.7, 95% CI = 1.5–9) and was the only significant risk factor for TIA or stroke in women under age 35 years (P = 0.003). A history of migraine was not relevant in men and in patients over 35 years; in these groups, recognized atherosclerotic risk factors were statistically significant, suggesting different risk profiles for cerebral ischaemic events in younger women and older men.[17]

Previous migraine with aura was more frequent in stroke patients compared to controls (OR = 8.6, 95% CI = 1–75). These epidemiological studies do not provide information on the temporal relationship of the stroke to a migraine attack or other confounding stroke mechanisms. This makes inferences about causality and mechanisms difficult.

Migraine-related stroke was evaluated as part of the prospective Physicians' Health Study, a randomized, double-blind, placebo-controlled trial of aspirin and beta-carotene. The study enrolled 22 071 male physicians.[18] In this study, 6.7% of the participants reported that they had migraine, but no distinction was made between migraine with or without aura. After adjusting for age, aspirin use, and other vascular risk factors, the relative risk of total stroke was 1.84 (95% CI = 1.06–3.20), comparing those who reported migraine with those who did not. For ischaemic stroke the relative risk was 2.00 (95% CI = 1.10–3.64). Since the diagnosis of migraine was based solely on self-report, migraine without aura may be underrepresented. In addition, the occurrence of stroke during migraine or the relationship of stroke to type of migraine was not ascertained.

Categories of migraine-related stroke

The International Headache Society (IHS) criteria include a disorder termed 'migrainous cerebral infarction' (IHS 1.6.2). It is defined as follows:

- Patients have previously fulfilled criteria for migraine with neurological aura.
- The present attack is typical of previous attacks but neurological deficits are not completely reversible within seven days and/or neuroimaging demonstrates ischaemic infarction in the relevant area.
- Other causes of infarction are ruled out by appropriate investigation.[19]

● **Table 13.1** Classification of migraine-related stroke[20]

Category	Feature
I	Coexisting stroke and migraine
II	Stroke with clinical features of migraine
	A Symptomatic migraine
	B Migraine mimic
III	Migraine-induced stroke
	A Without risk factors
	B With risk factors
IV	Uncertain

An expanded classification of migraine-related stroke that encompasses the full spectrum of the possible relationship between these conditions has been proposed (Table 13.1).[20]

Coexistent stroke and migraine
In this condition, 'a clearly defined clinical stroke syndrome must occur remotely in time from a typical attack of migraine'.[20] In this category, migraine may contribute to the risk of stroke through an unspecified mechanism. Mitral valve prolapse is comorbid with both migraine and stroke, which may help account for the association between migraine and stroke.

Stroke with clinical features of migraine
This is defined as a structural lesion, unrelated to migraine pathogenesis, that presents with clinical features of a migraine attack.[20] Two subtypes, symptomatic migraine and migraine mimic, are identified. In the symptomatic group, a structural central nervous system lesion, such as arteriovenous malformation, produces typical episodes of migraine with aura. The symptoms of migraine with aura may result from a mismatch between cerebral blood flow and neuronal activity.

Migraine mimic includes cases of acute stroke accompanied by both headache and focal neurological symptoms that are difficult to distinguish from migraine with aura. The differential diagnosis is difficult in patients who continue to have migraine with aura late in life, when the incidence of cerebrovascular disease increases. Carotid dissection, which occurs more commonly in migraineurs, can also produce symptoms that mimic a migraine attack but results in an ischaemic stroke.

Migraine-induced stroke
The criteria for migraine-induced stroke proposed by Welch and Levine[20] are:

- the neurological deficit must be identical to the migraine symptoms of previous attacks,
- the stroke must occur during the course of a typical migraine attack,
- all other causes of stroke must be excluded, although stroke risk factors may be present.

This condition corresponds closely to migrainous cerebral infarction as defined by the IHS.

Uncertain classification
Migraine and stroke appear related but a causal role is difficult to firmly establish. For example, a patient may have a typical migraine with aura, take a vasoactive drug such as sumatriptan or ergotamine, and then develop a cerebral infarction. In this sequence it is not clear if the stroke was a

consequence of the migraine itself, a result of the treatment with vasoconstrictive medication, or an interaction between the two. As a second example, consider a stroke that occurs during cerebral angiography in a patient with migraine and frequent or prolonged aura. Migraine-like headaches and stroke may also be associated with the antiphospholipid antibody syndrome, systemic vasculitides, oral contraceptive use, or mitochondrial encephalopathy with lactic acidosis and stroke-like episodes (MELAS). A causal relationship between migraine and stroke is difficult to prove in patients with these or other confounding variables.

Mechanisms of the comorbidity of migraine and stroke

Migraine can produce stroke in several ways:

- stroke may arise as a consequence of the migraine attack itself, due, for example, to reduced regional cerebral blood flow (rCBF)[21–23] or platelet dysfunction;[24–26]
- stroke may result from a condition comorbid with migraine such as carotid dissection,[27] mitral valve prolapse[28,29] or antiphospholipid antibody syndrome,[30,31] which are themselves risk factors for stroke, and
- both migraine and stroke may result from an underlying disorder such as MELAS[32,33] or cerebral autosomal dominant arteriopathy with subcortical infarcts and leukoencephalopathy (CADASIL).[34]

Migraine with aura is characterized by impaired cerebrovascular reactivity and decreased rCBF.[21,35–37] These haemodynamic changes are believed to be a consequence of primary neuronal events.[38] The process is thought to be analogous to the spreading cortical depression of Leão.[39] A wave of neuronal depression is associated with a reduction in rCBF (see Chapter 5). Olesen et al.[35,37] have described similar CBF changes, known as spreading oligaemia, during the aura of migraine in humans. Between attacks, CBF studies suggest that there may be cortical flow asymmetries and differences in cerebrovascular reactivity in migraine with aura patients versus control subjects.[40,41] It is uncertain whether this is part of the physiology or the result of repeated attacks of migraine with aura.

The decrease in rCBF secondary to arteriolar vasoconstriction may be accompanied by sluggish blood flow in dilated intracerebral conductance vessels. Perhaps these factors predispose to intravascular thrombosis and migraine-induced cerebral infarction. Increased platelet aggregability and elevated titres of antiphospholipid may contribute to the risk of enhanced coagulation. These conditions are shared risk factors for stroke and migraine with aura. Mitral valve prolapse, another condition comorbid with migraine, is also associated with platelet hyperaggregability and stroke in young adults.[28,42]

Structural changes of the cerebral arteries may contribute to the link between migraine with aura and stroke. Caplan[2] reviewed patients with migraine and vertebrobasilar ischaemia and concluded that posterior circulation ischaemia is common in migraine and is not always benign. Angiography in migraine sufferers revealed severe vasoconstriction in both the vertebral and basilar arteries and occlusion of the basilar or posterior cerebral arteries. The aetiology of the vascular occlusions is uncertain though no source of embolism could be identified. One possibility is that migraine produces 'pseudo-occlusion' due to vasoconstriction ('spasm') severe enough to prevent anterograde flow. Alternatively, prolonged vasoconstriction could also lead to haemostasis and in situ thrombosis. Moskowitz[43] has shown in his model of neurogenic inflammation that platelet aggregation occurs in the lumen of blood vessels. Thus, pathological activation of the trigeminovascular system could result in structural changes of the cerebral vessels, linking the mechanism for headache pain and the potential for cerebral ischaemia.

During migraine attacks, migraineurs may undergo severe vasoconstriction in the vertebral and basilar arteries.[2,44,45] Transcranial Doppler ultrasonography demonstrates persistent increased flow velocities, presumed secondary to focal arterial narrowing in migraineurs.[46,47] Migraine-induced vasoconstriction could lead to chronic structural changes in blood vessels. Levine and Ramadan[48] have suggested that repeated episodes of migraine-induced vasoconstriction and vasodilatation may weaken the internal elastic lamina of cerebral vessels and predispose to arterial dissection. Dissection is more common in migraineurs; therefore, migraine may be a risk factor for stroke because of morphologic changes in cerebral blood vessels.

It is also possible for stroke to produce migraine-like headache. Olesen et al.[49] analysed CBF changes in ischaemia-induced (symptomatic) migraine and migraine-induced ischaemic infarction. Olesen's symptomatic migraine is similar to migraine mimic. In a series of 15 consecutive patients, they concluded that symptomatic migraine may be more frequent than true migrainous infarction, although the distinction could not be made in all cases. Areas with decreased CBF may be more susceptible to spreading cortical depression giving rise to migraine aura. Although migraine is a risk factor for ischaemic stroke, more often cerebral ischaemia appears to trigger migraine-like headache. Recurrent migraine with aura may be a residual symptom of stroke due to a decreased migraine threshold. A genetic predisposition to migraine,[50] the location and extent of a stroke, and the persistence of small, marginally perfused cortical areas are possible factors to determine the development of migraine with aura after stroke.[49]

Both migraine and stroke produce cerebral metabolic derangements with elements in common. Both disorders produce elevated CBF levels of gamma-aminobutyric acid and cyclic adenosine monophosphate.[51] Migraine-like headaches and stroke-like episodes are both components of MELAS, a mitochondrial disorder due to a mutation in mitochondrial tRNA that results in abnormal oxidative metabolism.[32,33] It is possible that some cases of status migraine without other neurological manifestation may be a *forme fruste* of the mitochondrial disorders, although there are no reported cases published which establish this. More severe involvement may produce migrainous stroke due to endothelial dysfunction-induced cerebral angiopathy resulting from impaired energy metabolism.

CADASIL, an inherited arterial disease of the brain,[52] and familial hemiplegic migraine both map to chromosome 19.[53] Familial hemiplegic migraine is distinguished from CADASIL by its early onset, benign prognosis, and normal magnetic resonance imaging (MRI) findings. The main clinical presentation of CADASIL is recurrent subcortical ischaemic events, either transient or (more often) permanent.[54] The vascular presentation is not constant and other symptoms, such as dementia, depression or migraine with aura, can occur. Although these symptoms are usually associated with a history of recurrent strokes, they may be the prominent, or only, manifestation of the disease. Vascular dementia is found in one-third of affected family members and up to 90% of subjects before death. Attacks of migraine with aura occur in 22% of cases, while its prevalence in the general population is about 6% (see Chapter 6).

White matter abnormalities, possibly ischaemic in nature, have been reported in patients with migraine, particularly migraine with aura. Migraine with aura and white matter abnormalities could be a consequence of the same underlying pathophysiological mechanism that occurs in the mitochondrial diseases (see Chapter 6).

Spontaneous internal carotid artery dissection

Spontaneous internal carotid artery dissection (ICAD) is an uncommon but not altogether rare cause of headache and acute neurological deficit in younger patients. Headache, the most common symptom, is often unilateral and located in the orbital, periorbital and frontal regions. It is often accompanied by neck pain. The pain is usually moderate to severe and steady or throbbing in nature. A bruit or Horner's syndrome is often present. Focal cerebral symptoms such as TIA or stroke may precede the headache but frequently follow it by up to 2 weeks. These symptoms, seen in 60–75% of cases, point to a vascular aetiology for the headache. When focal cerebral symptoms are absent, Horner's syndrome, bruit, dysgeusia, and neck pain suggest the diagnosis, which can be confirmed by arteriography, MRI or carotid ultrasound.

Incidence

Dissection of the cervical segment of the internal carotid artery occurs predominantly in middle age. The mean age of 140 reported patients was 45 years (range 11–74 years); 70% were between the ages of 35 and 50 years.[55] The peak incidence is in the early forties in both sexes, but the exact incidence is unknown.

Pathogenesis

Spontaneous ICAD usually occurs without risk factors; the role of trivial trauma is uncertain. It has been reported after violent coughing, chiropractic manipulation,[55] nose-blowing, sports activities and even neck-turning.[57] Systemic arteriopathies associated with dissection include cystic medial necrosis, fibromuscular dysplasia, syphilis, and Marfan's and Ehlers–Danlos syndromes. In addition, migraine is a risk factor for dissection.

When haemorrhage into the anterior media occurs, subintimal or subadventitial dissection may result. Subintimal dissection causes stenosis and subadventitial dissection produces sac-like outpouchings of adventitia from the vessel wall.[58] The dissection may rupture back through the intima, forming a false lumen. Cerebrovascular symptoms, caused by tight stenosis or, more commonly, by embolization, can lead to stroke or TIA.

The pain of ICAD is due to arterial dilatation or distention, which stimulates nociceptors in the vessel wall. Electrical stimulation of the carotid bifurcation produces ipsilateral pain in the face and head.[59]

Clinical features

The IHS has established criteria for the diagnosis of dissection (Table 13.2). The sensitivity and specificity of these criteria have not been established. Since dissection can occur without Horner's syndrome, arterial bruit, tinnitus, TIA or stroke, sensitivity is probably low.[60]

Pain characteristics

Pain, the most common symptom of ICAD, usually presents as a unilateral headache that can involve any part of the head, face or neck. It often has no specific quality and is sudden in onset and variable in severity and location. It can present as carotodynia or as a headache suggestive of SAH with no associated features (Figure 13.1).[60]

A At least one of the following:

   1 TIA or ischemic stroke in territory of affected artery

   2 Horner's syndrome, arterial bruit, or tinnitus

B Dissection demonstrated by appropriate investigations or surgery

C Headache and cervical pain ipsilateral to arterial dissection

THE MOST FREQUENT REGIONS OF HEADACHE AND NECK PAIN ASSOCIATED WITH ICAD

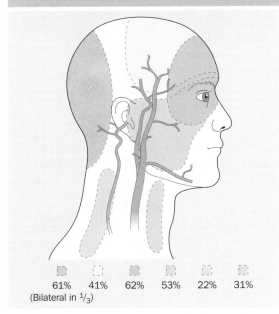

61%	41%	62%	53%	22%	31%

(Bilateral in ¹/₃)

● **Figure 13.1** *Schematic diagram showing the most frequent regions of headache and neck pain associated with ICAD.*

Biousse *et al.*[61] studied 67 patients with painful carotid dissection (38 men, 29 women; mean age 63 years). Five had bilateral extracranial carotid artery dissection. Diagnosis was based on the classical angiographic signs: irregular stenosis, tapered occlusion beginning distal to the cervical bifurcation and pseudoaneurysm.

Pain was present in 50 patients (75%): headache in 20 patients, neck pain in 6 patients, facial pain in 11 patients, and a combination of headache and neck pain in 12 patients. In 40 patients (60%), pain was the inaugural symptom of ICAD: headache in 23 patients, facial pain in 10 patients, and neck pain in 7 patients; in 10 patients, pain (headache, neck or facial pain) occurred after another local symptom such as tinnitus or Horner's syndrome, or after TIA or completed stroke.

Headache was unilateral and ipsilateral to the dissection in 20 patients (diffuse in 12 patients, localized in 8 patients) and bilateral in 12 patients, 2 of whom had bilateral extracranial carotid artery dissection. Neck pain and facial pain were always unilateral and ipsilateral to the dissection. Head pain was therefore on the side of the dissection in 38 patients (76%) and bilateral in 12 patients (18%). Pain was considered severe by 35 patients (70%). The pain lasted from 1 hour to 30 days (median 5 days) and usually resolved.[61,62] Cases of persistent pain have been reported,[63] particularly in patients with residual aneurysm.[64]

Migraine was present in 46% of patients with painful ICAD, but in only 18% with non-painful ICAD. Five patients described the headache of the ICAD as their 'usual migraine'.

In Mokri's[65] series of 36 patients with ICAD, 92% initially complained of headache; 85% were unilateral, and in all but 2 patients the headaches resolved. They were most often periorbital (60%), less often in the ear or mastoid area (39%), frontal area (36%), temporal area (27%) and least commonly in the angle of the mandible, face or occiput. Headache or neck pain often preceded the onset of cerebral ischaemic symptoms by several hours or days. This differs from cases of traumatic carotid dissection in which focal cerebral ischaemic symptoms are the most common.

Associated signs and symptoms

Retinal or cerebral ischaemia is the most common symptom of ICAD. Unilateral head or neck pain in a patient presenting with amaurosis fugax or TIA suggests an ICAD.[19,61,63,64,66–69] Ischaemic signs are often delayed and can occur up to one month after the onset of pain.[61] A key element is the presence of ipsilateral local signs associated with the pain in nearly half the patients with ICAD. The most frequent sign is Horner's syndrome, which has long been recognized as suggestive of ICAD.[61,64,66,67,69]

Fisher *et al.*[63] reported on seven patients with persistent hemiparesis or hemiplegia due to ICAD. All had a TIA or neurological prodrome of some kind.

Bogousslovsky *et al.*[70] suggested a much greater risk of initial severe infarction resulting from ICAD. Cervical ICAD was found in 2.5% of 1200 consecutive patients seeking treatment for a first stroke, seven of whom died. In this series, carotid dissection did not have its usual benign prognosis, but these patients had associated carotid occlusion and severe ischaemic symptoms.

Incomplete Horner's syndrome with ptosis and miosis but not anhidrosis is the third most common sign of ICAD. It occurred in 58% of one series of patients (25)[64] and in 31% of the patients reviewed by Fisher *et al.*[63] It may persist; in one series[64] it was present in 38% of the patients at late follow-up.

Less common symptoms of ICAD include neck-swelling, tearing, scintillation, syncope, dysgeusia, and ipsilateral tongue paresis from involvement of the hypoglossal nerve and chorda tympani, which course near the internal carotid artery.

ICAD can present with positive visual phenomena that partly resemble migraine visual aura but are associated with features not typical of migraine. In two cases the visual phenomenon lasted a few days; in a third it was maximal at onset and did not march.[71]

In Biousse's series,[61] associated symptoms included nausea and/or vomiting in 12% of patients, Horner's syndrome in 30%, tinnitus (at times pulsatile) in 16%, TIA in 26%, and completed stroke in 16%. A painful Horner's syndrome was the inaugural symptom of ICAD in 21%.

Radiological features

The gold standard test for dissection is arteriography. Cervical ICAD typically appears about 2 cm distal to its origin and extends a variable distance, usually terminating at or proximal to the entry of the artery into the petrous bone. Classic positive features on angiography include irregular stenosis ('string sign'), tapered occlusion beginning distal to the cervical bifurcation and pseudoaneurysm. In a compilation of reports, luminal stenosis was found in 65% of patients, occlusion in 28%, pseudoaneurysm in 26%, luminal irregularity in 13%, distal branch occlusion (emboli) in 13%, intimal flap in 12% and slow internal carotid artery/middle cerebral artery flow in 11% (Figures 13.2–13.4).[67]

A promising modality for demonstrating carotid dissections is MRI. High-resolution MRI, especially in the axial planes, can demonstrate the vessel lumina and changes in the arterial wall non-invasively and without contrast (Figure

13.5). We found this imaging modality very useful and it now often alleviates the need for formal angiography.

Duplex scanning (Table 13.3) may have several advantages over angiography. It can image the arterial lumen as well as the arterial wall and detect intracranial thrombosis. It

● **Table 13.3** *Duplex sonography: findings suggesting ICAD.*[74]

Indirect findings

No atheromatous plaques visible in carotid bifurcation

Bulb and proximal segment of ICA patent

No flow signal or high-resistance flow pattern (short, only systolic flow peak [stump flow] or bidirectional [reverberating] systolic flow) in proximal ICA

Lack of wall pulsations

Direct signs

Tapering of ICA lumen starting 2 cm distal to bulb

Irregular 'membrane' crossing ICA lumen

Demonstration of true lumen with flow and false (thrombosed) lumen without flow; unlike veins, true and false lumens are noncompressible by probe pressure; flow in false lumen resulting from more distal reentry into true lumen, as frequently found in CCA dissection associated with dissecting aortic aneurysm, is rare

Axial sections show 'membrane' as flap in lumen

Findings at follow-up examinations

Recovery of lumen patency

Flow recovery

Recovery of normal haemodynamics, when combined with TCD

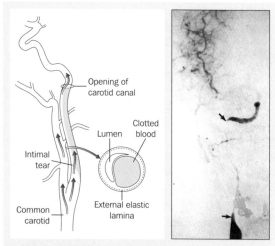

● **Figure 13.2** *Carotid angiograph and diagram showing elongated stenosis and abrupt reconstitution of the lumen at the carotid canal.*

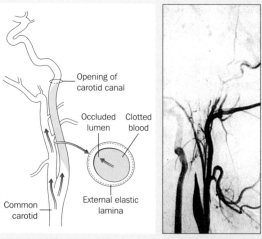

● **Figure 13.3** *Angiograph and diagram of internal carotid artery dissection in which the intramural hematoma is so enlarged that it has squeezed the true lumen to complete occlusion.*

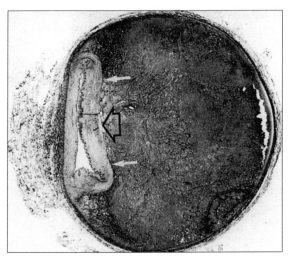

● **Figure 13.4** *Cross section of internal carotid artery dissection in which the intramural hematoma is clearly compressed and the true lumen of the vessel has been narrowed.*

Figures 13.2–13.5 are reproduced with permission from ref. 64.

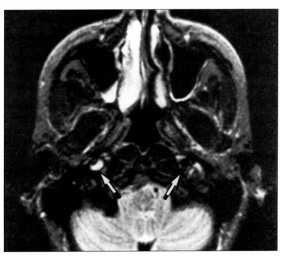

● **Figure 13.5** *MRI of the head of a patient with unilateral ICA dissection. The internal carotid artery on the right is normal in size, dark and the region of flow void is round. On the left, the region of flow void is significantly smaller and surrounded by a bright crescent reflecting the intramural hematoma.*

is non-invasive and can be easily repeated. Early *et al.*[75] reported six patients diagnosed by duplex scanning. Sturzenegger *et al.*[72] found duplex scanning, in combination with transcranial Doppler, to be a useful noninvasive modality for initial diagnosis and an excellent technique for serial follow-up examination. Rothrock *et al.*[73] used MRI and carotid duplex examination in two patients with ICAD and found both techniques helpful. Cox *et al.*[74] found MRI useful in two cases of ICAD.

Duplex scanning does have limitations, however (Table 13.4). Since most dissections occur distal to the carotid bifurcation, it is impossible to image a high dissection via duplex scanning. In addition, duplex scanning does not give information about intracerebral dissection or emboli.[75] Additional limitations include its inability to detect aneurysms and to identify the entire length of stenosis.

Angiography, MRI and carotid duplex findings are highly suggestive of, but not specific for, ICAD, unless a double lumen is present. Acute atherothrombotic occlusion of the intracranial internal carotid artery, emboli, temporal arteritis and radiation arteriopathy can produce a similar angiographic picture, and MRI and carotid duplex may not assist in their differentiation. Recent advances in magnetic resonance angiography may allow more accurate noninvasive diagnosis.

Outcome

Recurrent dissection in a previously dissected and healed vessel is rare. In a patient who had a prior dissection, a new dissection in the uninvolved internal carotid arteries or vertebral arteries is uncommon but not rare. The recurrence rate for second dissections is 2% for the first month and 1% per year for all age groups, more frequent for older patients. Most patients with spontaneous dissections experience excellent clinical and angiographic recovery. A complete or excellent clinical recovery occurs in about 85% of the patients with spontaneous ICAD. Angiographically, stenotic lesions either completely resolve or markedly improve in about 85% of the involved vessels. About 60% of the dissecting aneurysms resolve or diminish in size. Death from massive infarct and oedema may occur, but fortunately is

● **Table 13.4** *Limitations of duplex sonography*[74]

Anatomic
Short and/or fat neck, high cervical carotid bifurcation, goitre, calcification of atherosclerotic lesions (sound shadow)
Individual
Restless, agitated patients who continuously swallow air; emphysema; direct examination may be impossible
Methodologic
Occlusion cannot always be demonstrated directly because of its high cervical location
Usually, whole longitudinal extension of wall dissection and especially involvement of intracranial ICA segments (occurring in up to 20%) cannot be detected
Detection of aneurysms is usually not possible
Identification of fibromuscular dysplasia as underlying cause is hardly ever possible

quite uncommon (<5%). Studies that have drawn their cases from acute stroke registries have reported significantly higher death and disability rates. These, however, do not represent the usual disease profile.[76]

About 5% of patients with ICAD have severe strokes, and these individuals usually have symptomatic infarction as the initial manifestation. One compilation of 75 cases[71] showed that 75% of patients returned to normal, 16% were left with a minor, non-disabling deficit, and 8% suffered a major deficit or death.

Therapy

Although the natural history of extracranial spontaneous dissection appears to be relatively benign, a number of medical and surgical therapies have been used to treat these patients.

Medical therapy

Heparin is the medical modality that has been used most frequently. Although optimum timing is unclear, most practitioners delay heparin administration for several days. There is one report of a worsening ischaemic deficit occurring in a patient who received anticoagulants within several hours of the onset of symptoms; this may have been related to extension of the medial haemorrhage.[77] Anticoagulants can inhibit thrombosis in an aneurysmal sac. In patients, the optimal duration of coagulation is not clearly established. We often empirically treat with an anticoagulant for three months, although data are lacking.

Some patients treated with antiplatelet agents, such as aspirin and dipyridamole, have improved, with resolution of the condition and no haemorrhagic complications.

Surgical therapy

For cases refractory to medical therapy, as evidenced by progression or recurrence, acute or delayed surgical intervention may be warranted. Residual dissection, aneurysms and occlusions appear to be more common with trauma than spontaneous dissection.[65]

Summary

ICAD should be considered when any of the following symptoms are present: painful Horner's syndrome, head pain preceding ischaemic symptoms, or unilateral, severe, persistent neck pain of sudden onset with or without headache. Cephalic pain is a frequent symptom of dissection (75%), is often inaugural (60%), and is usually located on the side of the dissection (76%).

ICAD can also present with other varieties of head and neck pain, mimicking migraine,[61,65,69,78,79] cluster headache,[61,69] carotodynia,[60] SAH[60] or Raeder's syndrome.

Thunderclap headache and subarachnoid haemorrhage

Thunderclap headache is the sudden onset of a severe headache that reaches maximum intensity within one minute. Some further define it by the absence of a SAH. An acute neurological event must be ruled out in all patients who present with severe, acute-onset headache, although migraine can present in this manner.[80]

The first or worst attack of migraine may be very difficult to differentiate from SAH, particularly if the pain is of acute onset (thunderclap headache). SAH from a ruptured aneurysm occurs in 28 000 people a year in North America.[81] The classical presentation of an aneurysmal SAH is an acute-onset, severe headache associated with a stiff neck, photophobia, nausea, vomiting and perhaps obtundation or coma; it is easily differentiated from migraine. This catastrophic presentation is often preceded by a more minor haemorrhage that can signal the likelihood of a major rupture within hours, days or weeks, but which may be more difficult to diagnose.[81-86] In most series of patients with 'minor leaks' related to SAH, headache, nausea or vomiting are common; loss of conciousness is less common, and seizures or cranial nerve findings are rare. In one study, non-exertional activities preceeding the SAH were more frequent than exertional activities.[83] Harling et al.[87] could not clinically differentiate between SAH and other benign headaches in patients presenting with the sudden onset of their worst headache ever. Both the SAH and non-SAH groups had neck stiffness and photophobia, but the SAH group had significantly more vomiting.

An extensive neurological evaluation, including computed tomography (CT) and lumbar puncture, is indicated in patients presenting with their first or worst headache, particularly if it is associated with focal neurological signs, stiff neck or changes in cognition. Computed tomography, which would be performed by most physicians under these clinical circumstances, can miss subarachnoid blood in as many as 25% of cases, particularly if performed days after the onset of headache.[88] MRI is unreliable in detecting acute SAH. A lumbar puncture can confidently diagnose SAH and its omission can be detrimental to the patient.[89] Day and Raskin[90] have stated that all patients presenting with severe, sudden-onset headache should, in addition, be evaluated with angiography for an aneurysm, even if CT, MRI and lumbar puncture do not show evidence of SAH. They reported a case of thunderclap headache in which angiography showed an aneurysm and arterial spasm, but the CT scan was normal and the cerebrospinal fluid (CSF) bloodless. Several prospective studies had suggested that thunderclap headache is usually benign and angiography probably not necessary if neurological examination, CT or MRI, and CSF examination performed at the time of the ictus are normal.[87,91]

Wijdicks et al.[91] prospectively followed 71 patients with severe, sudden-onset thunderclap headaches who had normal CT and CSF findings. All but 2 patients were admitted to the hospital within two days of the headache; only 7 patients (10%) reported a previous similar headache. Neurological examination was normal except for questionable meningismus in 10 patients (14%). Four patients underwent angiography, which was normal. The patients were followed for a mean 3.3 years; none developed evidence of subsequent SAH. Recurrent headaches developed in 12 patients, beginning as early as one day and as long as four years after the initial one. Four patients were readmitted and still had normal CT and CSF studies; of these, 2 patients had normal angiography. A total of 31 patients (44%) developed tension headaches or migraine without aura during the follow-up period.

Harling et al.[87] prospectively followed 14 patients who presented to a regional neurosurgical unit with sudden headache suggestive of SAH but with normal CSF and CT scan. It was not possible, on clinical grounds alone, to distinguish these patients from those that had bled. These patients were followed for a minimum of 18 months. One had no further headache, 4 patients had musculoskeletal pain, 5 patients had psychogenic pain and 4 patients had migraine-type headaches. None developed an unequivocal SAH, and the investigators concluded that angiography cannot be justified in patients with thunderclap headache.

Markus[92] compared the clinical features of thunderclap headache to SAH in a prospective series of 55 patients who presented to a district general hospital with a provisional diagnosis of SAH. Criteria for thunderclap headache included a headache starting within seconds and reaching maximum intensity within one minute and a normal CSF examination within 48 hours of the onset of headache. The clinical features were compared to those of patients who presented to a regional neurosurgical unit with SAH without focal neurological symptoms or impairment of consciousness. The thunderclap headache was described as the worst headache they had ever experienced. Most common locations were occipital (50%) and frontal (38%). Three patients had previously experienced a similar thunderclap headache. No patient in the thunderclap group (n = 18) had developed a SAH at 24 months follow-up. This was the evidence for the absence of an unruptured aneurysm.

Hughes[93] reported two cases of thunderclap headache due to unruptured aneurysms. Case 1 was a healthy 32-year-old man who presented with a severe, abrupt-onset, left-sided headache. When evaluated 12 days after the ictus, the headache was gone, CT was negative and lumbar puncture showed nine red blood cells. A left middle cerebral artery trifurcation aneurysm was found; no evidence of recent haemorrhage was found at surgery. Case 2 was a 48-year-old woman who presented with a severe, abrupt-onset headache that was different from her usual migraine. She had a large left posterior cerebral artery aneurysm that showed no evidence of rupture at surgery.

Ng and Pulst[94] reported a 53-year-old woman who presented with the acute onset of the worst headache of her life. Examination, CT and lumbar puncture were normal. She was discharged after 36 hours of observation, but she was re-admitted two days later due to recurring persistent headaches. The next day she was found unresponsive. An angiogram showed a distal right internal carotid artery aneurysm. She died shortly thereafter.

Raps et al.[95] looked at the clinical spectrum of unruptured intracranial aneurysms, performing a retrospective study of 111 patients (with 132 unruptured aneurysms) who presented to a tertiary referral center. Aneurysms were defined as unruptured by the absence of visible hemorrhage on CT scan, lack of xanthochromia or red blood cells on CSF examination and by visual inspection at the time of surgery. The study included 85 women and 26 men with a mean age of 51.2 years. Fifty-four symptomatic patients were identified; 19 had acute symptoms: ischemia (n = 7), headache (n = 7), seizures (n = 3) and cranial neuropathy (n = 23). Thirty-five had chronic symptoms attributed to mass effect, including headache (n = 18) and visual loss (n = 10).

Acute severe thunderclap headache, comparable to SAH but without nuchal rigidity, was seen in 6.3% (7/111) of the patients with unruptured aneurysms, most of which were located in the anterior circle of Willis.[95] Thus cataclysmic headache may serve as the symptom of both a ruptured and an unruptured aneurysm. The mechanism for acute headache is likely to involve the vessel wall and may include acute expansion, intraluminal bleeding or occult haemorrhage. While this study shows conclusively that an unruptured aneurysm can cause thunderclap headache, it does not allow an estimate of the prevalence of this phenomenon in the population due to selection bias.

Intracranial berry aneurysm occurs in 1–2% of the adult population.[95] If <7% of these in a selected series present with thunderclap headache, the prevalence of this headache type in the general population is no more than 0.1%. The age range is 10–70 years and frequency of recurrence is uncertain. Migraine is an episodic disorder with a one year prevalence of about 12%. If 5% of migraineurs had an attack of acute-onset headache, prevalence would be about 0.6%, which is approximately an order of magnitude higher than that of thunderclap headache from unruptured aneurysm. This could, in part, account for the failure of clinical prospective series of thunderclap headache to detect large numbers of unruptured aneurysms. In addition, the criterion for detection is rupture, not angiography. Thus patients followed for three years still could have an unruptured aneurysm (the risk for rupture is only 1% annually.)

In summary, unruptured aneurysm can cause thunderclap headache. The true frequency of unruptured aneurysms among patients with thunderclap headache is unknown. All patients with a possible unruptured aneurysm should have magnetic resonance angiography. The routine use of cerebral angiography is proscribed by the risk of permanent (0.1%) and transient (1.2%) deficits in this low-yield population, but the issue can be a difficult clinical judgement.[96]

Implications for management diagnosis and treatment

The comorbidity of migraine and stroke has implications for patient management. TIA or stroke can be very similar to migraine aura without headache, creating diagnostic challenges. Episodes of TIA or stroke are often associated with headache; headache may precede or follow the onset of a thromboembolic event.[3] Differentiating TIA or stroke from migraine aura depends on the pattern of symptoms: a history of a slow march of aura symptoms with features that cross vascular territories suggests migraine. The gradual evolution of both positive and negative phenomena (i.e. scintillations scotoma) suggests migraine aura, in contrast to the acute onset of monocular or hemianoptic visual loss seen with stroke. Any patient with migraine and focal neurological signs or with symptoms that are not consistent with IHS migraine with simple aura requires a neuroimaging study to search for structural disease (i.e. mass lesion, arteriovenous malformation or stroke).

The epidemiological studies indicate that migraine is an independent risk factor for stroke (especially in young women). Certainly, migraine patients should be advised not to smoke. Vasoconstrictive medications should be limited or avoided in patients with hemiplegic migraine, basilar migraine and migraine with prolonged aura. Despite controlled trials that show they are safe and effective, there is some controversy about the use of beta-blockers in migraine with aura. Consider using β_1-selective blockers, which have no adverse effect on platelet function, in preference to nonselective beta-blockers, which can increase platelet aggregability. We prefer

to use calcium-channel blockers, such as verapamil, as preventive treatment in patients with migraine with aura. Divalproex sodium, a Food and Drug Administration-approved effective migraine medication, is not vasoactive and is an excellent drug of first choice for preventive therapy in migraineurs with aura, especially those in whom vasoactive medications are contraindicated.[97,98]

Shared risk factors for migraine and stroke include the antiphospholipid antibody syndromes, increased platelet aggregability and mitral valve prolapse. Since these conditions could potentially lead to migrainous infarction, antiplatelet therapy (low-dose aspirin) should be considered if there are no medical contraindications. Aspirin use should also be considered in patients with prolonged or atypical aura. Other cerebrovascular risk factors need to be identified. The use of low-dose oestrogen-containing oral contraceptives or hormonal replacement should be avoided in patients at high risk for stroke although their use in patients with typical migraine poses only a small absolute risk (Table 13.5). Patients with non-visual aura symptoms (aphasia, focal sensory motor symptoms or brainstem symptoms) or prolonged aura require aggressive preventive migraine treatment and an extensive evaluation for coexistent cerebrovascular or other central nervous system disease. Any change in migraine aura symptoms, especially atypical aura, requires urgent re-evaluation, as those symptoms may represent impending stroke rather than migraine.

● **Table 13.5** *Risk of stroke*

General	
Risk of stroke in a female age 20 years	2 per 100 000 women
Risk of stroke on oral contraceptives	3.6 per 100 000 women
Excess stroke risk during pregnancy and six weeks postpartum	8.1 per 100 000 pregnancies
Migraineurs	
Added risk (odds ratios) to a female migraineur under the age of 45 years from:	
Migraine without aura	3
Migraine with aura	6
Oral contraceptives and migraine	13.9
Smoking and migraine	10.2

References

1. Fere C. Contribution a l'etude de la migraine opthalmique. *Rev Med (Paris)* 1881; 1: 625–47.
2. Caplan LR. Migraine and vertebrobasilar ischemia. *Neurology* 1991; 41: 55–61.
3. Gorelick PB, Hier DB, Caplan LR, Langenberg P. Headache is acute cerebrovascular disease. *Neurology* 1986; 36: 1445–50.
4. Mitsias P, Ramadan NM. Headache in ischemic cerebrovascular disease. Part I: clinical features. *Cephalalgia* 1992; 12: 269–74.
5. Mitsias P, Ramadan NM. Headache in ischemic cerebrovascular disease. Part II: mechanisms and predictive value. *Cephalalgia* 1992; 12: 341–4.
6. Alvarez J, Matias-Guiu J, Sumalla J et al. Ischemic stroke in young adults, I; analysis of etiological subgroups. *Acta Neurol Scand* 1989; 80: 29–34.
7. Tatemichi TK, Mohr JP. Migraine and stroke. In: Barnett HJM, Mohr JP, Stein BM, Yarsu FM (eds). *Stroke: pathophysiology, diagnosis and management*. 2nd edition. New York: Churchill-Livingstone, 1992: 761–85.
8. Bougousslavsky J, Regli F. Ischemic stroke in adults younger than 30 years of age: cause and prognosis. *Arch Neurol* 1987; 44: 479–82.
9. Rothrock J, North J, Madden K et al. Migraine and migrainous stroke: risk factors and prognosis. *Neurology* 1993; 43: 2473–6.
10. Broderick JP, Swanson JW. Migraine-related strokes: clinical profile and prognosis in 20 patients. *Arch Neurol* 1987; 44: 868–71.
11. Sacquegna T, Andreoli A, Baldrati A et al. Ischemic stroke in young adults: the relevance of migrainous infarction. *Cephalalgia* 1989; 9: 255–8.
12. Bougousslavsky J, Regli F, VanMelle G et al. Migraine stroke. *Neurology* 1988; 38: 223–9.
13. Collaborative Group for the Study of Stroke in Young Women. Oral contraceptives and stroke in young women. *JAMA* 1975; 281: 718–22.
14. Henrich JB, Horowitz RI. A controlled study of ischemic stroke risk in migraine patients. *J Clin Epidemiol* 1989; 42: 773–80.
15. Tzourio C, Iglesias S, Hubert JB et al. Migraine and risk of ischemic stroke: a case controlled study. *Br Med J* 1993; 307: 289–92.
16. Tzourio C, Iglesias S, Tehindrazanarivelo A, Chedru F, Bousser MG, The AICSJ Group. Migraine and ischemic stroke in young women (abstract). *Stroke* 1994; 25: 15.
17. Carolei A, Marini C, DeMatteis G, Italian National Research Council Study Group on Stroke in the Young. History of migraine and risk of cerebral ischaemia in young adults. *Lancet* 1996; 343: 1503–6.

18. Baring JE, Hebert P, Romero J et al. Migraine and subsequent risk of stroke in the physicians' health study. *Arch Neurol* 1995; 42: 128–34.
19. Headache Classification Committee of the International Headache Society. Classification and diagnostic criteria for headache disorders, cranial neuralgias, and facial pain. *Cephalalgia* 1988; 8(Suppl. 7): 1–96.
20. Welch KMA, Levine SR. Migraine-related stoke in the context of the International Headache Society classification of migraine. *Arch Neurol* 1990; 47: 458–62.
21. Lauritzen M, Olesen J. Regional cerebral blood flow during migraine attacks by xenon 133 inhalation and emission tomography. *Brain* 1984; 107: 447–61.
22. Levine SR, Welch KMA, Ewing JR, Robertson WM. Asymmetric cerebral blood flow patterns in migraine. *Cephalalgia* 1987; 7: 245–8.
23. Olesen J. Cerebral and extracranial circulatory disturbances in migraine: pathophysiological implications. *Cerebrovasc Brain Metab Rev* 1991; 3: 1–28.
24. Joseph R, Welch KMA. Migraine and the platelet: nonspecific association. *Headache* 1987; 27: 375–80.
25. Kalendovsky Z, Austin JH. 'Complicated Migraine'; its association with increased platelet aggregability and abnormal plasma coagulation factors. *Headache* 1975; 15: 18–35.
26. Kalendowsky Z, Austin J, Steele P. Increased platelet aggregability in young patients with stroke. *Arch Neurol* 1975; 32: 13–20.
27. Ramadan NR, Tietjen GE, Levine SR, Welch KMA. Carotid artery dissection associated with scintillating scotomata. *Neurology* 1991; 41: 1084–7.
28. Pfaffenrath V, Pöllmann W, Autenrieth G, Rosmanith U. Mitral valve prolapse and platelet aggregation in patients with hemiplegic and nonhemiplegic migraine. *Acta Neurol Scand* 1987; 75: 253–7.
29. Herman P. Migraine and mitral valve prolapse. *Arch Neurol* 1989; 46: 1165.
30. Brey RL, Hart RG, Sherman DG, Tegeler CH. Antiphospholipid antibodies and cerebral ischemia in young people. *Neurology* 1990; 40: 1190–6.
31. Tietjen GE, Levine SR, Welch KMA. Migraine and antiphospholipid antibodies. In: Appel SH (ed). *Current Neurology, Volume 12*. Chicago: Mosby-Year Book 1992: 201–13.
32. Pavlakis SG, Rowland LP, DeVivo DL, Bonilla F, Divlauro S. Mitochondrial myopathies and encephalomyopathies. In: Plum F. (ed) *Advances in Contemporary Neurology*. Contemporary neurology series. Philadelphia: FA Davis, 1988: 95–134.

33. Ciafaloni E, Ricci J, Shanske S et al. MELAS; clinical features, biochemistry, and molecular genetics. *Ann Neurol* 1992; 31: 391–8.
34. Chabriat H, Vahedi K, Iba-Zizen MT et al. Clinical spectrum of CADASIL: study of 7 families. *Lancet* 1995; 346: 934–9.
35. Olesen J, Lauritzen M, Tfelt-Hansen Pk, Henriksen L, Larsen B. Spreading cerebral oligemia in classical- and normal cerebral blood flow in common migraine. *Headache* 1982; 22: 242–8.
36. Lauritzen M, Olesen TS, Lassen NA, Paulson OB. Changes in regional cerebral flood flow during the course of classic migraine attacks. *Ann Neurol* 1983; 13: 633–41.
37. Olesen J, Larsen B, Lauritzen M. Focal hyperemia followed by spreading oligemia and impaired activation of RCBF in classic migraine. *Ann Neurol* 1981; 9: 344–52.
38. Lauritzen M. Pathophysiology of the migraine aura: the spreading depression theory. *Brain* 1994; 17: 199–210.
39. Leão AAP. Spreading depression of activity in the cerebral cortex. *J Neurophysiol* 1944; 7: 359–90.
40. Levine SR, Welch KMA, Ewing JR, Joseph R, D'andrea G. Cerebral blood flow asymmetries in headache-free migraineurs. *Stroke* 1987; 18: 1164–5.
41. Lagreze HL, Dettmers C, Hartmann A. Abnormalities of interictal cerebral perfusion in classic but not common migraine. *Stroke* 1988; 19: 1108–11.
42. Scharf RE, Hennerici M, Bluschke V, Lueck J, Kladetzky RG. Cerebral ischemia in young patients: it is associated with mitral valve prolapse and abnormal platelet activity in vivo? *Stroke* 1982; 13: 454–8.
43. Moskowitz MA. The neurobiology of vascular head pain. *Ann Neurol* 1984; 16: 157–68.
44. Schon F, Harrison MJ. Can migraine cause multiple segmental cerebral artery constrictions? *J Neurol Neurosurg Psych* 1987; 50(4): 492–4.
45. Laurent B, Michel D, Antoine JC, Montagnon D. Migraine basilaire avec alexie sans agraphie; spasme arteriel a l'arteriographie et effet de la naloxone. *Rev Neurol (Paris)* 1984; 40: 663–5.
46. Schroth G, Gerber WD, Langohr HD. Ultrasonic doppler flow in migraine and cluster headache. *Headache* 1983; 23: 284–5.
47. Thie A, Spitzer K, Lachenmayer L, Kunze K. Prolonged vasospasm in migraine detected by noninvasive transcranial doppler ultrasound. *Headache* 1988; 28: 183–6.
48. Levine SR, Ramadan NM. The relationship of stroke and migraine. In: Adams HP (ed). *Handbook of Cerebrovascular Diseases*. New York: Marcel Dekker, Inc. 1993; 221–31.

49. Olesen J, Friberg L, Olsen TS et al. Ischemia-induced (symptomatic) migraine attacks may be more frequent than migraine-induced ischemic insults. *Brain* 1993; 116: 187–202.

50. Welch KMA. Migraine: a behavioral disorder. *Arch Neurol* 1987; 44: 323–7.

51. Welch KMA. Chabi E, Nell JH et al. Biochemical comparison of migraine and stroke. *Headache* 1976; 6: 160.

52. Tournier–Lasserve E, Joutel A, Melki J et al. Cerebral autosomal arteriopathy with subcortical infarcts and leukoencephalopathy maps to chromosome 19q12. *Nature Genet* 1993; 3: 256–7.

53. Ophoff RA, van Eijk R, Sandkuijl LA et al. Genetic heterogeneity of familial hemiplegic migraine, *Genomics* 1994; 22: 21–6.

54. Chabriat H, Tournier-Lasserve E, Vahedi K et al. Autosomal dominant migraine with MRI white-matter abnormalities mapping to the CADASIL locus. *Neurology* 1995; 45: 1086–91.

55. Hart RG, Easton JD. Dissections of cervical and cerebral arteries. *Neurol Clin* 1983; 1: 155–82.

56. Sherman DG, Hart RG, Easton JD. Abrupt change in head position and cerebral infarction. *Stroke* 1981; 12: 2–6.

57. Luken MG, Ascherl GF, Correll JW. Spontaneous dissecting aneurysms of the internal carotid arteries. *Am J Surg* 1971; 122: 549–51.

58. Friedman WA, Day AL, Quisling RG, Sypert GW, Rhoton AL. Cervical carotid dissecting aneurysms. *Neurosurgery* 1980; 7: 207–14.

59. Fay T. Atypical facial neuralgia, a syndrome of vascular pain. *Ann Otol Laryngol* 1932; 41: 1030–62.

60. Biousse V, Woimant F, Amarenco P, Touboul PJ, Bousser MG. Pain as the only manifestation of internal carotid artery dissection. *Cephalalgia* 1992; 12: 314–17.

61. Biousse V, D'Anglejan JD, Touboul P et al. Headache in 67 patients with extracranial internal carotid artery dissection. 5th International Headache Congress. *Cephalalgia* 1991; 11(Suppl 11): 349–50.

62. Mas JL, Bousser MG, Hasboun D, Laplane D. Extracranial vertebral artery dissections: a review of 13 cases. *Stroke* 1987; 18: 1037–47.

63. Fisher CM, Ojemann RG, Robertson GH. Spontaneous dissection of cervicocerebral arteries. *Can J Neurol Sci* 1987; 5: 9–19.

64. Mokri B, Sundt TM, Houser OW, Piepgras DG. Spontaneous dissection of the cervical internal carotid artery. *Ann Neurol* 1986; 19: 126–38.

65. Mokri B, Houser W, Sandok BA, Piepgras DG. Spontaneous dissections of the vertebral arteries. *Neurology* 1988; 38: 880–5.

66. D'Anglejan Chatillon J, Ribiero V, Mas JL, Bousser MG, Laplane D. Dissection de l'artère carotide interne extracranienne. Soizante duex observations. *Presse Méd* 1990; 19: 661–7.

67. Anson J, Crowell RM. Cervicocranial arterial dissection. *Neurosurgery* 1991; 29: 89–96.

68. Biller J, Hingtgen WL, Adams HP, Smiker WRK, Godersky JC, Toffol GJ. Cervicocephalic arterial dissections. A ten-year experience. *Arch Neurol* 1986; 43: 1234–8.

69. Fisher CM. The headache and pain of spontaneous carotid dissection. *Headache* 1982; 22: 60–5.

70. Bogousslavsky J, Despland PA, Regli F. Spontaneous dissection with acute stroke. *Arch Neurol* 1987; 44: 137–40.

71. Ramadan NM, Tietjen GE, Levine SR, Welch KMA. Scintillating scotomata associated with internal carotid artery dissection: report of three cases. *Neurology* 1991; 41: 1084–7.

72. Sturzenegger M. Ultrasound findings in spontaneous carotid artery dissection. *Arch Neurol* 1991; 48: 1057–63.

73. Rothrock JF, Lim V, Press G, Gosink B. Serial magnetic resonance and carotid duplex examinations in the management of carotid dissection. *Neurology* 1989; 39: 686–92.

74. Cox LK, Bertorini T, Laster RE. Headaches due to spontaneous internal carotid artery dissection: magnetic resonance imagng evaluation and follow up. *Headache* 1991; 31: 12–16.

75. Early TF, Gregory RT, Wheeler JR et al. Spontaneous carotid dissection: duplex scanning in diagnosis and management. *J Vasc Surg* 1991; 14: 391–7.

76. Mokri B. Headache in spontaneous carotid and vertebral artery dissections. In: Goadsby PJ, Silberstein SD (eds). *Blue Books of Practical Neurology: Headache.* Boston: Butterworth-Heinemann 1997: 327–54.

77. Chapleau CE, Robertson JT. Spontaneous cervical carotid artery dissection: outpatient treatment with continuous heparin infusion using a totally implantable infusion device. *Neurosurgery* 1981; 8: 83–7.

78. Bousser MG, Baron JC, Chiras J. Ischemic strokes and migraine. *Neuroradiology* 1985; 27: 583–7.

79. Shuaib A. Stroke from other etiologies masquerading as migraine-stroke. *Stroke* 1991; 22: 1068–74.

80. Silberstein SD. Evaluation and emergency treatment of headache. *Headache* 1992; 32: 396–407.

81. Leblanc R. The minor leak preceding subarachnoid hemorrhage. *J Neurosurg* 1987; 66: 35–9.

82. Waga S, Ohtsubo K, Handa H. Warning signs in intracranial aneurysms. *Surg Neurol* 1975; 3: 15–20.

83. Fontanarosa PB. Recognition of subarachnoid hemorrhage. *Ann Emerg Med* 1989; 18: 1199–1205.

84. Duffy GP. The "warning leak" in spontaneous subarachnoid hemorrhage. *Med J Aust* 1983; 1: 514–16.

85. King RB, Saba MI. Forewarnings of major subarachnoid hemorrhage. *NY State J Med* 72: 638–9.

86. Bartleson JD, Swanson JW, Whisnat JP. A migrainous syndrome with cerebrospinal fluid pleocytosis. *Neurology* 1981; 31: 1257–62.

87. Harling DW, Peatfield RC, Van Hille PT, Abbott RJ. Thunderclap headache: is it migraine? *Cephalalgia* 1989; 9: 87–90.

88. Adams HP, Kassell NF, Torner JC, Sahs AL. CT and clinical correlations in recent aneurysmal subarachnoid hemorrhage: a preliminary report of the cooperative aneurysm study. *Neurology* 1983; 33: 981–8.

89. Silberstein SD, Marcelis J. Headache associated with changes in intracranial pressure. *Headache* 1992; 32: 84–94.

90. Day JW and Raskin NH. Thunderclap headache: symptom of unruptured cerebral aneurysm. *Lancet* 1986; 2: 1247–8.

91. Wijdicks EFM, Kerkhoff H and Van Gijn J. Long-term follow-up of 71 patients with thunderclap headache mimicking subarachnoid hemorrhage. *Lancet* 1988; ii: 68–70.

92. Markus HS. A prospective follow up of thunderclap headache mimicking subarachnoid hemorrhage. *J Neurol Neurosurg Psychiatry* 1992; 54: 1117–25.

93. Hughes RL. Identification and treatment of cerebral aneurysms after sentinel headache. *Neurology* 1992; 42: 1118–19.

94. Ng PK, Pulst S-M. Not so benign "thunderclap headache." *Neurology* 1992; 260(Suppl. 3): 42.

95. Raps EC, Rogers JD, Galetta SL et al. The clinical spectrum of unruptured intracranial aneurysms. *Arch Neurol* 1993; 50: 265–8.

96. Leow K, Murie JA. New information on several painful conditions: thunderclap headache mimicking subarachnoid hemorrhage. *Neurology Alert* 1988; 7: 5–6.

97. Saper J, Matthew N, Silberstein S et al. Safety and efficacy of divalproex sodium in the prophylaxis of migraine headache: a multicentred double-blind, placebo-controlled study. *Neurology* 1993; 43: 401.

98. Hering R, Kuritzky A. Sodium valproate in the prophylactic treatment of migraine; a double-blind study vs placebo. *Cephalalgia* 1992; 12: 81–4.

Sinus headache

Sinusitis

Sinus infection is much less frequent today than in the pre-antibiotic era. Despite this, it is frequently overdiagnosed: the media would lead one to believe that most headaches are due to sinus disease. Recurrent episodic pain in the sinus areas is most likely migrainous in nature with secondary (neurovascular) changes in the sinuses producing local symptoms. Whether nasal obstruction can lead to chronic headache is very controversial.[1] Paradoxically, sinus disease also tends to be underdiagnosed, as sphenoid sinus infection is frequently missed.[2]

Sinusitis, which affects more than 31 million people in the United States, resulted in 16 million physician visits in 1989.[3] While sinusitis is generally more common in children than adults, frontal and sphenoid sinusitis are rare in children. In the pre-antibiotic era the sphenoid sinus was involved in up to 33% of cases of sinusitis. Today its incidence is about 3%.[2]

The maxillary and ethmoid sinuses, both present at birth, are the most common sites of clinical infection in children. The sphenoid sinus develops after the age of two years and starts to pneumatize at the age of eight years. The frontal sinuses develop from the anterior ethmoid sinus at about six years of age. The frontal and sphenoid sinuses become clinically important in the teens, and frequently become infected in pansinusitis. Isolated sphenoid sinusitis is rare.[4,5]

The clinical diagnosis of sinusitis is usually based on symptoms indicating maxillary or frontal sinus involvement. This may occur secondary to, and is frequently a result of, ethmoid disease. The ethmoid sinuses are the key to sinus infection. Obstruction of the sinus ostia is the usual precursor to sinusitis.[6,7]

Anatomy and physiology

The lateral nasal wall is composed of the ethmoid bone, a T-shaped structure that supports the bilateral ethmoid labyrinth. The horizontal limb of the T is formed by the cribriform plate, from which is suspended the ethmoid labyrinth, a complex structure with multiple bony septa and the medial projections of the superior and middle turbinates. Lateral to the uncinate process, a secondary projection of the ethmoid bone, is the infundibulum, a recess into which the maxillary sinus drains. The infundibulum drains into the hiatus semilunaris which in turn drains into the middle meatus, which is located between the uncinate process and the middle turbinate. The frontal sinus drains into the frontal recess, which may drain into the middle meatus or the ethmoidal infundibulum. This region is known as the osteomeatal complex[8] (maxillary sinus ostium,

infundibulum, hiatus semilunaris, middle turbinate, ethmoidal bulla and frontal ostium). The sphenoidal sinus and posterior ethmoidal cells drain into the sphenoethmoidal recess (Figure 14.1).

The primary functions of the nasal passages are humidification, warming and removal of particulate material from the inspired air. The paranasal sinuses are air-filled cavities that communicate with the nasal airway. They are lined with pseudostratified-ciliated epithelium, which is covered by a thin layer of mucus that receives the largest deposits of inhaled large particulate matter. The cilia and this mucous layer are in constant motion in a predetermined direction. Mucus and debris are transported towards the ostia by the beating of the cilia and are expelled into the nasal airway.[4,6,8]

Any bacterial contamination of the sinuses is effectively cleared by this mechanism. If the sinus ostia are obstructed, mucociliary flow is interrupted. Obstruction causes the oxygen tension within the sinus to decrease and the carbon dioxide tension to increase. This anaerobic, high-carbon dioxide, stagnant environment can facilitate bacterial growth.[8]

Surgical drainage of the sinuses, avoiding the region of the natural ostia, had been the treatment of choice for sinus infections for many years. This procedure alleviated the acute sinus infection but did not prevent reaccumulation of mucus within the sinus. Because the normal beat of the cilia transports mucus toward the natural ostium, creating a new ostium at a site distant from the natural ostium fails to direct the flow of mucus to the new opening.[8]

All sinuses normally contain anaerobic bacteria, and more than one-third harbour a mixed environment of anaerobic and

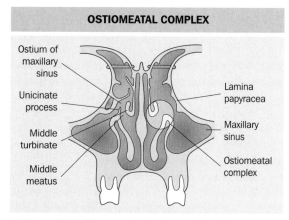

OSTIOMEATAL COMPLEX

● *Figure 14.1* *Diagram showing the position of the region known as the osteomeatal complex.*

aerobic organisms. Therefore, ciliary dysfunction and retention of secretions, commonly a result of ostia obstruction, is necessary for bacterial proliferation and the development of sinus infection. Aerobes present in both normal and disease states include the Gram-positive streptococci (alpha, beta and *Streptococcus pneumoniae*) and *Staphylococcus aureus*, and Gram-negative *Moraxella catarrhalis*, *Haemophilus influenzae* and *Escherichia coli*. Anaerobic organisms include the Gram-positive peptococci and *Propionibacterium* species. The *Bacteroides* and *Fusobacterium* species also play a role in chronic sinusitis.[4,9]

Systemic diseases which predispose to sinusitis include cystic fibrosis, immune deficiency, bronchiectasis and the immobile cilia syndrome. Local factors include upper respiratory infection (usually viral), allergic rhinitis, overuse of topical decongestants, hypertrophied adenoids, deviated nasal septum, nasal polyps, tumours and cigarette smoke.[4]

Unobstructed flow through the sinus ostia and its narrow communicating passage within the osteomeatal complex is integral to mucociliary clearance and ventilation. Persistent low-grade inflammation in the ethmoid sinus may cause few localizing symptoms but can predispose to recurrent maxillary and frontal sinus infections.[4,8]

Diagnostic testing
Standard radiography
This is inadequate for the clinical evaluation of sinusitis as it does not evaluate the anterior ethmoid air cells, the upper two-thirds of the nasal cavity, or the infundibular, middle meatus and frontal recess air passages.[6]

Computed tomography (CT)
This may demonstrate mucosal thickening, sclerosis, clouding, or air-fluid levels. Imaging must be performed in the coronal plane to adequately demonstrate the ethmoid complex. It can reveal the extent of mucosal disease in the osteomeatal complex. In a hundred CT examinations of patients with chronic sinusitis, the middle meatus was involved in 72%. Anterior ethmoid sinus infection was found in each patient who had frontal or maxillary sinusitis. Middle meatal disease was found in the rest of these patients; it extended to, and occluded, the frontal recess in the patients who had frontal sinusitis and extended to, and occluded, the infundibulum in all cases of maxillary mucoperiosteal disease.[3,7]

Magnetic resonance imaging (MRI)
The appearance of normal nasal mucosa during the oedematous phase of the nasal cycle on T2-weighted image can resemble pathological change. Despite these problems with specificity, MRI is more sensitive than CT in detecting fungal infection.[6]

Maxillary mucosal thickening >6 mm, complete sinus opacification and air-fluid levels on neuroimaging correlate to positive sinus cultures.[10] However, 30–40% of the normal population will have mucosal thickening on CT evaluation.[11]

Transillumination, ultrasonography and anterior rhinoscopy
Transillumination of the sinuses has low sensitivity and specificity.[12] Ultrasonography has lower sensitivity and specificity than sinus X-rays.[12] Routine anterior rhinoscopy performed with a headlight and nasal speculum allows only limited inspection of the anterior nasal cavity.

Diagnostic fibreoptic endoscopy
The flexible fibreoptic rhinoscope allows direct visualization of the nasal passages and sinus drainage areas (osteomeatal complex) and is complementary to CT or MRI. This procedure is easily performed by the trained operator and is readily tolerated by the patient. Infection is easily diagnosed if purulent material is seen emanating from the sinus drainage region. Mucosal sinus thickening is frequently present in normal, non-symptomatic patients. In these cases, endoscopy should be positive before a diagnosis of sinusitis can be made.[8,9] Sphenoid sinusitis is an exception to this generalization.

Endoscopy should be considered when a sinus-related problem is suspected in a patient who fails conservative medical treatment and whose CT or MRI is inconclusive. Some use endoscopy prior to neuroimaging. Negative neuroimaging and endoscopy usually, but not always, rules out sinus disease.[6]

Castellanos and Axelrod[13] evaluated 246 patients with undiagnosed headache and a negative neurological evaluation. Ninety-eight had only rhinoscopic evidence of sinusitis, 84 had both rhinoscopic and standard radiographic evidence of sinusitis and 64 had neither. Patients were treated with antibiotics for four weeks, at which time only those patients with rhinoscopic and/or radiological evidence of sinusitis reported headache improvement. This was an open uncontrolled study, but repeat rhinoscopic evaluation showed clearing of infection coincident with headache improvement.

Clinical findings
Acute sinusitis lasts from 1 day to 3 weeks. Subacute sinusitis lasts from 3 weeks to 3 months. Chronic sinusitis lasts more than 3 months.[12]

Facial tenderness and pain, nasal congestion and purulent nasal discharge are common manifestations of acute sinus infection. Other 'classic' signs and symptoms include anosmia, pain upon mastication and halitosis. An upper respiratory infection or a history of such infection may be present.[12] While fever is present in about 50% of adults and 60% of children and headache is common, the symptoms of headache, facial pain and fever are often of minimal value in the diagnosis of sinusitis. Williams *et al.*[14] looked at the sensitivity and specificity of individual symptoms in making the diagnosis of sinusitis. No single item was both sensitive and specific. Maxillary toothache was highly specific (93%), but only 11% of the patients had this symptom. Logistic regression analysis showed five independent predictions of sinusitis: maxillary toothache (odds ratio (OR) = 2.9), abnormal transillumination (OR = 2.7, sensitivity = 73%, specificity = 54%), poor response to decongestants (OR = 2.4), purulent discharge (OR = 2.9) and coloured nasal discharge (OR = 2.2). The data did not support the other textbook findings for sinusitis, an antecedent upper respiratory infection or history of facial pain. 'Headache' had an odds ratio of 1.0 with a 68% sensitivity and 30% specificity. The low specificity is due to lack of descriptive features of the headache. Facial pain and itchy eyes had an odds ratio of 1.0. Fever, sweats or chills were found in 48% with an odds ratio of 0.9 (sensitivity 45%, specificity 51%). In children, symptoms are often minimal even in the face of marked sinus involvement.[15]

Sinus infection can result in acute suppurative meningitis, subdural or epidural abscess, and brain abscess. In addition, osteomyelitis and subperiosteal abscess can occur. Infection of the ethmoid and, to a lesser extent, the sphenoid sinuses, is responsible for orbital complications, which include oedema, orbital cellulitis, subperiosteal and orbital abscess.[4]

A mucocele is a mucus-containing cyst located in the sinuses. These are most common (and benign) in the maxillary sinus (mucus retention cyst). Those located in the frontal, sphenoid or ethmoid sinus can enlarge and erode into the surrounding structures. A pyocele is an infected mucocele.[5,16]

Wolff[17] showed that the sinuses themselves are relatively insensitive to pain. The pain associated with sinusitis comes from engorged and inflamed nasal structures: nasofrontal ducts, turbinates, ostia and superior nasal spaces. Headache associated with paranasal sinus disease usually has a deeper, dull, aching quality combined with a heaviness and fullness. It is seldom associated with nausea and vomiting.

The International Headache Society (IHS) has established criteria for acute sinus headache (Table 14.1).[18] To qualify as acute sinus headache, there must be purulent discharge, abnormal neuroimaging, and simultaneous onset of headache and sinusitis. These criteria may not be valid for sphenoid sinusitis, however, as purulent discharge is often lacking, and headache may precede sinus drainage. Once drainage begins, obstruction is relieved and the headache may begin to abate.

All sinusitis pain is not the same. Maxillary sinusitis pain is most typically located in the cheek, the gums, and the teeth of the upper jaw. Ethmoid sinusitis pain is said to be felt between the eyes. The eyeball may be tender and pain may be aggravated by eye movement. Frontal sinusitis pain is felt mainly in the forehead. Sphenoid sinusitis pain is said to be felt in the vertex, but has more general localization. Ethmoid and maxillary sinusitis is usually associated with rhinitis.

Hypertrophic turbinates, atrophic sinus membranes and nasal passage abnormalities due to septal deflection are other conditions which may cause headache; however, they are not sufficiently validated as a cause of headache. Migraine and tension-type headache are often confused with true sinus headache because of similarity in location. In order to diagnose 'IHS' sinus headache, the above criteria must be strictly fulfilled.

The relationship between headache and subacute and chronic sinus disease is highly controversial. Radiographical evidence of sinus disease is very common and does not establish the headache's aetiology.[11] Headache associated with sinus disease is usually continuous, not intermittent. Chronic sinusitis is frequently associated with engorged and swollen nasal mucosa and a purulent or sanguinopurulent nasal discharge. The IHS has not validated chronic sinusitis as a cause of headache or facial pain unless it relapses into an acute stage.[19]

Faleck *et al.*[20] reported that 10% of 150 children and adolescents presenting with chronic, non-progressive headache, clinically indistinguishable from 'muscle contraction' headache, had radiographical evidence of sinus pathology. None had prominent respiratory symptoms. All improved with treatment directed towards the sinus pathology. Although some had complete sinus opacification, none had endoscopy to show the presence of active disease in the ostia.

Table 14.1 *Acute sinus headache. IHS diagnostic criteria*

A Purulent discharge in the nasal passage either spontaneous or by suction

B Pathological findings in one or more of the following tests:
- X-ray examination
- Computerized tomography or magnetic resonance imaging
- Transillumination

C Simultaneous onset of headache and sinusitis

D Headache location:
- In acute frontal sinusitis, headache is located directly over the sinus and may radiate to the vertex or behind the eyes
- In acute maxillary sinusitis, headache is located over the antral area and may radiate to the upper teeth or the forehead
- In acute ethmoiditis, headache is located between the eyes and may radiate to the temporal area
- In acute sphenoiditis, headache is located in the occipital area, the vertex, the frontal region, or behind the eyes.

E Headache disappears after treatment of acute sinusitis

Treatment

Management goals for the treatment of sinusitis include:

- Treatment of bacterial infection
- Reduction of ostial swelling
- Sinus drainage
- Maintenance of sinus ostia patency.

Uncomplicated sinusitis, other than sphenoid sinusitis, should be treated with a broad spectrum oral antibiotic for 10–14 days. Nasal culture does not correlate to sinus pathogens, thus initial treatment is empiric.[12] Steam and saline prevent crusting of secretions in the nasal cavity and facilitate mucociliary clearance. Locally active vasoconstrictor agents provide symptomatic relief by shrinking inflamed and swollen nasal mucosa. Their use should be limited to 3–4 days to prevent rebound vasodilation. Oral decongestants should be used if prolonged treatment (>3 days) is necessary. These agents are α-adrenergic agonists that reduce nasal blood flow without the risk of rebound vasodilation.[12]

Antihistamines are not effective in the management of acute treatment of rhinitis. Anti-inflammatory topical corticosteroids may help maintain patency of the ostia.

Treatment failure and recurrent infections are indications for neuroimaging and endoscopy to search for a source of obstruction. Sinus sampling for culture should be considered. Endoscopic nasal surgery may be necessary to reopen and maintain the patency of the sinus ostia and ostiomeatal complex.[12]

Treatment of complications consists of high doses of intravenous antibiotics and surgical drainage, if appropriate, of any enclosed space.

Sphenoid sinusitis

Sphenoid sinusitis, because of its rarity, unique location, and complications, is discussed separately. It is an uncommon infection that accounts for approximately 3% of all cases of acute sinusitis. It is usually accompanied by pansinusitis; less commonly it occurs alone. In contrast to other paranasal sinus infections, it is frequently misdiagnosed,[21] since the sphenoid sinus is not accessible to direct clinical examination even with the flexible endoscope and is not adequately visualized with routine sinus X-rays. While sphenoid sinusitis is an uncommon cause of headache, it is potentially associated with significant morbidity and mortality and requires early identification and aggressive management.[2,21,22]

The sphenoid sinus is contained within the body of the sphenoid bone deep in the nasal cavity and is divided in half by the intersphenoid septum. Each sinus communicates with the sphenoethmoidal recess, located at the posterior superior aspect of the superior concha. The sphenoidal sinuses are present as minute cavities at birth, and it is not until puberty that their main development occurs.[23]

The roof of the sphenoid sinus is related to the middle cranial fossa and the pituitary gland in the sella turcica; lateral is the cavernous sinus; posteriorly is the clivus and pons; anteriorly the posterior nasal cavity, posterior ethmoid cells and cribriform plate; and inferiorly the nasopharynx. The cavernous sinus, which is lateral to the sphenoid sinus, contains the internal carotid arteries and the IIIrd, IVth, Vth and VIth cranial nerves. The maxillary division of the Vth nerve may indent the wall of the sphenoid sinus. The sphenoid walls can be extremely thin, and sometimes the sinus cavity is separated from the adjacent structure by just a thin mucosal barrier. Because of the close proximity to the cortical venous system, cranial nerves and meninges, infection may spread to these structures and present as a CNS infection or neurological catastrophe.[2,24]

Symptoms (Table 14.2)

Headache is the most common symptom of acute sphenoid sinusitis: it is present in all patients who are able to complain about it. It is aggravated by standing, walking, bending or coughing, it often interferes with sleep and is poorly relieved by narcotics. Its location is variable: vertex headache is rare; frontal, occipital, or temporal headache or a combination of these locations is most common. Periorbital pain is common. This is in contrast to the common teaching that retro-orbital or vertex headache is the most common presenting symptom of sphenoid sinusitis.[2,21,22,25,26,27]

Nausea and vomiting frequently occur, but nasal discharge, stuffiness and postnasal drip are unusual. Fever occurs in over half the patients with acute sphenoid sinusitis.

● **Table 14.2** *Sphenoid sinusitis*

Symptom	Goldman[21]	Kibblewhite[22]	Lew[2]
Headache or facial pain	12/12	13/14*	30/30**
Pain worse with head movement	12/12	Most	?
Nasal discharge/ congestion	6/12	4/14	?
Fever	7/12	8/14	Most
Nausea or vomiting	?	8/14	?
Complications	0/12	8/14	10/14 acute, 3/15 chronic

* Patient comatose; ** 15 acute, 15 chronic

Diagnosis

The diagnosis of sphenoid sinusitis is frequently delayed. Sphenoid sinusitis should be included in the differential diagnosis of acute or subacute headache. It may be mistaken for frontal or ethmoid sinusitis, aseptic meningitis, brain abscess or septic thrombophlebitis. It can mimic trigeminal neuralgia, migraine, carotid artery aneurysm or brain tumour.[2,21,22]

The clinical features of a severe, intractable, new-onset headache that interferes with sleep and is not relieved by simple analgesics should alert one to the diagnosis of sphenoid sinusitis. Headache increases in severity with time and has no specific location. Pain or paraesthesias in the facial distribution of the Vth nerve and photophobia or eye tearing are suggestive of sphenoid sinusitis.[2,21,22,25,26,28]

The physical examination may not be helpful. Not all patients are febrile, sinus tenderness is rarely present and pus is not always seen, although Lew et al.[2] state that a careful examination of the nose and throat often demonstrated pus. Whether this reflects advanced disease or the presence of pansinusitis is uncertain. In a more recent series of 14 patients with acute sphenoid sinusitis, Kibblewhite et al.[22] found purulent exudate in only 3 patients.

Neuroimaging is necessary to definitively diagnose sphenoid sinusitis. All of Kibblewhite's cases were diagnosed by X-ray.[22] Some cases can be diagnosed by plain sinus X-rays, but, because of the superimposition of soft tissues, plain X-rays are non-diagnostic in about 25% of cases.[21] If sphenoid sinusitis is suspected and plain radiographs are non-diagnostic, CT or MRI is indicated (Figure 14.2).

In a high-risk group of 300 patients referred with a clinical diagnosis of sinusitis, 68% had abnormal plain radiographs but none had sphenoid sinus abnormalities, suggesting that the specificity of plain radiographs is very high.[29] The mucosa of the sinus approximates the bone so closely that it cannot be visualized on CT. Therefore any bulge of soft tissue seen in the sinus is abnormal.[30] Digre et al.[31] reviewed 300 CT or MRI radiographic studies. The sphenoid sinus was visualized in all cases. Abnormalities were detected in 7% of routine CT scans, 8% of posterior fossa scans and 6% of MRI scans. Of the 21 patients with sphenoid abnormalities, 24% in their highly selected sample had important clinical related disease.

Complications

Major complications of sphenoid sinusitis include bacterial meningitis,[2] cavernous sinus thrombosis,[2,21,22,24] subdural abscess,[2,21,22] cortical vein thrombosis,[2,21,22] ophthalmoplegia and pituitary insufficiency.[2,21,22] In addition, sphenoid sinusitis can present as an aseptic meningitis due to the presence of a parameningial focus.[32]

Patients can present with the complications of sphenoid sinusitis, including visual loss mimicking optic neuritis, multiple cranial nerve palsies or papilloedema. Sudden onset, as a result of cavernous sinus thrombosis, can mimic a subarachnoid haemorrhage.[33]

Øktedalen and Lilleås[34] reported on four patients who were admitted to an infectious disease department with meningitis, sepsis and orbital cellulitis. Diagnosis was difficult in all cases. All four patients had fever and headache. Three of the four had normal plain sinus radiographs. CT scan diagnosed all cases. Six of Lew's[2] 15 acute cases had meningitis, 5 had cavernous sinus thrombosis, 1 had cortical vein thrombosis, 1 had unilateral ophthalmoplegia and 1 had orbital cellulitis. Eight of Kibblewhite's[22] 14 patients had complications on admission. None of Goldman's[21] patients had complications. The difference in the complication rate is a result of selection bias: Goldman's[21] patients were retrieved from emergency room records, Lew's[2], Øktedalen and Lilleås' [34] and Kibblewhite's[22] from inpatient records.

Treatment

Sphenoid sinusitis without complications may be managed with high-dose intravenous antibiotics and topical and systemic decongestants for 10–14 days.[21,22] If the fever (if present) and the headache do not start to improve in 24–48 hours, or if any complications are present or develop, sphenoid sinus drainage is indicated.[21]

Nasal headache

Many rhinologists strongly hold the controversial belief that septal deformation, especially of traumatic origin, may exert pressure on the sensitive structure of the lateral nasal wall, causing referred pain and 'chronic headache'. McAntiffee et al.[16] studied the sensitivity of the nasal cavities and paranasal sinuses using touch, pressure and faradic stimulation. The

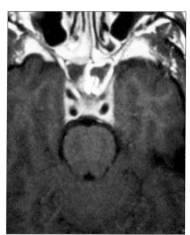

● *Figure 14.2*
MRI or CT neuroimaging can be used to diagnose sphenoid sinusitis.

nasal turbinates and sinus ostia were much more sensitive than the mucosal lining of the septum and the paranasal sinuses. Most of the pain elicited was referred pain. It was of increased intensity, longer duration and referred to larger areas in subjects with swelling and engorgement of the nasal turbinates and the sinus ostia.

Schønsted-Madsen et al.[1] followed up 444 patients with nasal obstruction, of whom 157 had headache. Treatment consisted of septoplastic surgery, reconstruction of the nasal pyramids or submucosal conchotomy. The headache was usually localized to the forehead, glabella or above and around the eyes. Thirty-six patients had constant, 48 daily, 56 weekly and 17 monthly headache. In 57, the headache was mild, in 66 moderate and in 34 severe. Many of these patients misused analgesics. Eighty per cent of the patients who underwent surgery were relieved of nasal obstruction (the primary reason for surgery) and 60% of the patients who underwent surgery were relieved of chronic headache. If the surgery relieved the nasal obstruction, 80% had headache relief; however, if the surgery failed, only 30% had headache relief.

This study does not account for the historical relationship between the onset of headache and the development of nasal obstruction, nor for the overuse of analgesics or decongestant which may produce daily headache. It does suggest that a minority of patients with nasal obstructions (157/444, or about one-third) have headache which is relieved if surgery is successful. Since the prevalence of migraine in the population is about 12%, the prevalence of episodic tension-type headache about 90%, and the prevalence of chronic tension-type headache about 3%, these data are difficult to interpret.

References

1. Schønsted-Madsen U, Stoksted P, Christensen P-H, Koch-Henriksen N. Chronic headache related to nasal obstruction. *J Laryngol Otol* 1986; 100: 165–70.
2. Lew D, Southwick FS, Montgomery WW, Weber AL, Baker AS. Sphenoid sinusitis: a review of 30 cases. *N Engl J Med* 1983; 19: 1149–54.
3. Moss AJ, Parsons VL. Current estimates from the National Health Interview Survey. United States, 1985. *Vital and Health Statistics. Series 10: Data from the National Health Survey.* 1986; i–iv: 1–182.
4. Reilly JS. The sinusitis cycle. *Otolaryngol Head Neck Surg* 1990; 103: 856–62.
5. Kennedy DW. Overview. *Otolaryngol Head Neck Surg* 1990; 103: 847–54.
6. Zinreich SJ. Paranasal sinus imaging. *Otolaryngol Head Neck Surg* 1990; 103: 863–9.
7. Zinreich SJ, Kennedy DW, Rosenbaum AE et al. Paranasal sinuses: CT imaging requirements for endoscopic surgery. *Radiology* 1987; 163: 769–75.
8. McCaffrey TV. Functional endoscopic sinus surgery: an overview. *Mayo Clin Proc* 1993; 68: 571–7.
9. Kennedy DW. Surgical update. *Otolaryngol Head Neck Surg* 1990; 103: 884–6.
10. Druce HM, Slavin RG. Sinusitis: a critical need for further study. *J Allergy Clin Immunol* 1991; 88: 675–7.
11. Havas TE, Motbey JA, Gullane PJ. Prevalence of incidental abnormalities on computed tomographic scans of the paranasal sinuses. *Arch Otolaryngol* 1988; 114: 856–9.
12. Stafford CT. The clinician's view of sinusitis. *Otolaryngol Head Neck Surg* 1990; 103: 870–5.
13. Castellanos J, Axelrod D. Flexible fiberoptic rhinoscopy in the diagnosis of sinusitis. *J Allergy Clin Immunol* 1989; 83: 91–4.
14. Williams JW, Simel DL, Roberts L, Samsa GP. Clinical evaluation for sinusitis. *Ann Intern Med* 1992; 117: 705–10.
15. Kogutt MS, Swischuk LE. Diagnosis of sinusitis in infants and children. *Pediatrics* 1973; 52: 121–4.
16. Hilger PA. Diseases of the nose. In: Adams GL, Pores LR, Hilger PA (eds). *Boies Fundamentals of Otolaryngology: a Textbook of Ear, Nose, and Throat Disease.* Philadelphia: WB Saunders 1989: 206–48.
17. Wolff HG. *Wolff's Headache and Other Head Pain.* 1st edition. New York: Oxford University Press, 1948.
18. Headache Classification Committee of the International Headache Society. Classification and diagnostic criteria for headache disorders, cranial neuralgia, and facial pain. *Cephalalgia* 1988; 8(Suppl. 7): 196.
19. Saunte C, Soyka D. Headache related to ear, nose, and sinus disorders. In: Olesen J, Tfelt-Hansen P, Welch JMA (eds). *The Headaches.* New York: Raven Press, 1993: 753–7.
20. Faleck H, Rothner AD, Erenberg G, Cruse RP. Headache and subacute sinusitis in children and adolescents. *Headache* 1988; 28: 96–8.
21. Goldman GE, Fonanarosa PB, Anderson JM. Isolated sphenoid sinusitis. *Am J Emerg Med* 1993; 11: 235–8.
22. Kibblewhite DJ, Cleland J, Mintz DR. Acute sphenoid sinusitis: management strategies. *J Otolaryngol* 1988; 17: 159–63.
23. Goss CM (ed.) *Gray's anatomy of the human body.* 27th edition. Philadelphia: Lea & Febiger, 1959.
24. Sofferman RA. Cavernous sinus thrombophlebitis secondary to sphenoid sinusitis. *Laryngoscope* 1983; 93: 797–800.
25. Deans JAJ, Welch AR. Acute isolated sphenoid sinusitis: a disease with complications. *J Laryngol Otol* 1991; 105: 1072–4.
26. Nordeman L, Lucid E. Sphenoid sinusitis, a cause of debilitating headache. *J Emerg Med* 1990; 8: 557–9.
27. Urquhart AC, Fung G, McIntosh WA. Isolated sphenoiditis: a diagnostic problem. *J Laryngol Otol* 1989; 103: 526–7.
28. Turkewitz D, Keller R. Acute headache in childhood: a case of sphenoid sinusitis. *Pediatr Emerg Care* 1987; 3: 155–7.
29. Axelsson A, Jensen A. The roentgenologic demonstration of sinusitis. *Am J Roentgenol Rad Ther Nuclear Med* 1974; 122: 621–7.
30. Schatz CJ, Becker TS. Normal CT anatomy of the paranasal sinuses. *Radiol Clin North Am* 1984; 22: 107–18.
31. Digre KB, Maxner CE, Crawford S, You WTC. Significance of CT and MR findings in sphenoid sinus disease. *AJNR* 1989; 10: 603–6.
32. Brook I, Overturf GD, Steinberg EA, Hawkins DB. Acute sphenoid sinusitis presenting as aseptic meningitis: a pachymeningitis syndrome. *Int J Pediatr Otorhinolaryngol* 1982; 4: 77–81.
33. Dale BAB, Mackenzie IJ. The complications of sphenoid sinusitis. *J Laryngol Otol* 1983; 97(7): 661–70.
34. Øktendalen O, Lilleås F. Septic complications to sphenoidal sinus infection. *Scand J Infect Dis* 1992; 24: 353–6.
35. Druce HM. Adjuncts to medical management of sinusitis. *Otolaryngol Head Neck Surg* 1990; 103: 880–3.

chapter 15

Headache associated with central nervous system infection

Introduction

Headaches are associated with a wide range of infections in both intracranial and extracranial structures. In the IHS system, infections are divided into those that are intracranial, those that are extracranial and those that effect the cranium and associated structures (Table 15.1). This chapter emphasizes selected intracranial and system infections including meningitis and encephalitis. We highlight issues related to Lyme borreliosis and the aquired immunodeficiency syndrome (AIDS), two disorders of increasing importance over the last decade.

Central nervous system (CNS) infections remain one of the great concerns of clinicians worldwide. CNS infections may be announced by headache and even after adequate treatment headache may remain as the final residua of treated infection. The importance of CNS infections has been considerably enhanced in recent years by the acquired immunodeficiency syndrome (AIDS) which may present as, or intercurrently have as a feature, intracranial infections. The International Headache Society defines the clinical problem as headache that occurs at the onset of intracranial infection and disappears after successful treatment of intracranial infection (Table 15.1).[1]

Meningitis

Meningitis is an inflammatory disorder of the meninges; here we will consider infective causes (the inflammatory conditions are dealt with previously in this book). Meningitis is classified according to the pathogen; it is most commonly viral or bacterial, with other infections being seen mainly in primary or secondary immune deficiency states. Bacterial meningitis was first described by Vieusseaux after an outbreak in Switzerland in 1805 and was named 'epidemic cerebrospinal fever'. 'Aseptic meningitis', a term introduced by Wallgren in 1925, describes a benign and self-limited variant of meningitis usually due to a viral infection, with headache a prominent feature of the illness. Quinke, who is responsible for introducing the lumbar puncture in 1881, originally described viral meningitis and encephalitis in 1896.[2]

The annual incidence of acute bacterial meningitis in the United States is 5–10 cases per 100 000.[3,4] It occurs somewhat more frequently in men than in women, for reasons that are unknown.[3,4,5] Children under the age of five years account for the majority of cases, with the highest risk during infancy. Other predisposing factors are sickle cell disease, alcoholism and AIDS and other immunocompromised states.

The annual incidence of viral meningitis in the USA is 10.9 per 100 000, with most cases occurring in the summer.[6] Most cases occur in children and young adults, with the incidence dropping significantly after the third decade of life. Again, the rate is higher in men than in women.

Clinical features

The clinical features of meningitis are similar for both bacterial and viral causes, although bacterial meningitis is generally more clinically fulminant. Headache pathophysiology is dealt with in Chapter 5, however, it is appropriate to comment that the pain is likely to be related to both the effects of the agent and, perhaps even more notably, to the host response. Headache is seen in many febrile illnesses and the headaches of interferons-α,[7] -β,[8] -γ,[9] and immunoglobulins[10] suggest that endogenously released substances may play a crucial role in headache generation in CNS infections. Typically, the headache of bacterial meningitis progresses in a short course from mild to severe and may often be the first symptom. It is usually a generalized headache with bilateral occipital and neck radiation and diffuse general discomfort. Patients tend to become withdrawn from sensory stimulation, avoiding light and sound, and they may have cognitive dysfunction, depending on the spread and nature of the infection. They may be nauseated and vomiting, and will have a fever and may look flushed. Physical examination will usually demonstrate a stiff neck, photophobia, and pain with eye movement. A rash may be seen in meningococcal infection.

● **Table 15.1** *Classification of headaches associated with infection*

7	Headaches associated with non-vascular intracranial disorders
	7.3 Intracranial infections
9	Headaches associated with non-cephalic infections
	9.1 Viral infection
	9.2 Bacterial infection
	9.3 Headache related to other infections
11	Headache or facial pain associated with disorders of the cranium, neck, eyes, ears, nose, sinuses, teeth, mouth or other facial or cranial structures

The signs and symptoms of acute bacterial meningitis include headache, fever, neck stiffness, nausea, vomiting, photophobia, alteration of consciousness, and (rarely) seizures. Kernig's and Brudzinski's signs are often present. Sufferers maintain a flexed posture with tense neck muscles and head extension.[11] Eye movements are often painful and cranial nerve palsies may be present.[11,12] Headache is the most common symptom of bacterial meningitis. It is severe and unremitting, usually generalized (but may be frontally predominant), and may radiate down the neck and back and into the extremities.[13] A thunderclap headache that increases in severity in minutes may be the first symptom of acute bacterial meningitis. Young children usually do not complain of headache.[11,14,15] Infants may present with fever and a bulging fontanelle.[14,15] The elderly have fewer headaches than do young adults.[12,14,] The signs and symptoms of meningitis may be accompanied by signs involving the original site of infection, such as an upper respiratory infection or otitis media.

In chronic meningitis, such as tuberculous meningitis, severe headache and fever evolving subacutely may occur in isolation.[14] A chronic headache increasing in severity over weeks to months, without fever or other neurological findings, is the most common symptom of cryptococcal meningitis.[16] A picture of chronic infection may also be seen with a modest fever and muscle pains or even milder deterioration in cognitive function over time. An infection producing hydrocephalus, such as CNS tuberculosis or a cryptococcal infection, may present as progressive ataxia or cognitive decline. More chronic syndromes may be seen with *Brucella* meningitis or Lyme disease.

A suspected CNS infection as the cause of headache demands neuroimaging followed by lumbar puncture. If meningitis is suspected, lumbar puncture may be performed without imaging if there are no contraindications or obstacles present. Contraindications to lumbar puncture include signs of increased intracranial pressure (papilloedema, coma, anisocoria, fixed pupils), a suspicion of a mass lesion in the CNS, a skin infection at the proposed lumbar puncture site, or a coagulopathy that cannot be even temporarily corrected. Obstacles include unstable vital signs and the need for ventilatory assistance. When bacterial meningitis is suspected and a mass lesion has been ruled out clinically or by neuroimaging, the cerebrospinal fluid (CSF) should be sent for Gram stain and culture and be examined for glucose (usually <40 mg/dl or <50% of the blood glucose), protein (significantly elevated), and cell counts (usually >1000 cells/mm^3 with polymorphonuclear predominance).[12,17,18] The CSF pressure is usually elevated. The CSF should also be sent for specific bacterial antigen and endotoxin assays.[15,17–19] Blood cultures should be drawn, since they are positive in >50% of cases of bacterial meningitis.[19,20] X-rays of the skull and sinuses may reveal a site of infection or portal of entry into the CNS, but they are not routinely used. Likewise, magnetic resonance imaging (MRI) may show meningeal enhancement,[21] but it is seldom necessary in typical cases. The peripheral white blood count will likely be elevated with a predominance of polymorphonuclear cells and immature forms, supporting the diagnosis of a bacterial process.[18]

The defining investigation in a suspected case of meningitis is a CSF examination. It is essential to have a sample and, moreover, to have an adequate sample. Many patients have been subjected to repeated lumbar punctures in chronic setting when inadequate samples are taken. This can be avoided if a microbiological differential diagnosis is carefully formulated, with advice from an infectious disease specialist when chronic meningitis is suspected. While it is generally the practice to image the brain prior to lumbar puncture to ensure that there is no mass lesion, treatment should not be delayed if acute bacterial meningitis is suspected. Treatment is directed to specific therapy, antibiotic, antiviral or antifungal agents, and supportive measures, such as fluids and antipyretics.

Bacterial meningitis

Bacterial meningitis remains a deadly disease. Rapid assessment is essential and can be life-saving. Bacterial infections present typically with fever, headache, and neck stiffness; the commonest causes are listed in Table 15.2. The most common organisms, causing approximately 80% of all cases of acute bacterial meningitis in adults in the USA, are *Haemophilus influenzae*, *Neisseria meningitidis* and *Streptococcus pneumoniae*.[4,5] *Eschericia coli* and *Listeria* are together responsible for approximately 10% of the cases. Neonatal meningitis is caused by Group B streptococci, *Listeria* and *E. coli* and other Gram-negative organisms.[4,14,15] If a CSF leak is present secondary to a skull

Table 15.2 Common causes of acute bacterial infections in the CNS

Haemophilus influenzae
Neisseria meningitidis
Streptococcus pneumoniae
Streptococcus (group B)
Listeria monocytogenes
Escherichia coli
Staphylococcus (aureus and epidermidis)

fracture, *Pneumococcus* is the most common causative organism, followed by skin flora.[5] Neurosurgical patients may be affected with a wide variety of organisms, particularly Gram-negative rods.[5,14] Patients who are receiving chemotherapy and are immunosuppressed, those who have lymphoma, leukaemia and malnutrition, and those with AIDS, may be infected with unusual pathogens. *Mycobacterium tuberculosis* causes both subacute and chronic meningitis, while *cryptococcus, nocardia, candida, histoplasma* and coccidiomycosis are common causes of chronic meningitis. Faced with immunocompromised patients, such as those with acquired immunodeficiency from malnutrition, human immunodeficiency virus (HIV) infection, leukaemia, lymphoma or anticancer treatments, a search for more unusual pathogens is mandatory. Bacterial meningitis may complicate sinusitis, skull fractures, mastoiditis or local cranial infections, as well as being a manifestation of a primary infection in any site, such as may be seen in osteomyelitis or pneumonia. In a bacterial infection there is a purulent exudate in the CNS that is reflected in a highly active CSF with neutrophils, protein and a low glucose when compared with a contemporaneous blood glucose level. Once suspected, there should be no delay in treating the infection with antibiotics that would cover the pathogens expected in the community or hospital setting in which the infection has been acquired.

Nonbacterial infections

Aseptic meningitis is characterized by a severe, rapid-onset headache, fever, malaise, anorexia, phonophobia, photophobia and nuchal rigidity. There may be altered sensorium, although this rarely progresses to obtundation or coma.[14,22,23] Again, the headache may be less prominent in children. All patients with aseptic meningitis experience a severe and bilateral headache.[24] Generally, although not invariably, non-bacterial intracranial infections follow a more benign clinical course. Many such patients when first seen with headache, fever, and neck stiffness, are managed with antibiotics, and the diagnosis is questioned when there is no obvious response. The CSF examination with an excess of lymphocytes, an unremarkable or modestly elevated CSF protein and a normal ratio of CSF to blood: plasma glucose suggests a non-bacterial infection. In viral meningitis, the CSF shows a mild pleocytosis (usually <100 cells/mm^3).[14,18,22,23] Early in the course there may be a predominance of polymorphonuclear cells, but this rapidly shifts to lymphocytic pleocytosis. The CSF pressure is normal or slightly elevated, the CSF protein is normal or slightly elevated, and the glucose is either normal or slightly reduced. If the diagnosis is still in doubt, antibiotics should be started and the lumbar puncture repeated after 12

● **Table 15.3** *Common viral pathogens in meningitis*

Enterovirus	Epstein–Barr virus
Coxsackie A and B	Rubella
Cytomegalovirus	Mumps
Herpes simplex	Adenovirus
Herpes zoster	Human immunodeficiency virus

hours to document the shift from polymorphonuclear cells to mononuclear cells. The CSF should be analysed for viral antigens and incubated for viral culture. Acute and convalescent serum viral titres will provide clues to the aetiology of the disease. The peripheral white blood count may be normal or elevated with a normal differential cell count. Virus can be isolated from other sites, such as the throat and stool, in certain cases.[14] Aseptic meningitis is usually viral in origin, with the enteroviruses (echo, coxsackie, polio), the mumps virus, and the arboviruses being the most common causative organisms (Table 15.3).[3,6,14] Less common viral causes are HIV, lymphocytic choriomeningitis virus, herpes simplex virus type 2, rubella, Epstein–Barr virus, herpes zoster, influenza, parainfluenza and adenovirus.[14,23,25] Virus prevalence is often geographic and seasonal. The causative virus is isolated in only 11–12% of cases.[3,6] Other conditions which can resemble aseptic meningitis include fungal meningitis, parameningeal infections, non-infectious conditions (malignant meningitis, sarcoidosis or chemical meningitis from spinal anaesthesia, myelography or intrathecal medications), and bacterial agents that are difficult to routinely culture (such as *Treponema palladium, Mycobacterium tuberculosis* and *Borrelia burgdorferi*).[23,25,26] Epstein–Barr virus may have a very chronic course, and it has been suggested that many cases of new persistent daily headache are triggered by an episode of Epstein–Barr infection. An interesting diagnosis of exclusion related to non-bacterial intracranial infections is the clinical syndrome of a migrainous headache, with prolonged aura, neck stiffness, fever and a lymphocytosis in the CSF.[27] The nature of this syndrome remains to be more clearly elucidated.

Lyme disease

One of the most remarkable intracranial infections that has been increasingly recognized in recent years is neuroborreliosis or Lyme disease. The neurologic clinical picture is pleomorphic with meningitis, cranial nerve lesions, particularly of the facial nerve and radiculopathy and neuropathy.[28] Lyme borreliosis is a multisystem infection caused by the spirochete *Borrelia burgdorferi*.[29] Early in the illness, patients may have a characteristic cutaneous infection, erythema migrans. Some patients develop disseminated and then chronic infections with prominent neurological, rheumatological and cardiac manifestations. During erythema migrans, headache occurs in from 38 to 54% of patients and presents few diagnostic challenges.[30,31] Headache may also accompany the causally related neurological syndromes described below. More problematic are the patients who present with headache as an isolated manifestation of Lyme disease.

The American Academy of Neurology 'Practice Parameters for the Diagnosis of Patients with Nervous System Lyme Borreliosis (Lyme Disease)' defines four causally related forms of neurological disease or dysfunction:[32]

- *Lymphocytic meningitis with or without cranial neuritis or painful radiculoneuritis or both*. This syndrome is common early in the course of Lyme borreliosis. Headache occurs in the majority of patients and is typically bilateral, gradual in onset and variably associated with migrainous features (throbbing quality, nausea). Meningism is uncommon in patients with Lyme meningitis.[31,33]
- *Encephalomyelitis*. This monophasic, slowly progressive, unifocal or multifocal inflammatory disease of the CNS occurs in about 0.1% of patients with Lyme borreliosis.[32] The disorder involves white matter more prominently than grey matter. Headache is common; it is often bilateral, and again variably associated with migrainous features.
- *Peripheral neuropathy*. The radiculoneuropathy, usually a mononeuropathy multiplex, occurs without meningitis and without evidence of CNS infection. Only a minority of patients complain of headache.[31]
- *Encephalopathy*. Cognitive complaints and cognitive dysfunction may develop in the absence of evidence of CNS infection. Encephalopathy may be an indirect effect of systemic infection, mediated by the action of cytokines and neuromodulators on the CNS. Headache may occur in the encephalopathy syndrome.

Headache as the most prominent manifestation of Lyme borreliosis

There are rare reports of headache as the most prominent neurological manifestation of CNS Lyme disease. Halperin *et al.*[33] reported a woman with chronic headache and a positive CSF Lyme antibody index whose headaches completely resolved after treatment with ceftriaxone. Brinck *et al.*[34] reported two patients with headaches resembling chronic tension-type headache. In both cases, the CSF Lyme antibody index was positive and the headaches resolved after intravenous antibiotic therapy. In addition to headaches, the first patient had constant nausea, vomiting, weight loss and episodes of paraesthesias in her fingertips. The second patient had double vision and a progressive paraparesis that evolved over a two-year period and eventually led to a work-up and diagnosis.

Brinck *et al.*[35] point out that neither of their patients had meningeal signs or fever. Both had headache symptoms that did not fully meet IHS criteria. Both went from having very few headaches to an almost constant headache over several days. They recommend considering a workup for Lyme borreliosis when headaches are atypical, especially if the onset is subacute.

Laboratory tests

The appropriate workup for patients with headache and suspected Lyme disease is problematic. The role of laboratory tests in neuroborreliosis was recently reviewed by Halperin *et al.*[32] We summarize information about selected tests.

Serologic testing (enzyme-linked immunosorbent assay, ELISA)

Serological diagnostic tests for Lyme and for other infectious agents demonstrate possible exposures to the causative agent, not current active infection.[35] In asymptomatic individuals, serological tests are positive in 5–10% of the population in endemic areas and in 1% of the population in non-endemic areas.[32,36] Thus, most positive serological tests in headache patients are likely to be false-positives.

If serological testing is performed in individuals with a characteristic Lyme-related illness (a high prior probability of Lyme disease), the positive predictive value goes up.[32]

Western blot

While serological tests detect antibody, Western blots characterize the specific *B. burgorferi* antigens. This test serves primarily to confirm a positive ELISA or identify false-positives.[32]

Demonstration of intrathecal antibody production

The demonstration of antibody production within the CNS relies on the ratio of antibody in CSF to antibody in serum. These procedures have high specificity (95%) and sensitivity (90%) and may rarely be positive despite negative peripheral serological tests.[37,38]

Culture and polymerase chain reaction

These have high specificity but most likely have modest sensitivities.[32,39]

Preliminary recommendations

Routine testing for Lyme disease is not recommended in patients presenting with headache. The false-positive tests would most likely lead to inappropriate evaluation or treatment. If a headache is accompanied by apparent systemic or neurological manifestations suggestive of Lyme disease, serum antibody testing by ELISA is suggested. Evaluation should proceed as recommended in the AAN practice guidelines.[32] In patients with atypical headaches (rapid increase to near-daily headache, unusual associated symptoms or poor response to treatment), serological testing for Lyme disease should be considered. Suspected false-positive ELISA should be confirmed by a Western blot for *Borrelia*-specific antigens. Patients with headache as the sole neurological manifestation and a positive ELISA and Western blot should be treated with oral doxycycline 100 mg p.o., b.i.d. for three to four weeks. If the headache does not remit, lumbar puncture should be considered. In patients with headache and evidence of Lyme-related neurological disorders/dysfunction (such as encephalopathy, cognitive deficits, focal deficits), neuroimaging and lumbar puncture for cell count, protein glucose and Lyme antibody index should be performed. If CNS disease is present, intravenous therapy should be considered, as discussed in the AAN practice guidelines.[32]

Encephalitis

Encephalitis is an infection involving the brain parenchyma. Generally, encephalitic processes are due to viral infections; and the common causes are listed in Table 15.4. The causative agent in encephalitis is identified approximately 15% of the time in large population studies.[3,6] In one study of a very select group of patients (summarized by Johnson),[39] the aetiology was determined in two-thirds of the cases. Mumps was isolated 15% of the time, arbovirus 11%, enteroviruses 10%, lymphocytic choriomeningitis virus 9% and herpes simplex virus 95%. Other causes included Epstein–Barr virus, measles, influenza virus and *Mycoplasma*. The larger studies reported a somewhat higher incidences of measles and varicella-zoster virus, especially in children. Measles, mumps and varicella-zoster virus can cause postinfectious encephalomyelitis as well

● **Table 15.4** *Common causes of encephalitis*

Mumps	Toxoplasmosis
Arbovirus	Epstein–Barr virus
Herpes simplex	Adenovirus
Herpes zoster	

as infectious encephalitis. In the USA, the incidence of viral encephalitis is 7.4 per 100 000 per year, with most occurring in the summer and early fall.[3,6] The incidence is highest in infancy and gradually drops, to attain a steady rate by the age of forty. Males are more often affected than females. Encephalitis is characterized by headache, fever, alteration of consciousness, focal neurological deficit and seizures (usually focal). Meningeal signs may be present as well. Thunderclap headache alone may be the initial manifestation of encephalitis.[40] A prodrome of a less severe but constant headache associated with malaise, mild fever and myalgia may precede the onset of the neurological deficit by several days.[23] Herpes simplex virus encephalitis typically has no identifiable systemic prodrome and may present with behavioural changes or memory disturbance.[23,41] In one series of patients with herpes simplex virus encephalitis, half had presented with headache, two-thirds with signs of meningeal irritation, almost all with fever, about 90% with focal neurological deficits and 61% with seizures. Over one-third were comatose on admission.[42] When there is mass effect, which commonly involves the temporal cortex, a localized headache may be present. Subacute encephalopathy that progresses over several months with headache, lethargy, and possibly focal neurological signs is another presentation of herpes simplex virus encephalitis.[43] The symptomatology may recur after antiviral therapy, although this is rare and may be due to a postinfectious encephalitis.[44]

Encephalitis is marked clinically by impaired cognition and sometimes by distinct anatomically-resolvable clinical syndromes. Patients usually have headache, fever and neck stiffness, although headache and impaired consciousness may be the only clinical manifestation. The cerebral picture may be predated by a prodrome of feeling generally unwell, with fever, malaise or myalgia for up to a week prior to the more acute presentation. While some encephalitides are clinically mild, some, such as herpes simplex, can be devastating. Very often involving temporal cortex bilaterally and being accompanied by an abnormal electroencephalogram almost invariably, patients with suspected herpes simplex encephalitis require early treatment with antiviral agents in adequate doses. In immunosuppressed patients certain pathogens, such as toxoplasmosis, cryptococcoses and cytomegalovirus, are more common and must be borne in mind and actively sought.

During an encephalitis epidemic, diagnosis is not difficult. The sporadic case is easily confused with encephalopathy, however. The presence or absence of fever, headache and focal neurologic signs help in the diagnosis. Peripheral leukocytosis, CSF pleocytosis and regional abnormalities on neuroimaging or electroencephalogram favour the diagnosis of encephalitis.[23] The CSF protein may be normal or elevated and the glucose is normal or slightly depressed.[18] The CSF cell count is usually <200 cells/mm³, predominantly lymphocytes. In herpes simplex virus encephalitis, the CSF may be xanthochromic and may contain red blood cells, reflecting the haemorrhagic necrosis taking place in the brain.[18] Antigen may be detected in the CSF.[45] The ability of MRI to detect herpes simplex virus encephalitis at an earlier stage than CT scanning has made it the imaging procedure of choice;[21,46] however, a brain biopsy may be rarely needed to establish a definite diagnosis. Virus may be isolated from the brain specimen, but the culture results may not be available for several days. Since acyclovir is effective against only a small number of encephalitides and is not innocuous, the indiscriminate use of this drug must be avoided. If a brain biopsy is going to be performed the patient can be given acyclovir up to 24 hours before surgery without affecting herpes simplex virus isolation from the specimen.[23] In the near future, polymerase chain reaction assays for herpes simplex virus in the CSF may expedite the diagnosis[47] and obviate the need for brain biopsy; CSF assays for herpes simplex virus glycoproteins are also being developed.

Special problems

Acquired immunodeficiency syndrome

Of all the conditions that predispose to intracranial infection and thus produce headache, HIV disease is perhaps one of the most challenging. Headache can occur in HIV-positive patients in the acute phase of the infection, as part of a HIV meningitis or encephalitis, and in the setting of secondary infections, which is seen frequently in patients with AIDS. A particularly common infection is toxoplasmosis, which is often seen as multiple contrast-enhancing parenchymal lesions on computed tomographic brain scans. This condition generally responds to treatment and biopsy diagnosis is not necessary unless there is no therapeutic response or the lesion is in some way atypical. Meningitis in AIDS can involve all of the common pathogens but rarer infections are frequent. Cryptococcal infection is common and relatively easily diagnosed via CSF examination with India ink stain and cryptococcal antigen testing. Similarly, tuberculous meningitis is often seen in AIDS patients and must be sought diligently with CSF examination using polymerase chain reaction (PCR) techniques.

Brain abscess

The signs and symptoms of a brain abscess depend on the location of the abscess and the amount of mass effect it produces. Although headache is the most common presenting symptom, the presenting symptom may be a seizure.[48,49] Focal neurological signs and altered mental status are common.[50,51]

Signs of an antecedent infection, such as otitis media, sinusitis, a dental infection or endocarditis, may be present. Fever and leukocytosis are less likely to be present. Nausea and vomiting often begin a week after headache onset.[51] These symptoms may result from increased intracranial pressure, although less than half the patients have papilloedema at presentation.[51,52] With a cerebellar abscess, the headache is often suboccipital and there is associated cervical pain and rigidity.[13]

In 1893, Sir William Macewen described the successful treatment of brain abscess by surgical drainage. The development of antibiotics, advances in neurosurgical techniques, and the use of CT scanning and MRI have all contributed to the significant reduction in mortality that has occurred.

The overall incidence of brain abscess is approximately 1 per 100 000, with peak incidence in chilhood and after the age of sixty.[3,51,52] In one series, abscesses were multiple in 27% of those affected.[51] It is three times as likely to occur in men than in women. Risk factors include neurosurgery, penetrating brain trauma, and, particularly in children, otitis media.

Brain abscesses may be caused by aerobic or anaerobic bacteria and often contain multiple organisms that come from the source of the infection.[50,51,53,54] Those arising from otitis media, mastoiditis, or sinusitis contain aerobic or anaerobic streptococci, *Staphylococcus aureus* and *Bacteroides*. Those arising from open head trauma or neurosurgery are associated with streptococci, staphylococci or Gram-negative rods. Bacterial endocarditis yields abscesses with *Staphylococcus aureus* or *Streptococcus viridans*. Pulmonary infections are associated with staphylococci, streptococci, *Actinomyces*, Gram-negative rods or fusobacteria, and, less commonly, *Nocardia* (especially in a immunocompromised host).[50,51] Abscess formed by *Candida, Aspergillus*, or *Toxoplasma* may also be found in an immunocompromised host. Overall, there is a high incidence of *Streptococcus milleri* isolated from brain abscesses of all causes.[50,52]

Neuroimaging is the diagnostic procedure of choice for brain abscesses. CT scan shows a central area of decreased attenuation surrounded by a ring of intense contrast enhancement, which may then be surrounded by oedema.[21,50,51,53] The presence of gas within the lesion supports the diagnosis. Prior to capsule formation, a low density region, reflecting early cerebritis, may be seen. MRI may be superior to CT scanning in its ability to detect early cerebritis, oedema, minor haemorrhage and disruption of the blood–brain barrier,[21,48] but this imaging procedure is not always readily available. Since a brain tumour, a cerebral infarct and radiation necrosis may appear identical to an abscess on CT scan, diagnostic (and therapeutic) neurosurgical intervention is often necessary,[50,53] although with the growing availability of MRI, *diagnostic* intervention is seldom necessary. The abscess should be incised and its contents drained and sent for bacterial culture and biopsy. Routine blood tests are rarely helpful in the diagnosis of brain abscess; the peripheral white blood count is usually normal or only slightly elevated. Blood cultures should be drawn if endocarditis is suspected.

A brain abscess must be differentiated from a brain tumour. Their appearance on CT may help differentiate them, although both may 'ring-enhance'. A brain abscess with early cerebritis may produce fever, headache and meningeal signs that mimic meningitis. A subdural haematoma or an empyema can mimic a brain abscess. A history of closed head trauma and the appearance of the lesion on imaging studies will help distinguish between these entities. When there is no history of fever or prior infection, a brain abscess may be confused with a cerebral infarction or a subdural haematoma; imaging studies will differentiate between them.

Headache treatment

The headache associated with intracranial infections should resolve with treatment of the underlying condition. Until the infection has cleared, the headache can be treated with non-narcotic analgesics or, if severe, with narcotics, bearing in mind that the use of narcotics may obscure certain aspects of the neurological examination (e.g. level of consciousness, pupillary size). If the headache persists long after the infection and its complications have resolved, the patient may require evaluation and treatment of a chronic type of headache. The evaluation includes neuroimaging to rule out the sequelae of intracranial infections, such as obstructive or communicating hydrocephalus, residual cerebral oedema, or mass effect. Once these entities have been excluded, a lumbar puncture may be necessary to rule out increased intracranial pressure, even in the absence of papilloedema.

References

1. Headache Classification Committee of the International Headache Society. Classification and diagnostic criteria for headache disorders, cranial neuralgias and facial pain. *Cephalalgia* 1988; 8(7): S1–96.
2. Silberstein SD. Headache associated with meningitis, encephalitis, and brain abscess. *Neurobase* (in press).
3. Nicolosi A, Hauser WA, Beghi E, Kurland LT. Epidemiology of central nervous system infections in Olmsted County, Minnesota, 1950–1981. *J Infect Dis* 1986; 154: 399–408.
4. Schlech WF. The epidemiology of bacterial meningitis. *Antibiot Chemother* 1992; 45: 517.
5. Schlech WF, Ward JI, Band JD, Hightower A, Fraser DW, Broome CV. Bacterial meningitis in the United States, 1978 through 1981. *JAMA* 1985; 253: 1749–54.
6. Beghi E, Nicolosi A, Kurland LT et al. Encephalitis and aseptic meningitis, Olmsted County, Minnesota, 1950–1981: I. Epidemiology. *Ann Neurol* 1984; 16: 283–94.

7. Schiller JH, Hank J, Storer B et al. A direct comparison of immunologic and clinical effects of interleukin 2 with and without interferon-alpha in humans. *Cancer Res* 1993; 53: 1286–92.
8. Yung WK, Castellanos AM, VanTassel P, Moser RP, Marcus SG. A pilot study of recombinant interferon beta (IFN-beta ser) in patients with recurrent glioma. *J Neurol Oncol* 1990; 9: 29–34.
9. Gluszko P, Undas A, Amenta S, Szceklik A, Schmaier AH. Administration of gamma interferon in human subjects decreases plasminogen activation and fibrinolysis without influencing C1 inhibitor. *J Lab Clin Med* 1994; 123: 232–40.
10. Watson JD, Gibson J, Joshua DE, Kronenberg H. Aseptic meningitis associated with high dose intravenous immunoglobulin therapy. *J Neurol Neurosurg Psychiatr* 1991; 54: 275–6.
11. Isenberg H. Bacterial meningitis: signs and symptoms. *Antiobiot Chemother* 1992; 45: 79–95.
12. Carpenter RR, Petersdorf RG. The clinical spectrum of bacterial meningitis. *Am J Med* 1962; 33: 262–75.

13. De Marinis M, Kurdi AA, Welch KMA. Headache associated with intracranial infection. In: Olesen J, Tfelt-Hansen P, Welch KMA (eds). *The Headaches.* New York: Raven Press, 1993: 697–704.
14. Franke E. The many causes of meningitis. *Postgrad Med* 1987; 82: 175–88.
15. Lipton JD, Schafermeyer RW. Evolving concepts in pediatric bacterial meningitis. Part I: pathophysiology and diagnosis. *Ann Emerg Med* 1993; 22: 1602–15.
16. Tija TL, Yeow YK, Tan CB. Cryptococcal meningitis. *J Neurol Neurosurg Psychiatry* 1985; 48: 853–8.
17. Benson CA, Harris AA, Levin S. Acute bacterial meningitis: general aspects. In: Vinken PJ, Bruyn GW, Klawans HL, Harris AA (eds). *Handbook of Clinical Neurology: Microbial Disease.* Amsterdam: Elsevier Science Publishers, 1988: 119.
18. Fishman RA. *Cerebrospinal fluid in diseases of the nervous system.* 2nd edition. Philadelphia: W.B. Saunders, 1992.
19. Oliver LG, Harwood-Nuss AL. Bacterial meningitis in infants and children: a review. *J Emerg Med* 1993; 11: 555–64.

20. Pohl CA. Practical approach to bacterial meningitis in childhood. *Am Fam Physician* 1993; 47: 1595–1603.

21. Smith RR. Neuroradiology of intracranial infection. *Pediatriatr Neurosurg* 1992; 18: 92–104.

22. Lepow ML, Coyne N, Thompson LB, Carver DH, Robbins FC. The clinical, epidemiologic and laboratory investigation of aseptic meningitis during the four-year period, 1955–1958. II. The clinical disease and its sequelae. *N Engl J Med* 1962; 266: 1188–93.

23. Davis LE. Acute viral meningitis and encephalitis. In: Kennedy PGE, Johnson RT (eds). *Infections of the Nervous System*. London: Butterworths, 1987: 155–76.

24. Lamonte M, Silberstein SD, Marcelis JF. Headache associated with aseptic meningitis. *Headache*, 1995; 35: 520–6.

25. Connolly KJ, Hammer SM. The acute aseptic meningitis syndrome. *Infect Dis Clin North Am* 1990; 4: 599–622.

26. Bharucha NE, Bhaba SK, Bharucha EP. Infections of the nervous system. B. Viral infections. In: Bradley WG, Daroff RB, Fenichel GM, Marsden CE (eds). *Neurology in Clinical Practice*. Stoneham: Butterworth-Heinemann, 1991: 1085–97.

27. Pachner AR, Steere AC. The triad of neurological manifestation of Lyme disease: meningitis, cranial neuritis, and radiculoneuritis. *Neurology* 1985; 35: 47–53.

28. Schraeder PL, Burns RA. Hemiplegic migraine associated with an aseptic meningeal reaction. *Arch Neurol* 1980; 37: 377–9.

29. Steere AC. Lyme disease. *N Engl J Med* 1989; 321: 586–96.

30. Berger BW. Cutaneous manifestations of Lyme borreliosis. *Rheum Dis Clin North Am* 1989; 15: 635–47.

31. Scelsa SN, Lipton RB, Sander H, Herskovitz S. Headache characertistics in hospitalized patients with Lyme disease. *Headache* 1995; 35: 125–30.

32. Halperin JJ, Logigian EL, Finel MF, Pearl RA. Practice parameters for the diagnosis of patients with nervous system Lyme borreliosis (Lyme disease). *Neurology* 1996; 46:619–27.

33. Hansen K, Lebech A. The clinical and epidemiological profile of Lyme neuroborreliosis in Denmark 1985–1990: a prospective study of 187 patients with Borrelia burgdorferi specific intrathecal antibody production. *Brain* 1992; 115: 399–423.

34. Halperin JJ, Luft BJ, Anand AK *et al*. Lyme neuroborreliosis central nervous system manifestations. *Neurology* 1989; 39: 753–9.

35. Brinck T, Hansen K, Olesen J. Headache resembling tension-type headache as the single manifestation of Lyme neuroborreliosis. *Cephalalgia* 1993; 13: 207–9.

36. Luger SW, Krauss E. Serologic tests for Lyme disease. *Arch Inter Med* 1990; 150: 761–8.

37. Steere AC, Taylor E, Wilson ML, Levine JF, Spielman A. Longitudinal assessment of the clinical and epidemiologic features of Lyme disease in a defined population. *J Infect Dis* 1986; 154: 295–300.

38. Steere AC, Berardi VP, Weeks KB, Logigian EL, Ackermann R. Evaluation of the intrathecal antibody response to Borrelia burgdorferi as a diagnostic test for Lyme neuroborreliosis. *J Infect Dis* 1990; 161: 1203–9.

39. Hansen K, Lebech AM. Lyme neuroborreliosis: a new sensitive diagnostic assay for intrathecal synthesis of Borrelia burgdorferi — specific immunoglobulins G, A and M. *Ann Neurol* 1991; 30: 197–205.

40. Karlsson M, Hovind HK, Svenungsson B, Stiernstedt G. Cultivation and characterization of spirochetes from cerebrospinal fluid of patients with Lyme borreliosis. *J Clin Microbiol* 1990; 28: 473–9.

41. Johnson RT. *Viral Infections of the Nervous System*. New York: Raven Press, 1982.

42. Silberstein SD. Evaluation and emergency treatment of headache. *Headache* 1992; 32: 396–407.

43. Young CA, Humphrey DM, Ghadiali EJ, Klapper PE, Cleator GM. Short-term memory impairment as a presentation of Herpes simplex encephalitis. *Neurology* 1992; 42: 260–1.

44. Kennedy PGE. A retrospective analysis of forty-six cases of Herpes simplex encephalitis seen in Glasgow between 1962 and 1985. *Q J Med* 1988; 68: 533–40.

45. Sage JL, Weinstein MP, Miller DC. Chronic encephalitis possibly due to Herpes simplex virus: two cases. *Neurology* 1985; 35: 1470–2.

46. Davis LE, McLaren LC. Relapsing Herpes simplex encephalitis following antiviral therapy. *Ann Neurol* 1983; 26: 192–5.

47. Lakeman FD, Koga J, Whitley RJ. Detection of antigen to Herpes simplex virus in cerebrospinal fluid from patients with Herpes simplex encephalitis. *J Infect Dis* 1987; 155(6): 1172–8.

48. Takahashi M. Infections of the central nervous system. *Curr Opin Neurol Neurosurg* 1992; 5: 849–53.

49. Rowley AH, Whitley RJ, Lakeman FD, Wolinsky SM. Rapid detection of Herpes simplex virus DNA in cerebrospinal fluid of patients with Herpes simplex encephalitis. *Lancet* 1990; 335: 440–1.

50. Kaplan K. Brain abscess. *Med Clin North Am* 1985; 69(2): 345–60.

51. Chun CH, Johnson JD, Hofstetter M, Raff MJ. Brain abscess: a study of 45 consecutive cases. *Medicine* 1986; 65: 415–31.

52. Molavi A, Dinubile MJ. Brain abscess. In: Vinken PJ, Bruyn GW, Klawans HL, Harris AA (eds). *Handbook of Clinical Neurology: Microbial Disease*. Amsterdam: Elsevier Science Publishers, 1988: 143–66.

53. Nicolosi A, Hauser WA, Musicco, Kurland LT. Incidence and prognosis of brain abscess in a defined population: Olmsted County, Minnesota, 1935–1981. *Neuroepidemiology* 1991; 10: 122–31.

chapter 16

Pregnancy, breast feeding and headache

Pregnancy

Migraine can occur for the first time during pregnancy; pre-existing migraine may worsen, particularly during the first trimester, or migraine may disappear or there may be no change in some women.[1] The true incidence of migraine in pregnancy is uncertain and most reported cases have been of migraine with aura or prolonged aura.

Tension-type headache and other primary headache disorders also occur during pregnancy. However, conditions that mimic them may also occur at this time. Vasculitis, brain tumour, or occipital arteriovenous malformation (AVM) occur and may mimic the primary headache disorders.[2,3] Sinusitis, meningitis, idiopathic intracranial hypertension and subarachnoid haemorrhage (SAH) are headache disorders that occur during pregnancy.[3] These symptomatic conditions require neuroimaging and/or a lumbar puncture to diagnose them. Some disorders that produce headache occur more frequently or exclusively during pregnancy. These include stroke, cerebral venous thrombosis, eclampsia, SAH, pituitary tumour and choriocarcinoma.[4,5] Idiopathic intracranial hypertension does not occur more commonly than expected during pregnancy (Table 16.1).

Diagnostic testing serves to exclude organic causes of headache, to confirm the diagnosis and to establish a baseline before treatment. If neurodiagnostic testing is indicated, the study that will provide the most information with the least fetal risk is the study of choice.

Although drugs are commonly used during pregnancy, there is insufficient knowledge about their effects on the growing fetus. Most drugs are not teratogenic. Adverse effects, such as spontaneous abortion, developmental defects, and various postnatal effects, depend on the dose and route of administration and the timing of the exposure relative to the period of fetal development.

While medication use should be limited, it is not absolutely contraindicated in pregnancy. In migraine, the risk of status migrainosus may be greater than the potential risk of the medication use to treat the pregnant patient. Non-pharmacological treatment is the ideal solution; however, analgesics such as acetaminophen (paracetamol) and narcotics can be used on a limited basis. Preventive therapy is a last resort.

Neurodiagnostic testing: radiology

The effect of radiation on the developing conceptus is a major concern for the pregnant patient. At the time of implantation, the most common radiation effect is death of the conceptus, with a threshold of ≥ 5 rad. Radiation exposure during embryogenesis and organogenesis may result in developmental anomalies or growth retardation, with threshold doses of ≥ 5 rad. A radiation dose of ≥ 15 rad is necessary to produce deformities that might warrant pregnancy termination. The dose to the uterus from a skull or cervical spine film is <1 mrad, ≤ 1000 mrad from a thoracic spine series, and 1500 mrad from a lumbar spine series.[6] A standard head or cervical spine computed tomography (CT) exposes the uterus to <1 mrad, and thoracic CT exposure is about 20 mrad. However, the dose from a lumbar spine CT is approximately 700 mrad.[6]

The radiation dose for a typical cervical or intracranial angiogram is <1 mrad. Fluoroscopy delivers 1 rad per minute to the skin.[6] Unless an aneurysm, an AVM, or vasculitis is suspected, there is little reason to perform angiography in a patient who has a normal neurological examination, a normal CT or magnetic resonance imaging (MRI), and a history consistent with a benign primary headache disorder, particularly if she is pregnant.

The potential risk of MRI in pregnancy is still controversial. Magnetic resonance magnets induce an electric field and raise the core temperature by $<1^{\circ}C$. While high body temperature may increase the incidence of neural tube defects, the effects of MRI are unknown. Gadolinium crosses the placental barrier and is excreted through the fetal kidneys, although no ill effects have been demonstrated, gadolinium injection should be avoided, as should CT contrast.[6]

Head CT is relatively safe during pregnancy and is the study of choice for head trauma and possible non-traumatic subarachnoid, subdural or intraparenchymal haemorrhage. For all other non-traumatic or non-haemorrhagic craniospinal pathology, MRI is preferred. Use MRA first to evaluate any

• **Table 16.1** *Headache disorders and pregnancy*

Less common	As common	More common
Migraine	Idiopathic intracranial hypertension	Stroke
Menstrual headache	Tension-type headache	Cerebral venous thrombosis
	Sinusitis	Eclampsia
	Meningitis	Subarachnoid haemorrhage
	Vasculitis	Pituitary tumour
	Brain tumour	Choriocarcinoma

- Determine the necessity and the potential risks of the procedure
- If possible, perform the examination during the first 10 days postmenses, or if the patient is pregnant, delay the examination until the third trimester or preferably postpartum
- Pick the procedure with the highest accuracy balanced by the lowest radiation
- Use MRI if possible
- Avoid direct exposure to the abdomen and pelvis
- Avoid contrast agents
- Do not avoid radiologic testing purely for the sake of the pregnancy
- If significant exposure is incurred by a pregnant patient, consult a radiation biologist
- Consent forms are neither required nor recommended

*Adapted from R.B. Schwartz's Neurodiagnostic Imaging of the Pregnant Patient that appeared in 'Neurologic complications of pregnancy'.[6]

suspected vascular pathology, but when necessary, angiography is reasonably safe in the pregnant patient (Table 16.2).

Potential indications for CT or MRI in headache investigation during pregnancy include: the first or worst headache of the patient's life, particularly if it is of abrupt onset (thunderclap headache); a change in the frequency, severity or clinical features of the headache attack; an abnormal neurological examination; a progressive or new daily persistent headache; neurological symptoms that do not meet the criteria of migraine with typical aura; persistent neurological defects; definite EEG evidence of a focal cerebral lesion; an orbital or skull bruit suggestive of AVM; and new comorbid

partial (focal) seizures.[3] In each case a judgement must be made about the risk of not diagnosing the condition compared to the minor risk of radiation

Mechanisms

Rising or sustained high oestrogen levels have been proposed as the mechanism of migraine relief that often occurs during pregnancy; this mechanism, however, cannot explain the worsening or new appearance of migraine that sometimes occurs.[7] The rapid fall of oestrogen levels may be responsible for menstrual and postpartum migraine. Women with a prior history of migraine are more likely to develop postpartum migraine.[8] Migraine relief during pregnancy is not dependent on adequate 'protective' levels of progesterone.

Course of migraine during pregnancy

Approximately 60–70% of migraineurs will improve during pregnancy, while some women without prior migraine will experience their first migraine headache (Table 16.3). Case reports[7,9] of migraine that occur for the first time during pregnancy emphasize the presence of focal neurological symptoms (migraine with aura), probably because patients with these dramatic presentations are more likely to be referred to a neurologist.

Series (Table 16.3)

Migraine improved in 58% of women, while 42% worsened or had no change with pregnancy in Lance's study.[10] Sixty-four percent of women with menstrual migraine had relief during pregnancy, compared to 48% relief in those without menstrual migraine (Table 16.4).

● **Table 16.3** *Migraine and pregnancy*

Parameter	Lance (1966)	Callaghan (1968)	Somerville (1970)	Bousser (1990)	Granella et al. (1993)	Rasmussen (1993)	Chen and Leviton (1994)	Maggioni et al. (1995)
Women studied		200	200	703	1300	975	55,000	428
History of migraine and pregnancies	120	41	38	116	943	80	484	80
Number of pregnancies	252	200	200	147	943		484	?
New migraine during pregnancy	0	33/41 (80%)	7/38 (18%)	16/147 (11%)	12 (1.3%)	?	0	1/428
New migraine postpartum				?	42 (4.5%)	?	0	?
Prior migraine	252	8	31	131	571	80	484	91
Prior migraine improved	145/252 (58%)	4 (50%)	24/31 (77%)	102/131 (78%)	384/571 (67.3%)	48%	382/484 (79%)	80%
Prior migraine unchanged or worsened	107/252 (42%)	3 (38%)	7/31 (23%)	29/131 (22%)	187/571 (32.7%)	52%	102/484 (21%)	20%
Type series	R, H	R, H	R, H	R, O	R, H	R, POP	P, O	R, H

H = headache or neurologic; P = prospective; R = retrospective; POP = population base

● **Table 16.4** *Menstrual migraine and migraine improvement with pregnancy*

Menstrual/non-menstrual	Lance (1966)	Bousser (1990)
Menstrual		
Disappeared or improved	64%	86%
Worsened	36%	7%
Non-menstrual		
Disappeared or improved	48%	60%
Worsened	52%	15%

Pre-existing migraine improved or disappeared in 77.9%, worsened in 7.6%, was unchanged in 8.4% and was variable in 6.1% in Bousser's series of 131 pregnancies.[11] Migraine appeared for the first time in 16 women. Disappearance or improvement did not differ significantly in migraine with or without aura, but worsening was much more common in migraine with aura. Women with menstrual migraine showed the most improvement (Table 16.4).

Granella *et al.* found significant improvement in 17.4% and worsening in 3.5%.[12] Women whose migraine started with menarche had a higher remission rate (36.4% vs. 13.99%) than women whose headaches began at other times. Migraine began during pregnancy in 1.3% of the patients and postpartum in 4.5%.

Rasmussen found 49% of pregnant women had disappearance or significant improvement in their headache, and only 4% worsened.[13] Chen and Leviton found that 17% had a complete remission and another 62% showed some improvement with pregnancy.[14] Maggioni *et al.* found one new case of migraine without aura began during pregnancy.[15] Of the migraineurs, 80% had at least a 50% decrease in attack frequency, usually after the first trimester.

Outcome of pregnancy in migraineurs

Miscarriage, toxaemia, congenital anomalies or stillbirth are not increased in migraineurs when compared to national averages or controls.[16] However, in Chancellor's small series, four of nine patients developed complications, including pre-eclampsia in two.[7]

Postpartum migraine

Postnatal headache (PNH) occurs in about 39% of women and is most frequent on days 3 to 6 postpartum.[8] PNH is commonly associated with a personal or family history of migraine (58% of migraineurs developed PNH). PNH, while less severe than the patients' typical migraine, was bifrontal, prolonged, and associated with photophobia, nausea and anorexia.

Newly occurring frequent headache occurred in 3.6% of women and migraine in 1.4% of 11 701 women by three months postpartum.[17] Two of Wright and Patel's cases of focal neurological migraine presented postpartum.[9] Both had a history of migraine with aura. Migraine frequently restarts in the postpartum period and can begin *de novo*.

Most women's migraine improves during pregnancy. Some women have their first migraine attack during pregnancy. Migraine often recurs or begins for the first time postpartum. Migraineurs are not different than non-migraineurs in miscarriages, toxaemia, congenital anomalies or stillbirth.

Treatment
Risk of drug treatment (Table 16.5)

The recognition of the teratogenicity of aminopterin and thalidomide and the rubella epidemic of 1963–1964 resulted in extremely conservative drug use during pregnancy. In 1977 the Food and Drug Administration (FDA) developed a policy against phase I and early phase II testing in pregnant women or in women of child-bearing potential, and many practitioners now avoid drug treatment in pregnancy even when it is indicated. Over 3000 drugs have been tested by the FDA and only 20 are known human teratogens. There is insufficient knowledge about the birth defect risks from drug exposure despite the fact that 67% of women take drugs during pregnancy and 50% take them during the first trimester.[18]

Most drugs cross the placenta and have the potential to adversely affect the fetus, and, although studies have not absolutely established the safety of any medication during pregnancy, some are believed to be relatively safe (see Tables 16.7–16.17).[19–22]

● **Table 16.5** *Definitions and drug effects*

Spontaneous abortion:	Death of the conceptus. Most due to chromosomal abnormality.
Embryotoxicity:	The ability of drugs to kill the developing embryo.
Congenital anomalies:	Deviation from normal morphology or function.
Teratogenicity:	The ability of an exogenous agent to produce a permanent abnormality of structure or function in an organism exposed during embryogenesis or fetal life.
Fetal effects:	Growth retardation, abnormal histogenesis (also congenital abnormalities and fetal death). The main outcome of fetal drug toxicity during the second and third trimesters of pregnancy.
Perinatal effects:	Effects on uterine contraction, neonatal withdrawal, or haemostasis.
Postnatal effects:	Drugs may have delayed long-term effects: delayed oncogenesis, and functional and behavioural abnormalities.

In 1966 the FDA replaced the Multigeneration Continuous Feeding Reproductive Study with a three-segment design, identified as Segment I (Fertility and General Reproductive Performance), Segment II (Teratology) and Segment III (Perinatal and Postnatal Evaluations), for testing drugs. These studies were designed to detect agents that specifically interrupt reproduction. More than 3300 chemicals have been tested; of these, 37% are teratogenic. These studies frequently used very high doses of drugs, which then produced maternal toxicity, not fetal teratogenicity. Currently 19 drugs, or drug groups, and two chemicals have been established as human teratogens. Negative results in other species cannot predict a lack of teratogenicity in humans, and drugs that are teratogenic at high doses in these species may not be teratogenic in humans at lower doses.[23] Thalidomide, which has no teratogenic effect in mice and rats, has profound teratogenic effects in humans.[19,24]

A negative pregnancy test is often a condition of enrolment in a study, while post-enrolment pregnancy can lead to termination of participation. This poses a problem for pregnant women who are sick and in need of treatment. If the drug has not been tested in pregnant women during the research phase, information is lacking about the safety and efficacy of the drug for the women as well as the fetus.[25] The Institute of Medicine Committee on Research in Women made the controversial recommendation that pregnant and lactating women be considered eligible for enrolment in clinical studies on a routine basis.[25] This report reversed the existing exclusion of pregnant women and the severely restricted enrolment of women of 'child-bearing potential' from most clinical studies. With regard to enrolment, the Committee recommended that women who are or may become pregnant in the course of a study should be viewed as any other potential research subject.

If women of childbearing age participated in clinical trials, more information will be gained about the risks of birth defects, but uncertainty will still persist. If a drug is associated with a very high level of birth defects (e.g. thalidomide), very few exposures need to be followed to detect this risk; if a drug is associated with a slight increase in birth defects, approximately 300 exposed pregnancies need to be followed to detect a doubling of risk; and if a drug is associated with an increase of a rare specific defect (e.g. 1/1000), approximately 10 000 exposed pregnancies need to be followed to detect a doubling of risk.[18]

The World Health Organization (WHO) surveyed drug utilization during pregnancy. Eighty-six percent of 14 778 pregnant women took medication, each receiving an average of 2.9 prescriptions. Over-the-counter drugs were not considered. Of a total of 37 309 prescriptions, 73% were given by obstetricians, 12% by general practitioners and 5% by midwives. Forty percent of pregnant women at Parkland Memorial Hospital in Dallas took some type of medication other than iron or vitamin supplements and up to 20% used an illicit drug or alcohol.[26] There was a 576% increase in discharges of drug-using parturient women and a 456% increase in discharges of drug-affected newborns in the United States between 1979 and 1990.

While no medication is absolutely safe, some are believed to be relatively safe.[18] Most drugs cross the placenta and potentially can adversely affect the fetus. Drugs are routinely tested in animals for teratogenicity, but these findings cannot always be extrapolated to women.

Adverse drug effects depend on the dose and route of administration, concomitant exposures, and the timing of the exposure relative to the period of development (Table 16.6), which consist of the pre-implantation period, embryogenesis, and fetal development. The pre-implantation period lasts from conception to one week postconception, during which time the conceptus is relatively protected from drugs.[26] Embryogenesis is the time of organogenesis, which occurs from the time of implantation to 60 days postconception.[26] Most congenital malformations arise during this time. Placental transport is not well established until the fifth week after conception. This protects the embryo from maternal drugs. The final phase, fetal development, follows embryogenesis. The fetus grows mainly in size, although structural changes such as neuronal arrangement also occur. Malformations can develop at this time in normally formed organs due to their necrosis and reabsorption.[26]

Death to the conceptus, teratogenicity, fetal growth abnormalities, perinatal effects, postnatal developmental abnormalities, delayed oncogenesis and functional and behavioural changes can result from drugs or other agents (Table 16.5). According to the Perinatal Collaborative Project, a prospective and concurrent epidemiological study of more than 50 000 pregnancies, many drugs have little or no human teratogenic risk.[27]

Spontaneous abortion

Nearly half of early pregnancies spontaneously abort, most due to chromosomal abnormalities. Prior to the time of organogenesis, exposure to a potential teratogen or toxic

● **Table 16.6** *Periods of development*

Preimplantation period

   Conception to one week postconception
   Conceptus is relatively protected from drugs

Embryogenesis

   Time of organogenesis
   From implantation to 60 days postconception

Fetal development

   Follows embryogenesis

drug has an all-or-none effect. An exposure around the time of conception or implantation may kill the conceptus, but if the pregnancy continues, there is no increased risk of congenital anomalies.

Developmental defects

Developmental defects may result from genetic or environmental causes, or from interactions between them. Teratogenic drug effects are generally visible anatomic malformations but are defined as the production of a permanent alteration of structure or function in an organ due to intrauterine exposure (Figure 16.1). These are dose- and time-related, with the fetus at greatest risk during the first trimester of pregnancy. Drug exposure accounts for only 23% of birth defects: approximately 25% are genetic and the causes of the remainder are unknown. The incidence of major malformations either incompatible with survival (e.g. anencephaly) or requiring major surgery (e.g. cleft palate or congenital heart disease) is approximately 2–3% in the general population. If all minor malformations are included (ear tags or extra digits), the rate may be as high as 7–10%. The risk of malformation after drug exposure must be compared with this background rate. The classic teratogenic period in the human is a critical six weeks, lasting from approximately 31 days to 10 weeks from the last menstrual period. A teratogenic effect is dependent on the timing of the exposure as well as the nature of the teratogen. Early exposure, when the heart and central nervous system are forming, may result in an anomaly such as congenital heart disease or neural tube defect, while later exposure may result in malformation of the palate or ear. Once the teratogenic period has passed, the major risk of congenital anomaly is gone, but other abnormalities can occur. These include fetal effects, neonatal effects and postnatal effects.

Fetal effects

Fetal effects include damage to normally formed organs, damage to systems undergoing histogenesis, growth retardation or fetal death. Growth retardation is most common.

Neonatal and postnatal effects

Adverse drug effects include withdrawal, neonatal hypoglycaemia, and disorders of uterine contracture and haemostasis. Chronic exposure to psychoactive medications, such as alcohol, during the second and third trimester may cause mental retardation, which may not be recognized until later in life.

Delayed oncogenesis

Exposure to diethylstilboestrol as late as 20 weeks' gestation may cause reproductive organ anomalies that are not recognized until after puberty.

Maternal physiology (Table 16.7)[28]

Profound structural and physiological changes occur during pregnancy. The uterus rapidly increases in size, transformed from an almost-solid structure weighing 70 g into a relatively thin-walled, muscular organ large enough to accommodate the fetus, placenta and amniotic fluid.[29] Uterine growth depends on oestrogen and, to a lesser extent, progesterone, during the first few months of pregnancy. After 12 weeks, growth results from the pressure exerted by the expanding products of conception. Cell and tissue growth is dependent on increased synthesis of polyamines (including spermidine and spermine and their immediate precursor, putrescine).[29]

Metabolic changes occur in response to the rapidly-growing fetus and placenta. Weight gain, due to the increase in the uterus and its contents, the breasts, the blood volume and the extravascular extracellular fluid, averages about 11 kg, with about 1 kg occurring during the first trimester.[29] Water retention (about 6.5 litres by term) is a normal occurrence, mediated, in part, by a fall in plasma osmolality of 10 mOsm/kg, due to a resetting of the osmoreceptor. The fetus, placenta, and amniotic fluid contain about 3.5 litres of water. Another 3.0 litres of water results from increased maternal blood volume and the increase in uterine and breast size. Near term, blood volume is about 45% above baseline. Weight loss during the first 10 days postpartum averages about 2 kg.[29]

While pregnancy is potentially diabetogenic, in healthy pregnant women the fasting plasma glucose concentration may fall due to increased plasma insulin levels. Progesterone,

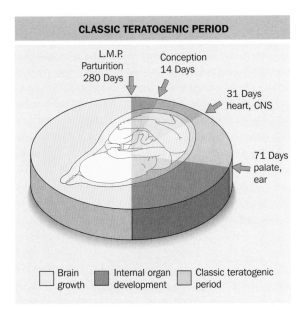

CLASSIC TERATOGENIC PERIOD

L.M.P.
Parturition
280 Days

Conception
14 Days

31 Days
heart, CNS

71 Days
palate,
ear

☐ Brain growth
■ Internal organ development
☐ Classic teratogenic period

● *Figure 16.1* The fetus is at greatest risk from tetatogenic drug effects during the first trimester of pregnancy.

● **Table 16.7** *Physiological changes during pregnancy*

Parameter	Change	Potential implications for toxicology
Extracellular volume	↑4–6 litres	Dilution of substances in circulation
Plasma volume	↑by 40%	Same
Plasma renin/ aldosterone	↑↑	Renal retention/ excretion
Renal blood flow	↑ 30–50%	Same
Glomerular filtration rate	↑30–50%	Same
Sodium and calcium retention	↑↑	Retention of other divalent cations
Cardiac output	↑by 40%	Increased sensitivity to cardiotoxins (?)
Increased blood flow to skin	↑	↑Dermal uptake
Food intake	↑70 kcal/day (average)	Increased dose
Energy demand*	↑~300 kcal/day	Increased dose and metabolic shift
Lipid stores*	↑~3–4 kg over pregnancy	Same
Oxygen consumption*	↑51 ml O2/min	Metabolic shift (?)
Basal metabolic rate	↑13%	Metabolic shifts
Hepatic triglyceride synthesis	↑	Redistribution

*Dependent on nutrition, activity levels, and gestational state.
Table adapted from Metcalfe et al.[28]

when administered to a non-pregnant adult in an amount similar to what is produced during pregnancy, results in an increased basal insulin concentration and response to an oral glucose challenge similar to that of a normal pregnant woman. Additionally, oestradiol induces hyperinsulinism in both control and ovariectomized rats.[29]

Lipid, lipoprotein and apolipoprotein plasma concentrations increase during pregnancy. There is a positive correlation between lipid concentrations and levels of oestradiol, progesterone and human placental lactogen.

The kidneys barely increase in size during pregnancy.[30] Early in pregnancy, at the beginning of the second trimester, the glomerular filtration rate and renal plasma flow increase by about 50%.[31,32] The elevated glomerular filtration rate persists to term, whereas the renal plasma flow decreases during late pregnancy.[32] The human liver does not increase in size during pregnancy and we are not certain whether or not hepatic blood flow increases.

The profound physiological changes that occur during pregnancy can alter drug pharmacokinetics: plasma volume increases by half, cardiac output increases by 30–50% and renal plasma flow and glomerular filtration rate increase by 40–50%. Serum albumin decreases by 20–30%, resulting in decreased drug binding and increased drug clearance. Increased extracellular fluid and adipose tissue increases the volume of drug distribution. Drug metabolism may also be increased, modulated, in part, by the high concentration of sex hormones.[33]

Drug risk categories

The FDA lists five categories of labelling for drug use in pregnancy (Table 16.8).[34] These categories provide therapeutic guidance, weighing the risks as well as the benefits of the drug. An alternate rating system is TERIS, an automated teratogen information resource wherein ratings for each drug or agent are based on a consensus of expert opinion and the literature (Table 16.9).[35] TERIS was designed to assess the teratogenic risk to the fetus from a drug exposure. A recent study found that the FDA categories have little, if any, correlation to the TERIS teratogenic risk. This discrepancy results in part from the fact that the FDA categories were designed to provide therapeutic guidance and the TERIS ratings are useful for estimating the teratogenic risks of a drug and not vice versa.[36]

A woman's risk of having a child with a neural tube defect is associated with early pregnancy red cell folate levels in a continuous dose–response relationship.[37] Low serum and red blood cell folate levels are associated with spontaneous abortion and fetal malformations in animals and in humans.[38–41] Treatment with some drugs, including phenytoin, carbamazepine and barbiturates, can impair folate absorption. Valproic acid does not

● **Table 16.8** *FDA risk categories*

Category A:	Controlled human studies show no risk
Category B:	No evidence of risk in humans, but there are no controlled human studies
Category C:	Risk to humans has not been ruled out
Category D:	Positive evidence of risk to humans from human and/or animal studies
Category X:	Contraindicated in pregnancy.

● **Table 16.9** *TERIS risk rating*

- Undetermined (C)
- None (A)
- None–minimal (A)
- Minimal (B)
- Minimal–small (D)
- High (X)

Equivalent FDA ratings in parentheses.

produce folate deficiency, but it may interfere with the production of folinic acid by inhibiting glutamate formyl transferase.[42] In a small study, women with epilepsy taking phenytoin needed 1 mg of folate supplementation a day to maintain a normal serum level.[43] The current guidelines suggest increasing folic acid intake by 4 mg, which would result in a 48% reduction in neural tube defects.[38] Supplementing this by fortifying food with folate would benefit all women.

Headache treatment

The major concerns in the management of the pregnant patient are the effects of both medication and migraine on the fetus. Because of the possible risk of injury to the fetus, medication use should be limited; however, it is not contraindicated during pregnancy.[18] Since migraine usually improves after the first trimester, many women can manage their headaches with this reassurance and non-pharmacological means of coping, such as ice, massage and biofeedback.[18] Some women, however, will continue to have severe, intractable headaches, sometimes associated with nausea, vomiting and possible dehydration. Not only are these conditions disruptive to the patient, they may pose a risk to the fetus that is greater than the potential risk of the medications used to treat the pregnant patient.[18]

Symptomatic treatment, designed to reduce the severity and duration of symptoms, is used to treat an acute headache attack (Tables 16.10 and 16.11). Individual attacks should be treated with rest, reassurance and ice packs. For headaches that do not respond to non-pharmacological treatment, symptomatic drugs are indicated. The non-steroidal anti-inflammatory drugs (NSAID), acetaminophen (paracetamol)(alone or with codeine), codeine alone, or other narcotics can be used during pregnancy. Aspirin in low intermittent doses is not a significant teratogenic risk, although large doses, especially if given near term, may be associated with maternal and fetal bleeding. Aspirin should probably be reserved unless there is a definite therapeutic need for it (other than headache). Barbiturate and benzodiazepine use should be limited. Ergotamine, dihydroergotamine, and sumatriptan should be avoided.

The associated symptoms of migraine, such as nausea and vomiting, can be as disabling as the headache pain itself. In addition, some medications that are used to treat migraine can produce nausea. Metoclopramide, which decreases the gastric atony seen with migraine and enhances the absorption of co-administered medications, is extremely useful in migraine treatment. Mild nausea can be treated with phosphorylated carbohydrate solution (emetrol) or doxylamine succinate and vitamin B_6 (pyridoxine). More severe nausea may require the use of injections or suppositories. Trimethobenzamide, chlorpromazine, prochlorperazine and promethazine are available orally, parenterally and by suppository and can all be used safely. We frequently use promethazine and prochlorperazine suppositories. Corticosteroids can be utilized occasionally. Some use prednisone in preference to dexamethasone (which crosses the placenta more readily).

● Table 16.10 *Some therapeutic medications*

Drug class		Fetal risk	
		FDA	TERIS
Simple analgesics	Aspirin	C (D)	None–minimal
	Acetaminophen	B	None
	Caffeine	B	None–minimal
NSAID	Ibuprofen	B (D)	None–minimal
	Indomethacin	B (D)	None
	Naproxen	B (D)	Undetermined
Narcotics	Butorphanol	C (D)	None–minimal
	Codeine	C (D)	None–minimal
	Meperidine	B (D)	None–minimal
	Methadone	B (D)	None–minimal
	Morphine	B (D)	None–minimal
	Propoxyphene	C (D)	None–minimal
Ergots and serotonin agonists	Ergotamine	X	Minimal
	Dihydroergotamine	X	Undetermined
	Sumatriptan	C	Undetermined
Corticosteroids	Dexamethasone	C	None–minimal
	Prednisone	B	None–minimal
Barbiturates	Butalbital	C (D)	None–minimal
	Phenobarbital	D	None–minimal
Benzodiazepam	Chlordiazepoxide	D	None–minimal
	Clonazepam	D	Uncertain
	Diazepam	D	None–minimal

* Risk factor if used at end of third trimester given in parentheses.

● Table 16.11 *Neuroleptics/antiemetics*

Drug class		Fetal risk	
		FDA	TERIS
Antihistamines	Cyclizine (Marezine)	B	Undetermined
	Cyproheptadine	B	Undetermined
	Dimenhydrinate (Dramamine)	B	None–minimal
	Meclizine (Antivert)	B	None–minimal
Neuroleptics	Phenothiazines		
	Chlorpromazine (Thorazine)	C	None–minimal
	Prochlorperazine (Compazine)	C	None
	Butyrophenones Haloperidol	C	None–minimal
	Metoclopramide (Reglan)	B	None–minimal
Other	Emetrol	B	Unknown
	Doxylamine succinate	–	None
	Vitamin B_6 (pyridoxine)	B	None

Severe acute attacks of migraine should be treated aggressively.[18] We start intravenous fluids for hydration and then use prochlorperazine 10 mg i.v. to control both nausea and head pain. This can be supplemented by intravenous narcotics or intravenous corticosteroids. This is an extremely effective way of handling status migrainosus during pregnancy.

Preventive treatment

Increased frequency and severity of migraine associated with nausea and vomiting may justify the use of daily prophylactic, or preventive, medication. This treatment option should be a last resort and used only with the consent of the patient and her partner after the risks have been completely explained. Preventive therapy is designed to reduce the frequency and severity of headache attacks. Consider prophylaxis when patients experience at least three or four prolonged, severe attacks a month that are particularly incapacitating or unresponsive to symptomatic therapy and may result in dehydration and fetal distress. Beta-adrenergic blockers such as propranolol have been used under these circumstances, although adverse effects, including intrauterine growth retardation, have been reported. If the migraine is so severe that drug treatment is essential, the patient should be told of the risks posed by all the drugs that are used (Table 16.12). If the patient has a coexistent illness that requires treatment, pick one drug that will treat both disorders. For example, propranolol can be used to treat hypertension and migraine while fluoxetine can be used to treat comorbid depression.

Drug exposure

If a woman inadvertently takes a drug while she is pregnant or becomes pregnant while taking a drug, it is important to determine the dose, timing and duration of the exposure(s). Ascertain the patient's past and present state of health and the presence of mental retardation or chromosomal abnormalities in the family. Using a reliable source of information (such as TERIS), determine if the drug is a known teratogen (although for many drugs this is not possible).[24,26,35,44]

If the drug is teratogenic or the risk is unknown, have the obstetrician confirm the gestational age by ultrasound. If the exposure occurred during embryogenesis, then high-resolution ultrasound can be performed to determine whether damage to specific organ systems or structures has occurred. If the high-resolution ultrasound is normal, it is reasonable to reassure the patient that the gross fetal structure is normal (within the 90% sensitivity of the study).[26] However, fetal ultrasound cannot exclude minor anomalies or guarantee the birth of a normal child. Delay in achieving developmental milestones, including cognitive development, are potential risks, especially for children born to epileptics, that cannot be predicted or diagnosed prenatally. Have the obstetrician discuss the results of these studies with the mother and her partner; formal prenatal counselling may be helpful in uncertain cases.[26]

Breast feeding

Milk is a suspension of fat and protein in a carbohydrate–mineral solution. A nursing mother secretes 600 ml milk/day containing sufficient protein, fat and carbohydrate to meet the nutritional demands of the growing and developing infant.[20] The transport of a drug into milk depends on its lipid solubility, molecular weight, degree of ionization, protein binding and the presence or absence of active secretion. Species differences in the composition of milk can result in differences in drug transfer. Since human milk has a much higher pH (pH usually >7.0) than cows' milk (pH usually <6.8), bovine drug transfer data may not be accurate in humans.

Many drugs can be detected in breast milk at levels that are not of clinical significance to the infant. The concentration

● **Table 16.12** *Guidelines for prophylactic treatment*

Drug class	Dose	Fetal risk	
		FDA	**TERIS**
β-blockers			
Atenolol	50–120 mg/day	C	Undetermined
Metoprolol	50–100 mg/day	B	Undetermined
Nadolol	40–240 mg/day	C	Undetermined
Propranolol	40–320 mg/day	C	Undetermined
Timolol	10–30 mg/day	C	Undetermined
Antidepressants			
Tricyclics			
Amitriptyline	10–250 mg/day	D	None–minimal
Doxepin	10–150–mg/day	C	Undetermined
Nortriptyline HCl	10–100 mg/day	D	Undetermined
Protriptyline		C	Undetermined
SSRIs			
Fluoxetine	10–80 mg/day	B	None
Paroxetine	10–50 mg/day	C	Undetermined
Sertraline		B	Unknown
Calcium-channel blockers			
Verapamil	240–720 mg/day	C	Undetermined
Nifedipine	30–180 mg/day	C	Undetermined
Diltiazem	120–360 mg/day	C	Undetermined
Serotonin agonists			
Methysergide	2–8 mg/day in divided doses up to 14 mg/day	D	Undetermined
Methylergonovine maleate (Methergine)	0.2–0.4 mg q.i.d.	C	Undetermined
Pizotifen	1–6 mg/day	C	Undetermined
Anticonvulsants			
Divalproex sodium	500–3000 mg/day	D	Small–moderate

of drug in breast milk is a variable fraction of the maternal blood level. The infant dose is usually 1–2% of the maternal dose, which is usually trivial. Any exposure to a toxic drug or potential allergen may be inappropriate.

Drug concentration in breast milk depends on drug characteristics (pK$_a$, lipid solubility, molecular weight, protein binding) and breast milk characteristics (composition and volume). Breast milk is given its unique physicochemical properties by the active transport of electrolytes and the formation and excretion of lactose and proteins by glandular epithelial cells in the breast with passive diffusion of water. The volume produced depends on nutritional factors, the amount of milk removed by the suckling infant and the increase in mammary blood flow that occurs with breast feeding. Volume production

slowly increases from an average of 600 ml/day to 800 ml/day by the time the infant is six months old, and undergoes a diurnal variation, with the greatest quantity occurring in the morning. For the first 10 days of production, milk composition is characterized by a gradual increase in fat and lactose from a milk that is higher in protein content (colostrum).

Since most drugs are either weak acids or bases, the transfer across a biological membrane will be greatly influenced by the ionization characteristics (pK$_a$) and pH differences across the membrane. Because the pH of breast milk (7.0) is slightly lower than that of plasma (7.4), there is a tendency toward ion-trapping of basic compounds.

Classification of drugs used during lactation

The American Academy of Pediatrics Committee on Drugs has reviewed drugs in lactation and categorized the drugs as shown in Table 16.13.[45] When prescribing drugs to lactating women, the guidelines in Table 17.14 should be followed.[45]

The migraineur who is breast feeding should avoid bromocriptine, ergotamine and lithium, and use sumatriptan, benzodiazepam, antidepressants and neuroleptics cautiously. Acetaminophen (paracetamol) is compatible with breast feeding and is preferred to aspirin (Tables 16.15–16.17). Moderate caffeine use is compatible with breast feeding. However, accumulation may occur in infants whose mothers use excessive amounts. Narcotic use is compatible with breast feeding. Phenobarbital has caused sedation in some nursing infants and it should be given to nursing mothers with caution.

● **Table 16.13** *Drug categories and breastfeeding*[45]

- Contraindicated
- Require temporary cessation of breast feeding
- Effects unknown but may be of concern
- Use with caution
- Usually compatible

● **Table 16.14** *Prescribing guidelines and breastfeeding*[45]

- Is the drug necessary?
- Use the safest drug (e.g. acetaminophen (paracetamol) instead of aspirin).
- If there is a possibility that a drug may present a risk to the infant (e.g. phenytoin, phenobarbital), consider measuring the blood level in the nursing infant.
- Drug exposure to the nursing infant may by minimized by having the mother take the medication just after completing a breast feeding.

● **Table 16.15** *Drugs and breast feeding*[45]

Drug class		Breast feeding
Simple analgesics	Aspirin	Caution*
	Acetaminophen	Compatible
	Caffeine	Compatible
	NSAID	Compatible
Narcotics		Compatible
Barbiturates		Caution**
Benzodiazepam		Concern***
Antihistamines	Cyproheptadine	Contraindicated
Neuroleptics	Phenothiazines	
	Chlorpromazine	Concern
	Prochlorperazine	Compatible
	Metoclopramide	Concern

* Metabolic acidosis, platelet function abnormality;
** Sedation;
*** Effects unknown but of concern.

● **Table 16.16** *Drugs and breast feeding*[45]

Ergot/serotonin agonists	Breast feeding
Ergotamine	Contraindicated
Dihydroergotamine	Contraindicated
Methylergonovine maleate	Caution
Methysergide	Caution
Sumatriptan	Caution

● **Table 16.17** *Drugs and breast feeding*[45]

Drug class		Breast feeding
Antihypertensives	Beta-blockers	Compatible
	Adrenergic blockers	Compatible
	Calcium-channel blockers	Compatible
Antidepressants	Tricyclic antidepressants	Concern
	Selective serotonin reuptake inhibitors	Caution
Other drugs	Carbamazepine	Compatible
	Valproic acid	Compatible
	Corticosteroids	Compatible
	Bromocriptine	Contraindicated

References

1. Uknis A, Silberstein SD. Review Article: Migrain and Pregnancy. *Headache* 1991; 31: 372–374.

2. Silberstein SD, Saper J. Migraine: Diagnosis and treatment. In: Dalessio D, Silberstein SD (eds). *Wolff's Headache and Other Head Pain, (6th Edition)*. New York: Oxford University Press, 1993: 96.

3. Silberstein SD. Evaluation and emergency treatment of headache. *Headache* 1992; 32: 396–407.

4. Fox MW, Harms RW, Davis DH. Selected neurologic complications of pregnancy. *Mayo Clin Proc* 1990;65:1595–1618.

5. Hainline B. Headache. *Headache* 1994;12(3):443–60.

6. Schwartz RB. Neurodiagnostic imaging of the pregnant patient. In: Devinsky O, Feldmann E, Hainline B (eds). *Neurologic complications of pregnancy*. New York: Raven Press, 1994: 243–8.

7. Chancellor MD, Wroe SJ. Migraine occurring for the first time in pregnancy. *Headache* 1990;30:224–7.

8. Stein GS. Headaches in the first postpartum week and their relationship to migraine. *Headache* 1981;21:201–5.

9. Wright DS, Patel MK. Focal migraine and pregnancy. *BMJ* 1986;293:1557–1558.

10. Lance JW, Anthony M. Some clinical aspects of migraine. *Arch Neruol* 1966;15:356–361.

11. Bousser MG, Ratinahirana H, Darbois X. Migraine and pregnancy: a prospective study in 703 women after delivery. *Abstr Neurology* 1990;40(1):437.

12. Granella F, Sances G, Zanferrari C et al. Migraine without aura and reproductive life events: a clinical epidemiologic study in 1300 women. *Headache* 1993;33:385–389.

13. Rasmussen BK. Migraine and tension-type headache in a general population: precipitating factors, female hormones, sleep pattern, and relation to lifestyle. *Pain* 1993;53:65–72.

14. Chen TC, Leviton A. Headache recurrence in pregnant women with migraine. *Headache* 1994;34:107–110.

15. Maggioni F, Alessi C, Maggino T et al. Primary headaches and pregnancy (abstr). *Cephalalgia* 1995;15:54.

16. Wainscott G, Volans GN. The outcome of pregnancy in women suffering from migraine. *Postgrad Med J* 1978;54:98–102.

17. MacArther C, Lewis M, Know EG. Health after childbirth. *Brit J Obstet Gynecol* 1991;98:1193–1204.

18. Pitkin RM. Drug treatment of the pregnant woman: the state of the art. *Proceedings from the Food and Drug Administration conference on regulated products and pregnant women, November 1995,* VA (abstr).

19. Blake DA, Niebyl JR. Requirements and limitations in reproductive and teratogenic risk assessment. In: Niebyl JR (ed). *Drug Use in Pregnancy (2nd ed)*. Philadelphia: Lea & Febiger, 1988:19.

20. Briggs GG, Freeman RK, Yaffe SJ (eds). *Drugs in Pregnancy and Lactation (4th ed)*. Baltimore: Williams & Wilkins, 1994.

21. Niebyl JR. Tertology and drugs in pregnancy and lactation. In: Winters R (eds). *Danforth's Obstetrics and Gynecology (6th ed)*. New York: Lippincott, 1990.

22. Rayburn WF, Lavin JP. Drug prescribing for chronic medical disorders during pregnancy: an overview. *Am J Obstet Gynecol* 1986;155:565–569.

23. Cavagnaro JA. Traditional reproductive toxicology studies and their predictive value. *Proceedings from the Food and Drug Administration conference on regulated products and pregnant women. November 1994,* Va.

24. Silberstein SD. Headaches and women: treatment of the pregnant and lactating migraineur. *Headache* 1993;33(10):533–540.

25. Macklin R. Ethical conflicts and practical realities. *Proceedings from the Food and Drug administration conference on regulated products and pregnant women, November 7–8, 1994,* VA.

26. Gilstrap LC III, Little BB (eds). *Drugs and Pregnancy*. Elsevier: New York, 1992:23–29.

27. Heinonen OP, Slone S, Shapiro S. *Birth defects and drugs in pregnancy*. Littleton MA: Publishing Sciences Group, 1977.

28. Metcalfe J, Stock MK, Barron DH. Maternal physiology during gestation. In: Knobel E, Neill J (eds). *The Physiology of Reproduction*. New York: Raven Press, 1988:2145–2174.

29. Cunningham FG, MacDonald PC, Leveno KJ, Gant NF, Gilstrap III LC (eds). Maternal adaptations to pregnancy. In: *William's Obsteterics (19th ed)*. Connecticut: Appleton and Lange, 1993:209–246.

30. Bailey RR, Rolleston GL. Kidney length and ureteric dilatation in the puerperium. *Br J Obstet Gynaecol* 1971;78:55.

31. Chesley LC. Renal function during pregnancy. In: Carey HM (ed). *Modern Trends in Human Reproductive Physiology*. London: Butterworth, 1963.

32. Dunlop W. Serial changes in renal haemodynamics during normal human pregnancy. *Br J Obstet Gynaecol* 1981;88:1.

33. Chaudhuri G. Pharmacokinetics in pregnancy (abstr). *Proceedings of the Food and Drug administration conference on regulated products and pregnant women.* 11/7–8/1994, VA.

34. Barnhart ER (ed.). *Physicians' desk reference (45th ed)*. Oradell NJ: Medical Economics Inc, 1991.

35. Friedman JM, Polifka JE (eds). *Teratogenic effects of drugs: a resource for clinicians (TERIS)*. Baltimore: Johns Hopkins University Press, 1994.

36. Friedman JM, Little BB, Brent RL et al. Potential human teratogenicity of frequently prescribed drugs. *Obstet Gynecol* 1990;75:594–599.

37. Daly LE, Kirke PN, Molloy A, Weir DG, Scott JM. Folate levels and neural tube defects: implications for prevention. *JAMA* 1995;274:1698–1702.

38. Ogawa Y, Kaneko S, Otani K, Fukushima Y. Serum folic acid levels in epileptic mothers and their relationship to congenital malformations. *Epilepsy Res* 1991;8(Suppl 1):75–78.

39. Jordan RL, Wilson JG, Shumacher HJ. Embryotoxicity of the folate antagonist methotrexate in rats and rabbits. *Teratology* 1977;15:73–80.

40. Dansky LV, Andermann E, Rosenblatt D, Sherwin AL, Andermann F. Anticonvulsants, folate levels, and pregnancy outcome: a prospective study. *Ann Neurol* 1987;21(Suppl 2):176–182.

41. Reynolds EH. Anticonvulsants, folic acid and epilepsy. *Lancet* 1973;i:1376–1378.

42. Wegner C, Nau H. Alteration of embryonic folate metabolism by valproic acid during organogenesis: implications for mechanisms of teratogenesis. *Neurology* 1992;42(S5):17–24.

43. Berg MJ, Stumbo PJ, Chenard CA et al. Folic acid improves phenytoin pharmacokinetics. *J Am Diet Assoc* 1995;95(3):352–356.

44. Shepard TH. *Catalog of Teratogenic Agents (8th ed.)* Baltimore: Johns Hopkins University Press, 1973.

45. American Academy of Pediatrics Committee on Drugs. The transfer of drugs and update other chemicals into human milk. *Pediatrics* 1994;93:137–150.

chapter 17

Geriatric headache

Introduction

Headache prevalence is age-dependent.[1] Although less common in the elderly, 10% of women and 5% of men still report severe headaches at the age of 70 years.[2] Headache aetiology is also age-dependent. The incidence of primary headache disorders declines while the incidence of secondary headache disorders (such as mass lesions and temporal arteritis) increases with advancing age. Some secondary headache disorders, such as giant cell arteritis, occur almost exclusively in the elderly (Table 17.1).[3] At least one primary headache disorder, the hypnic headache syndrome, is unique to the elderly. Older patients are also more likely to have comorbid medical illness.[4]

Frequent headache was found in 11% of elderly women and 5% of elderly men participating in a health screening programme;[5,6] these patients commonly had other medical disorders.[7] Table 17.2 summarizes the major causes of headaches that begin late in life, divided into secondary and primary headache disorders. Headaches that begin after the age of 65 years are more likely to be due to serious conditions.[1,6] Systemic illnesses or medications that produce headache become increasingly common with advancing age. Mass lesions and giant cell arteritis (GCA; temporal arteritis) have devastating, but often avoidable, consequences. For these reasons, more testing is indicated when older patients present with headache, particularly if the headaches are atypical, of recent onset or associated with neurological findings.[1]

The initial evaluation of an elderly patient with a new-onset headache should be directed towards identifying or excluding secondary headache etiologies. Patients with headaches beginning after the age of 50 years usually require a neuroimaging procedure (computed tomography or magnetic resonance imaging) and an erythrocyte sedimentation rate (ESR) as part of the initial workup to identify or rule out structural lesions and GCA. After secondary causes of headache have been excluded, the primary headache disorder should be identified and treated. Although the common primary headache disorders (migraine; cluster headache; and tension-type headache, TTH) usually begin earlier in life, their prevalence in the elderly is significant and they may have unusual presentations, as exemplified by late-life migraine accompaniments.

In this chapter, we will first discuss the major secondary headache disorders as they present in later life. The discussion of primary headache disorders will emphasize the diagnostic and treatment dilemmas encountered in elderly patients.

● **Table 17.1** *Headache prevalence as a function of age*

Decrease in prevalence	Equally common	Increase in prevalence	Typically only in the elderly
Migraine	?Cluster headache	Intracranial lesions	Giant cell arteritis
Tension-type headache		Medication-induced (except rebound)	Hypnic headache
		'Metabolic headache' anaemia hypoxia hypercalcemia hyponatremia chronic renal failure	Headache of Parkinson's disease
		Cerebrovascular disease	

Note: Modified from ref. 6.

● **Table 17.2** *Common causes of headache beginning in late life*

Secondary headache disorders	Primary headache disorders
Mass lesions	Migraine
Giant cell arteritis	Tension-type headache
Medication-related headaches	Cluster headache
Trigeminal neuralgia	Hypnic headache
Postherpetic neuralgia	
Systemic disease	
Disease of the cranium, neck, eyes, ears and nose	
Cerebrovascular disease	
Parkinson's disease	

Secondary headache disorders

Mass lesions

Brain tumours (primary and metastatic) and subdural haematomas (SDH) occur with increased frequency in the elderly.[8,9] In the International Headache Society (IHS) criteria, mass lesions are included in the category called 'headache associated with nonvascular intracranial disorders'. The most frequent primary brain tumours are gliomas, meningiomas (especially common in elderly women) (Figure 17.1) and pituitary adenomas.[8,9] The most frequent metastatic tumours are lung and breast cancer, followed by malignant melanomas and carcinomas of the kidney and gastrointestinal tracts.[8]

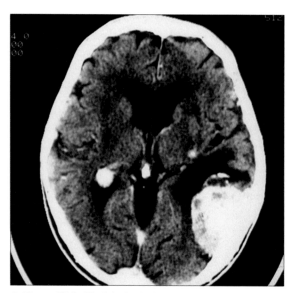

● **Figure 17.1** *CT of the brain illustrates meningioma arising in the left parietal region of an elderly woman. Because meningiomas arise from the dura mater, the tumours typically have a dural base as illustrated here.*

Tumour-associated pain patterns are highly variable because pain is generated by diverse mechanisms and depends upon the tumour location and the pattern of radiation. The headache profile most often resembles that of TTH; the 'brain tumour triad' of severe pain, early morning awakening and nausea occurs in only 17% of patients with brain tumours.[10] Headaches can antedate the development of focal neurological features; thus, early detection requires neuroimaging procedures in elderly patients with new-onset headaches.

Chronic subdural hematomas, grouped by the IHS with 'headaches associated with vascular disorders',[11] often act as mass lesions and may present with headache symptoms similar to symptoms of brain tumours. The elderly are at greater risk for subdural hematomas, due, in part, to brain atrophy, which decreases the support of bridging veins, allowing for tears and bleeding. Subdural hematomas are extra-axial (outside the brain parenchyma) and less likely to produce early neurological deficits. Even large lesions may produce headache with no focal neurological dysfunction. Some patients present with headache and confusion or a fluctuating level of consciousness. SDH may present long after trauma. A history of an antecedent head injury is often absent, perhaps because a minor injury was forgotten.

Giant cell arteritis

Giant cell arteritis (GCA) is a systemic vasculitis that primarily affects medium size arteries. Signs and symptoms include headache, visual loss, fatigue and myalgias. Rare before the age of 50 years, it has a dramatic age-related increase in incidence after the age of 50 years, when it occurs in 3–9 per 100 000 population per year, with women affected three times as often as men.[3,12,13]

GCA should be suspected in any elderly patient with new-onset headaches or a change in headache pattern. Headache is the most frequent symptom and is present in 70–90% of patients. The pain can be intermittent or constant. It is often located over the temples and is associated with scalp tenderness, especially over inflamed arteries. Local pressure, such as wearing a hat or resting the head on a pillow, may exacerbate the pain (Table 17.3).[14,15]

Polymyalgia rheumatica, whose symptoms include muscle pain and joint stiffness, is present in 25% of patients.[14] Other common symptoms of GCA include fever, weight loss, night sweats, masseter claudication, amaurosis fugax (which may be bilateral in half of patients), permanent blindness (often without warning) or partial visual loss.[16] GCA should be included in the differential diagnosis of amaurosis fugax.[17] Dysphoric mood, anorexia and weight loss are common in GCA and may lead to the primary diagnosis of depression. Patients or physicians may mistakenly relate the onset of symptoms to a coincidental painful life event.

Visual loss is the most feared complication of GCA, occurring in 7–60% of untreated patients, with a pooled incidence of 36% in 819 cases.[18] Visual loss is usually sudden and irreversible; however, gradual visual loss and recovery of vision with treatment have been reported.[19-23] Visual loss is usually due to ischaemic optic neuropathy secondary to arteritis of the short posterior ciliary arteries (the blood vessels that supply the anterior optic nerve).[15,19,20,24,25] Visual loss may also occur secondary to posterior ischaemic optic neuropathy, central retinal artery occlusion or bilateral occipital lobe infarction.[15,18,21,24,25] In untreated cases, monocular visual loss may be followed by loss of vision in the other eye.[8,19]

● **Table 17.3** *Symptoms and signs in giant cell arteritis*

Headache

Fatigue

Myalgia

Arthralgia

Depressed mood

Jaw claudication

Features of the temporal artery
• tenderness
• induration
• diminished or absent pulse

Other ischaemic symptoms can occur. Jaw claudication is characterized by the gradual onset of pain resulting from chewing for several minutes.[18] This gradual onset contrasts with the rapid onset of lancinating pain with chewing that characterizes trigeminal neuralgia. Temporomandibular joint dysfunction is typified by the rapid onset of a dull ache. Ischaemia of the extraocular muscles and/or the oculomotor nerves may produce diplopia due to ocular motor paresis. Coronary, mesenteric, hepatic and renal artery ischaemia has also been reported. Aortic arch syndrome may occur with rupture.[26]

Stroke and transient ischaemic attack (TIA) can occur in GCA. Stroke is usually associated with extracranial thrombus formation at sites of inflammation in the internal carotid or vertebral arteries leading to distal embolization or propagation of extracranial clot. Intracranial vasculitis is rare, perhaps because cerebral arteries lose their internal elastic lamina (which is the site of pathology) after they pierce the dura mater.[27]

The physical examination may support the diagnosis of GCA. Induration and tenderness of the temporal or occipital scalp arteries are the most common signs of temporal arteritis (Figure 17.2). The visual fields and visual acuity should be carefully assessed. In patients without visual loss, the funduscopic examination is normal. In acute anterior ischaemic optic neuropathy, optic disc oedema and visual loss may occur.[18,24] Altitudinal defects and central scotomas breaking into the periphery are frequent. In posterior ischaemic optic neuropathy, the normal initial funduscopic examination is replaced over weeks by optic disc pallor.[25] Diplopia is rare, and, when present, is usually due to ischaemia of the extraocular muscle, the cranial nerves, or both. True cranial nerve palsy is rare. Arterial bruits or diminished pulses are present in one-third of patients.

The most consistent laboratory abnormality is an elevation of the Westergren ESR. In one series, 41% of patients had a value >100 mm/h and 89% had a value >31 mm/h. Elevated C-reactive protein, mild liver function abnormalities and mild anaemia are also common. Occasionally GCA is diagnosed despite a normal ESR. In some cases, a normal ESR at presentation is followed by an elevated ESR as the disease progresses.[19,22,28] The ESR may be reduced in patients who are taking aspirin, non-steroidal anti-inflammatory drugs (NSAID), or systemic steroids, leading to a false-negative test.

Temporal artery biopsy is the diagnostic gold standard and should be performed within 48 hours of initiating steroid treatment if possible. Diagnostic yield on biopsy can be optimized by selecting a clinically symptomatic arterial segment based on tenderness, induration or a diminished pulse. If the biopsy appears negative, multiple sections should be examined to improve yield. GCA is characterized pathologically by skip lesions; affected and unaffected segments may be adjacent. If the biopsy is negative and the index of suspicion remains high, a second temporal artery biopsy is sometimes diagnostic.[26,29]

In patients who have the characteristic GCA profile and an elevated ESR, treatment should be initiated promptly while awaiting the results of a temporal artery biopsy (Figure 17.3). A short course of steroids prior to biopsy should not produce false-negative results. The major goal of treatment is to prevent sudden, irreversible visual loss. Initial doses of prednisone range from 60 to 80 mg daily. The headache and systemic symptoms typically remit shortly after treatment is started. After several weeks of therapy, the prednisone dose can be gradually reduced. A maintenance dose that controls

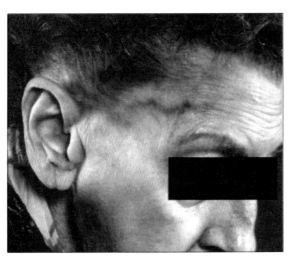

● **Figure 17.2** *Prominent temporal artery in a patient with giant cell arteritis. (Reproduced from ref. 90, with permission.)*

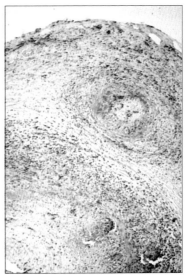

● **Figure 17.3**
Micrograph of a temporal artery biopsy in a patient with giant cell arteritis. (Reproduced from ref. 90, with permission.)

symptoms should be maintained for six months to one year. Steroids commonly produce minor side effects and may produce major side effects. Steroid therapy is often complicated by gastrointestinal side effects, osteoporosis, steroid myopathy, weight gain and other ill effects.

Medication-induced headache

Medications are an important cause of headache in the elderly (Table 17.4). The fact that a drug is associated with a headache, however, does not prove that it has a causal role for a particular patient, nor does it preclude the need to evaluate other causes. The IHS groups medication-induced headaches under the rubric 'headaches associated with substances or their withdrawal'.[11] Drugs may initiate a new type of headache or exacerbate a preexisting headache disorder.[30] In addition, medication withdrawal or rebound headaches may occur. Pre-existing headaches triggered by medication are properly classified as primary, not secondary, headache disorders.[11]

When medications trigger a pre-existing headache disorder, the provoked headaches are usually similar to the pre-existing headaches. Perhaps the most important pharmacological triggers of headaches are alcohol and nitrate compounds. Nitroglycerin can induce both migraine and cluster attacks. Oral contraceptives, hormonal replacement therapy and food additives, such as monosodium glutamate, aspartate, caffeine and tyramine, may all increase headache frequency.[31–35]

Medication withdrawal headaches (rebound headaches) are very common in headache subspecialty practices. They may be less common in the elderly than in young adults.[36] The typical patient has a prior history of episodic migraine. Over the years, medication use and headache frequency increase, while the severity of the pain and associated features (e.g.

nausea or photophobia) decrease. Finally, nearly continuous headaches without prominent migrainous features and superimposed interval headaches with typical migrainous features may occur. Medication that was initially administered as a headache treatment may become a cause of headache. The drugs that cause rebound include opioid analgesics, caffeine or barbiturate-containing combination-of-ingredient products, and vasoactive compounds such as ergot alkaloids, sumatriptan, isometheptene and caffeine (Table 17.4).

Trigeminal neuralgia

Trigeminal neuralgia is the most common neuralgic syndrome in the elderly, with a peak incidence of 155 cases per million and a female:male ratio of 3:2 (Table 17.5).[37] Trigeminal neuralgia is typically unilateral, but it can be bilateral in 4% of patients.[38] It is characterized by brief paroxysms of unilateral pain, similar to a spasm or an electric shock, in the distribution of one or more divisions of the trigeminal nerve. The mandibular or maxillary branches of the nerve are most frequently involved. The pain may be provoked by stimulation of specific trigger points, or by stimuli such as washing, shaving, talking, or brushing the teeth. The pain may precipitate facial muscle spasms, hence the term *tic douloureux*. Between paroxysms, a sustained, deep, dull ache may be present.[39]

Pretrigeminal neuralgia is a dull, continuous, aching-type pain in the jaw. It may be provoked by pressure about the face or mouth and may evolve into true trigeminal neuralgia. These non-specific clinical features may lead to dental evaluation and procedures. Hence dental procedures may be a response to pretrigeminal neuralgia rather than a cause of trigeminal neuralgia.[40]

● **Table 17.4** *Selected medications reported to cause headaches*

Amantadine	Monoamine oxidase inhibitors
Calcium-channel blockers	Nonsteroidal antiinflammatory agents
Caffeine	
Cimetidine	Nitrates
Corticosteroids	Nicotinic acid
Cyclophosphamide	Phenothiazines
Dipyridamole	Ranitidine
Estrogens	Sympathomimetic agents
Ethanol	Tamoxifen
Hydralazine	Theophyllines (thioxanthines)
Indomethacin	Tetracyclines
L-Dopa	Trimethoprim

● **Table 17.5** *Idiopathic trigeminal neuralgia*[11]

Diagnostic criteria

A Paroxysmal attacks of facial or frontal pain which last a few seconds to less than 2 minutes.

B Pain has at least 4 of the following characteristics:

    1 Distribution along one or more divisions of the trigeminal nerve.

    2 Sudden, intense, sharp, superficial, stabbing, or burning in quality.

    3 Pain intensity severe.

    4 Precipitation from trigger areas, or by certain daily activities such as eating, talking, washing the face or cleaning the teeth.

    5 Between paroxysms the patient is entirely asymptomatic.

C No neurologic deficit.

D Attacks are stereotyped in the individual patient.

E Exclusion of other causes of facial pain by history, physical examination, and special investigations.

The aetiology of trigeminal neuralgia varies with age (Table 17.6). When trigeminal neuralgia begins in the twenties and thirties, causes include demyelinating disease (multiple sclerosis), compression of the trigeminal nerve root at its exit foramen (e.g. myeloma or metastatic carcinoma of the sphenoid bone), and other mass lesions, such as meningiomas, acoustic neuromas, trigeminal neuromas, cholesteatomas, chordomas, aneurysms (especially of the basilar artery) and other vascular abnormalities.

In the elderly, trigeminal neuralgia commonly is a result of vascular compression of the trigeminal nerve due to abnormal arterial loops near the trigeminal nerve root entry zone. Vascular compression leads to demyelination and aberrant neuronal activity, which may produce sensitization in the trigeminal nucleus caudalis.[41] Other causes of trigeminal neuralgia in the elderly are the same as in young adults, as outlined above.

The diagnosis of trigeminal neuralgia is established by its typical clinical features. The physical examination is negative except for positive trigger points. Diagnostic studies are generally normal. Impaired sensation in the distribution of the Vth nerve suggests a structural, demyelinating or compressive trigeminal nerve lesion (Table 17.6). The initial evaluation should include magnetic resonance imaging, with special attention to the region of the cerebellopontine angle and the exit foramen of the trigeminal nerve.

In the absence of structural disease, medical therapy is initiated (Table 17.7). The initial drug of choice is carbamazepine,[42] followed by divalproex, baclofen and clonazepam.[39,42] If medication fails to adequately control symptoms, ablative procedures should be considered. Alcohol or glycerol injections may be used, with more proximal injections producing better long-term results. Gasserian ganglion injections have a five-year recurrence rate of 41–86%. Retrogasserian glycerol injections can produce mild

facial numbness, but painful dysaesthesias (impairment of any senses, especially touch) are rare and anaesthesia dolorosa (pain in an area or region that is anaesthetic) is absent. Mean recurrence time varies from 6 to 47 months. Radiofrequency gangliolysis provides relief in 82–100% of patients, with a recurrence rate of 9–28%. Major complications are rare: loss of corneal reflex occurs in 70% of patients; masseteric weakness occurs in approximately half of patients, but this improves over a three- to six-month period.[42] Minor paraesthesias (abnormal sensation, i.e. burning, prickling) occur in about 10% of patients, but anaesthesia dolorosa is rare.

The Janetta procedure (microvascular decompression), performed via an occipital craniotomy, removes any aberrant blood vessels from the trigeminal nerve root. Long-term benefit is reported in over 80% of patients, with recurrence rates of 1–6%. Surgical mortality is 1% and serious morbidity 7%.

● **Table 17.6** *Causes of trigeminal neuralgia*

A Decreased facial sensation
- Intracranial aneurysms
- Giant cell arteritis
- Intracranial tumours
- Dental mandibular malignancy
- Cranial malignancy

B Normal facial sensation
- Idiopathic trigeminal neuralgia (due to vascular compression)
- Multiple sclerosis
- Dental pathology
- Dental procedures

● **Table 17.7** *Drug treatment of trigeminal neuralgia*

Drug	Bioavailability (%)	Time to maximum concentration (h)	Half-life (h)	Time to steady-state concentration (days)*	Therapeutic 'target' range (mmol/l)
Baclofen	–	3–8	3–4	1	–
Carbamazepine	>70	2–8	11–27	5	24–43
Clonazepam	100	1–2	24–48	12	30–270
Lamotrigine	100	2–3	18–30	8	4–16
Oxcarbazepine	100	1–2	14–26	7	5–110
Phenytoin	98	4–8	15–20	14	20–80
Valproic acid	99	1–4	6–17	5	200–700

Note: modified from Refs. 42,43.

Because of these high rates of surgical morbidity, we start with the other, less invasive, procedures, such as percutaneous glycerol injection and radiofrequency rhizotomy, and reserve microvascular decompression for refractory patients.[43]

Glossopharyngeal neuralgia

Glossopharyngeal neuralgia (Table 17.8) is less common than trigeminal neuralgia. Unilateral pain occurs in the distribution of the glossopharyngeal and vagus nerves in and around the ear, jaw, throat, tongue or larynx. Radiation from the oropharynx to the ear is common. Paroxysms of jabbing or electric pain last for about one minute and may be accompanied by deep, continuous pain between paroxysms. Patients may have as many as thirty to forty attacks a day and may be awakened from sleep by the attacks.[44]

Paroxysms of pain may be triggered by chewing, talking, yawning, coughing or swallowing cold liquids. Stimulation of the external auditory canal and postauricular area may also provoke pain. In approximately 2% of cases, syncope (secondary to bradycardia or asystole) and seizures (from cerebral ischemia) have occurred. Atropine prevents syncope, suggesting a vagal afferent mechanism.[45]

The diagnosis of glossopharyngeal neuralgia is based on history. The neurological examination is usually normal. Other disorders are ruled out by history, physical examination, and diagnostic testing. The assumed cause of glossopharyngeal neuralgia is nerve compression from aberrant blood vessels. Symptomatic causes of a glossopharyngeal neuralgia-like syndrome include cerebellopontine angle tumour, nasopharyngeal carcinoma, carotid aneurysm, peritonsillar abscess and compression from an osteophytic stylohyoid ligament lateral to the glossopharyngeal nerve.[46]

The best diagnostic test is anaesthetization of the tonsil and pharynx, which can temporarily terminate a painful paroxysm and confirm the diagnosis. Pharmacotherapy is identical to the approach outlined for trigeminal neuralgia (Table 17.7). Surgical treatment involves intracranial sectioning of the glossopharyngeal nerve and the upper rootlets of the vagus nerve at the jugular foramen.[46]

Postherpetic neuralgia (Table 17.9)

Postherpetic neuralgia, a significant cause of head pain in the elderly, is defined by the presence of pain after the eruption of herpes zoster.[47] Acute herpes zoster often begins with paraesthesias and pain in the affected region, followed four or five days later by a vesicular eruption. Most patients have a deep aching or burning pain, paraesthesias and dysaesthesia. Some patients also report electric shock-like pains. Typical involvement in the head occurs unilaterally in the distribution of the ophthalmic or maxillary divisions of the trigeminal nerve, or at the occipitocervical junction.[47] Ophthalmic herpes may be associated with diplopia due to involvement of cranial nerves III, IV and VI. Geniculate herpes is associated with facial palsy (cranial nerve VII). Vesicles are often seen in the external auditory canal.

Pain persists after the eruption clears in many people. Opinions vary on how long the pain must persist before the term postherpetic neuralgia is applied. Most authors favour intervals varying from one to six months. Age is a risk factor for postherpetic neuralgia. It occurs in 5% of patients with acute zoster who are under the age of 40 years, 50% of those with zoster in their sixties, and 75% of those with zoster over the age of 70 years. Postherpetic neuralgia may be more common when the acute attack of zoster is intense. Other risk factors include diabetes mellitus, an ophthalmic location for the eruption and immunological compromise.[47]

The pain of postherpetic neuralgia has three components:

- constant, deep burning and pain,
- repetitive stabs and needle-pricking sensations, and
- superficial, sharp or radiating pain or itching provoked by light touch.

● **Table 17.8** *Idiopathic glossopharyngeal neuralgia*

Diagnostic criteria

A Paroxysmal attacks of facial pain which last a few seconds to less than two minutes.

B Pain has at least 4 of the following characteristics:

  1 Unilateral location

  2 Distribution within the posterior part of the tongue, tonsillar fossa, pharynx, or beneath the angle of the lower jaw, or in the ear

  3 Sudden, sharp, stabbing, or burning in quality

  4 Pain intensity severe

  5 Precipitation from trigger areas or by swallowing, chewing, talking, coughing, or yawning

C No neurologic deficit.

D Attacks are stereotyped in the individual patient.

E Other cause of pain ruled out by history, physical and special investigations.

● **Table 17.9** *Chronic postherpetic neuralgia*

Diagnostic criteria

A Pain is restricted to the distribution of the affected cranial nerves or divisions thereof.

B Pain persists more than 6 months after the onset of herpetic eruption.

The prominence of each of these components varies from individual to individual. Sleep is often interrupted. Postherpetic neuralgia is a deafferentation pain syndrome sometimes accompanied by increased sympathetic activity. The pain typically remits: after three years, 56% of patients are free of troublesome pain.[48]

Topical therapies such as compresses of Burow's solution, colloidal oatmeal, or calamine lotion are used to treat acute zoster. Oral glucocorticoids may speed the resolution of acute zoster pain,[49] but it is not clear if they prevent postherpetic neuralgia.[47] Antiviral agents may attenuate acute herpes zoster in immunocompromised patients. A 21-day course of acyclovir may ameliorate pain in the acute phase. Famciclovir, a new antiviral drug, may shorten the duration of postherpetic neuralgia. Acyclovir has not been proven to reduce the risk of postherpetic neuralgia.[47] The most effective treatment of the pain of acute herpes zoster is neuroblockade, but it is uncertain if this will reduce postherpetic neuralgia.[47]

Postherpetic neuralgia should be treated as soon as the diagnosis is made. Amitriptyline is commonly used, but nortriptyline or desipramine may be preferable, since they have fewer anticholinergic side effects. Capsaicin, a topical agent that depletes substance P, is helpful, but the burning pain that sometimes accompanies its application may limit its usefulness. Topical NSAID may be useful. Local anaesthetic preparations have been used with limited success. Peripheral and central surgical techniques are of little, if any, value.

Headaches associated with systemic disease

Headache can be a symptom of a systemic disease, some of which are more common in the elderly. The IHS groups these disorders as 'headaches associated with noncephalic infections' and as 'headaches associated with metabolic diseases'.[11] Infections are the most common systemic cause of headaches. Systemic viral and bacterial infections may produce headaches that are not necessarily age-related. Lyme disease and other spirochaetes can produce chronic headache, usually with associated abnormalities on neurological examination.[50] Headache may be associated with both acute Epstein–Barr virus infection and chronic fatigue syndrome.

Other systemic diseases that can cause headaches include acute, but not chronic, hypertension, hypercalcaemia, severe anaemia and both renal disease and its treatment (dialysis). Hypoxia or hypercarbia are more common in the elderly and may produce headache regardless of cause (e.g. primary pulmonary disorders, sleep apnoea or high altitude). Involvement of the mediastinum by tumour or during the course of pacemaker insertion may produce pain referred to the head through the autonomic nervous system.[52,53] Angina may present with exertional headache without thoracic pain.

Headache associated with disorders of the cranium, neck, eyes, ears and nose

Primary disorders of the cranial bones are rare. Abnormalities of the cervical spine have been reported to produce anterior or posterior head pain, perhaps by direct involvement of the cervical nerve roots or indirect involvement of the descending tract of the trigeminal nerve. The existence of cervicogenic headache as a distinct neurological disorder is controversial. The IHS recognizes a narrowly defined disorder termed 'headache associated with disorder of the cervical spine'.[11]

Typical clinical features of cervicogenic headache include:

- occipital or suboccipital pain, sometimes reproduced or augmented by suboccipital pressure,
- neck tenderness and muscle spasms that may produce pain with neck motion, limitation of movement or unusual postures, and
- sensory abnormalities in the distribution of the upper cervical roots.

These headaches are usually unilateral.[11,54] On imaging, cervical spine abnormalities are similar to those found in age-matched control subjects without pain complaints. Upper cervical spine radiographical abnormalities are common in the elderly, thus, the positive predictive value of any given abnormality is low.[54] Many patients who receive a diagnosis of cervicogenic headache meet criteria for migraine or tension-type headache.

Primary open-angle glaucoma, the most common cause of glaucoma, is rarely painful. Miotic eyedrops such as pilocarpine used in its treatment may produce brow ache. Acute angle closure glaucoma is less common; acute attacks produce intense eye pain that radiates widely; it is often associated with a red eye, corneal cloudiness, a red sclera and nausea. Laser iridotomy is curative. Secondary angle closure glaucoma resulting from diabetes or carotid insufficiency may produce a deep, boring unrelenting pain associated with a red eye and poor vision.[55]

Inflammation or infection can produce headache. Middle or external ear infection can usually be diagnosed on routine examination.[56] Acute sinusitis produces headache, usually in association with sinus tenderness, purulent nasal discharge, and, perhaps, fever.[57] The pattern of pain referral varies with the infected sinus. Nasopharyngeal malignancies may cause the sensation of nasal congestion and pain behind the nose. If this condition is suspected, an otolaryngologic examination is warranted.

Infection of the teeth or the mucous membranes of the mouth may cause pain in the adjacent areas of the mouth or face and can also produce pain beyond the site of disease, evoking head and facial pain.

Headaches associated with other neurological disorders

Several neurological disorders, including cerebrovascular disease, Parkinson's disease and postherpetic neuralgia, may produce headache in the elderly. Cerebrovascular disease may give rise to headaches before, during, or after the onset of stroke or TIA.[11] The headaches may occur with large vessel thrombotic stroke (20–40%), embolic stroke (20–40%), lacunar infarction (18%), subarachnoid haemorrhage (>95%) or intracerebral haemorrhage (80%). Headaches associated with stroke have been described in a series of studies.[58–60] Headache may also occur following carotid endarterectomy.[61,62]

Parkinson's disease

The association between Parkinson's disease[63] and headache is controversial. In one series, headache occurred in 41% of Parkinson's disease patients and 13% of controls. Another controlled series found no difference in headache prevalence.[64] Possible headache mechanisms include comorbid depression and muscle rigidity. In one study of early morning occipital headache in patients with Parkinson's disease, the headache failed to improve with treatment directed at muscle spasm, but it did improve with levodopa.[65] These headaches may respond to amitriptyline.[66]

Primary headache disorders in the elderly

Migraine headache

Migraine prevalence peaks in mid-adult life, near the age of 40 years, but migraine continues to occur even in elderly patients. Migraine prevalence is 5% in women and 2% in men over the age of 70 years. Migraine incidence also declines: only 2% of all migraine cases begin after the age of 65 years.[67] Thus, caution is advised when making the diagnosis of new-onset migraine in the elderly.

In one study, only 1 of 193 patients with headache beginning after the age of 65 year had migraine.[3] Cull,[68] however, collected ten patients with migraine onset after the age of 60 years, two of whom had strokes on computed tomography. The ratio of migraine with aura to migraine without aura was reversed (86%:14%) among new-onset migraine patients over the age of 40 years. Whether this is due to referral patterns or biological factors is uncertain.

Anecdotal information and clinic-based reports suggest that headache characteristics may change with advancing age. Several patterns have been described. Migraine attacks may remit[4] or evolve into chronic daily headache, with or without medication overuse.[36,69] Migraine with aura may transform into a periodic neurological deficit with little or no headache pain.[70,71] This phenomenon of 'aura without headache' has been termed late-life migraine accompaniments.[70,71]

Features of late life migraine accompaniments are listed in Table 17.10. The features most consistent with migrainous accompaniments are: scintillations or other visual displays; a slow evolution of the neurologic deficit, typically over a period of minutes; and the serial progression from one symptom to another.[70,71] Fisher stressed that it is best to regard the diagnosis as one of exclusion. The neurological examination and neuroimaging studies are normal. Alternative diagnoses include cerebral thrombosis, embolism, TIA, carotid or vertebral dissection, subclavian steal syndrome, epilepsy, thrombocythemia, polycythemia, hyperviscosity syndrome and lupus. Patients with late-life migraine accompaniments have normal angiograms and rarely develop permanent neurological deficits.

Medications that are commonly used in older patients can exacerbate preexisting migraine or precipitate new migraine-like headaches. Common offenders include nitroglycerin compounds and oestrogen replacement therapy.[72] Reducing the dose of the offending agent may ameliorate the headaches.

There are several acute migraine treatments that should be used cautiously in elderly patients. Ergot alkaloids and 5-hydroxytryptamine-1 agonists (sumatriptan and similar drugs) may exacerbate pre-existing hypertension, coronary artery disease, peripheral vascular disease, or cerebrovascular disease, and, in some instances, may provoke ischemic complications, including angina, myocardial infarction, or claudication.[73–75]

● **Table 17.10** *Migraine equivalents*

- Gradual appearance of focal neurologic symptoms — spread or intensification over a period of minutes.
- Positive visual symptoms characteristic of 'classic' migraine, specifically fortification spectra (scintillating scotoma), flashing lights, dazzles.
- Previous similar symptoms associated with a more severe headache.
- Serial progression from one accompaniment to another.
- The occurrence of two or more identical spells.
- A duration of 15 to 25 minutes.
- Occurrence of a 'flurry' of accompaniments.
- A generally benign course without permanent sequelae.

NSAID are more likely to cause peptic ulcer disease in elderly patients than in younger ones and can potentially interact with anticoagulants, hypoglycaemics, digoxin, antihypertensive agents and diuretics.[76,77] They may cause cognitive side effects and are associated with an increased risk of gastrointestinal bleeding. Antiemetic agents, such as metoclopramide and chlorpromazine, are more likely to be associated with extrapyramidal syndromes in the elderly.[18] Benzodiazepines and barbiturates may cause excessive sedation; the long-acting benzodiazepines, in particular, may cause excessive side effects due to slowed metabolic clearance.

Preventive treatments cause more side effects in the elderly than in younger patients.[1,4,6,78] The distribution and excretion of many medications are altered in the elderly patient, generally resulting in higher blood levels for a given dose of drug.[77,79] Elderly patients are also more sensitive to anticholinergic, orthostatic, sedative and cardiac side effects. For these reasons, medication should be started at a low dose and increased slowly. The tertiary amine tricyclic antidepressant agents, such as amitriptyline and doxepin, which are potent anticholinergic agents, should be used with caution. They can exacerbate glaucoma, produce visual blurring and cause cognitive problems. Agents with minimal anticholinergic and sedative side effects that do not cross the blood–brain barrier may be a better choice. Nortriptyline, a secondary amine, is a reasonable alternative and generally has less pronounced side effects. The selective serotonin reuptake inhibitors, while not as effective, are well tolerated in the elderly. Antihypertensive drugs may cause more hypotension or lethargy in the elderly, while divalproex sodium has a particularly good benefit-to-side-effect profile. Methysergide and methylergonovine are relatively contraindicated because they are vasoconstrictors and may cause cardiac ischaemia.[78] The principles of migraine treatment outlined in Chapter 6 apply to the elderly.

Non-pharmacological treatment in the elderly, as in all patients, is attractive because it avoids medications that may present risks or cause excessive side effects. Eliminating triggers, maintaining a proper diet and a regular sleep pattern, and avoiding excess caffeine are strategies that are useful in all patients. Biofeedback may not be as effective in the elderly patient. The most important non-pharmacological approach involves identifying and treating comorbid medical and psychiatric conditions. These techniques deserve careful consideration in light of the particular susceptibility of the elderly to medication side effects.

Tension-type headache

Tension-type headache (TTH) can begin at any age, but its onset is most common prior to the fourth decade. Headache prevalence declines with increasing age; headache severity decreases in the women who continue to report headaches but does not change in men.[6,80] In approximately 10% of patients, TTH begins after the age of 50 years. One community-based study reported a 27% prevalence rate in subjects over the age of 65 years.[5] Medical disorders that are common in the elderly may be mistaken for TTH, inflating prevalence estimates and leading to misdiagnosis in individual cases. The differential diagnosis includes mass lesions, temporal arteritis, visual acuity problems and chronic daily headache evolving from migraine.[4,81]

Treatment of TTH should be modified in elderly patients. Combination analgesics contain sedatives or caffeine, and their use should be limited, as overuse may cause dependence and more side effects. Preventive therapy should be administered when a patient has frequent headaches that produce disability or may lead to acute medication overuse. Antidepressants, the medication of choice, should be started at a very low dose and increased slowly every three to seven days.[78] Selective serotonin reuptake inhibitors may be preferable to tricyclics.

Cluster headache

Cluster headache typically begins between the age of 20 and 50 years, although onset in the eighth decade has been reported.[82] Both the episodic and chronic varieties of cluster may occur for the first time in the elderly. Cluster attacks may recur after many years of remission, or persist into senescence. Long-duration disease helps account for the continued presence of cluster headache in the elderly, despite its low incidence at advanced age. Of the many medications utilized in this age group, sublingual or transdermal nitroglycerin are potent precipitators of cluster attacks.[82]

Pharmacological treatment of cluster headache [83–86] in the elderly is influenced by the presence of comorbid medical conditions and their treatments. In the absence of chronic obstructive pulmonary disease, oxygen inhalation may be the safest and most effective method of aborting attacks. The other mainstays of abortive treatment, sumatriptan or ergotamine compounds, must be used very cautiously,[73–75] even in the absence of peripheral vascular disease, coronary heart disease or hypertension.

We do not recommend methysergide for elderly patients. Verapamil, lithium and prednisone should be used with caution.

Hypnic headaches

The hypnic headache syndrome is a rare primary headache disorder of the elderly.[87–89] The age of onset ranges from 65 to 84 years, and there is no clear gender preponderance. Patients present with headaches that awaken them from sleep at the same time almost every night. The headache duration ranges from 15 to 60 minutes. The pain is typically diffuse, often throbbing in quality, and not associated with the autonomic features of cluster headaches.[88,89] The headaches may be associated with rapid eye movement sleep (Table 17.11).[87]

Hypnic headache must be differentiated from a mass lesion, which may also present with nocturnal pain, and from temporal arteritis. Cluster headaches also present with nocturnal attacks, but can be differentiated from hypnic headaches by their unilaterality, their periorbital and temporal location, and their prominent autonomic features.

After excluding organic disease with an imaging procedure and an ESR, treatment with lithium carbonate at a dose of 300 mg at bedtime usually produces a prompt remission. If headaches recur, higher doses of lithium may be required. Lithium should be used with caution in the elderly, especially in the presence of renal disease, dehydration or diuretic therapy.

Conclusions

The approach to the elderly patient with a new-onset headache begins with a systematic search for an underlying cause. If one is identified, treatment should address both the underlying cause and the specific pain syndrome. If secondary headaches are excluded, a specific primary headache disorder should be diagnosed. Treatment goals include pain prevention, pain relief and optimal functioning and quality of life.

● **Table 17.11** Suggested IHS diagnostic criteria for hypnic headache[11]

4.7 Hypnic headache

A Headaches occur at least 15 times per month for at least one month.

B Headaches awaken patient from sleep.

C Attack duration of 5–60 minutes.

D Pain is generalized or bilateral.

E Pain not associated with autonomic features.

F At least one of the following:

- There is no suggestion of one of the disorders listed in groups 5–11.
- Such a disorder is suggested but excluded by appropriate investigations.
- Such a disorder is present, but the first headache attacks do not occur in close temporal relation to the disorder.

Note: Modified from Goadsby and Lipton (Brain, 1997).

References

1. Lipton RB, Pfeffer D, Newman L, Solomon S. Headaches in the elderly. *J Pain Symp Mgt* 1993; 8: 87–97.
2. Stewart WF, Lipton RB, Celentano DD, Reed ML. Prevalence of migraine headache in the United States. *JAMA* 1992; 267: 64–9.
3. Hauser KA, Ferguson RH, Holley KE et al. Temporal arteritis in Rochester, Minnesota, 1951–67. *Mayo Clin Proc* 1971; 46: 597–602.
4. Baumel B, Eisner LS. Diagnosis and treatment of headache in the elderly. *Med Clin N Amer* 1991; 75: 661–75.
5. Solomon G, Kunkel RS, Frame J. Demographics of headache in elderly patients. *Headache* 1990; 30: 273–6.
6. Edmeads J, Takahashi A. Headache in the elderly. In: Olesen J, Tfelt-Hansen P, Welch KMA (eds). *The Headaches*. New York: Raven Press, Limited, 1993, pp. 809–13.
7. Cook NR, Evans DA, Funkenstein H et al. Correlates of headache in a population-based cohort of elderly. *Arch Neurol* 1989; 46: 1338–44.
8. Salcman M, Kaplan R. Intracranial tumors in adults. In: Moossa A, Robson M, Schimpff S (eds). *Comprehensive Textbook of Oncology*. Baltimore: Williams and Wilkins, 1986, pp. 617–29.
9. Schoenberg B. Nervous system. In: Schotterfeld D, Joseph F (eds). *Cancer epidemiology and prevention*. Philadelphia: WB Saunders, 1982, pp. 969–83.
10. Forsyth PA, Posner JB. Headaches in patients with brain tumors. A study of 111 patients. *Neurology* 1993; 43: 1678–83.
11. Headache Classification Committee of the International Headache Society. Classification and diagnostic criteria for headache disorders, cranial neuralgia, and facial pain. *Cephalalgia* 1988; 8(suppl 7): 196.

12. Bengtsson BA, Malmvall BE. Giant cell arteritis. *Acta Medica Scand* 1982; (Suppl 658); 1102.

13. Machado EB, Michet CJ, Ballard DJ, Hunder GG, Beard CM, Chu CP, O'Fallon WM. Trends in incidence and clinical presentation of temporal arteritis in Olmsted County, Minnesota, 1950–1985. *Arthritis Rheum* 1988; 31(6): 745–9.

14. Solomon S, Cappa KG. The headache of temporal arteritis. *Am Geriatr Soc* 1987; 35: 163–5.

15. Chisolm H. Cortical blindness in cranial arteritis. *Br J Ophthalmol* 1975; 59: 332–3.

16. Caselli RJ, Hunder GG, Whisnant JP. Neurologic disease in biopsy-proven giant cell (temporal) arteritis. *Neurology* 1988; 38: 352–9.

17. Keltner JL. Giant-cell arteritis: signs and symptoms. *Ophthalmology* 1982; 89: 1101–10.

18. Goodman BW. Temporal arteritis. *Am J Med* 1979; 67: 839–52.

19. Graham E. Survival in temporal arteritis. *Trans Ophthalmol Soc UK* 1980; 100: 108–10.

20. Boghen DR, Glaser JS. Ischemic optic neuropathy: the clinical profile and natural history. *Brain* 1975; 92: 689–708.

21. Lipton RB, Solomon S, Wertenbaker C. Gradual loss and recovery of vision in temporal arteritis. *Arch Int Med* 1985; 145: 2252–3.

22. Schneider HA, Weber AA, Ballen PH. The visual prognosis in temporal arteritis. *Ann Ophthalmol* 1971; 3: 1215–30.

23. McLeod D, Oji EO, Kohner EM. Fundus signs in temporal arteritis. *Br J Ophthalmol* 1978; 62: 591–4.

24. Wagner KP, Hollenhorst RW. The ocular lesions of temporal arteritis. *Surv Ophthalmol* 1976; 20: 247–60.

25. Hayreh SS. Posterior ischemic optic neuropathy. *Ophthalmologica* 1981; 182: 29–41.

26. Raskin NH. Giant cell arteritis. In: Olsen J, Tfelt–Hansen P, Welch KMA (eds). *Headache (2nd ed)*. New York: Churchill Livingstone, 1988, pp. 317–332.

27. Goodwin J. Temporal arteritis. In: Vinken PJ, Bruyn GW (eds). *Handbook of Clinical Neurology (Vol. 39)*. Amsterdam: North Holland, 1980, pp. 313–347.

28. Wong RL, Korn JH. Temporal arteritis without an elevated erythrocyte sedimentation rate: case report and review of the literature. *Am J Med* 1986; 80: 959–64.

29. Wall M, Corbett JJ. Arteritis. In: Olesen J, Tfelt-Hansen P, Welch KMA (eds). *The Headaches*. New York: Raven Press, Limited, 1993, pp. 653–62.

30. Mathew NT, Reuveni U, Perez F. Transformed or evolutive migraine. *Headache* 1987; 27: 102–6.

31. Lipton RB, Newman LC, Cohen JS, Solomon S. Aspartamine as a trigger of migraine. *Headache* 1989; 29: 90–3.

32. Peatfield RC, Gover V, Littlewood JT, Sandler M, Rose FC. The prevalence of diet-induced migraine. *Cephalalgia* 1984; 4: 179–83.

33. Dalton K. Food intake prior to a migraine attack: study of 2313 spontaneous attacks. *Headache* 1975; 15: 188–93.

34. Selby G, Lance JW. Observations on 500 cases of migraine and allied vascular headache. *J Neurol Neurosurg Psychiatry* 1960; 23: 23–32.

35. Bergh VV, Anery WK, Waelkens J. Trigger factors in migraine: a study conducted by the Belgian Migraine Society. *Headache* 1987; 27: 191–6.

36. Mathew NT. Drug-induced headache. *Neurol Clin* 1990; 8: 903–12.

37. Penman J. Trigeminal neuralgia. In: Vinken PJ, Bruyn GW (eds). *Handbook of Clinical Neurology (Vol. 5)*. Amsterdam: North Holland,Publishing Co. 1968, pp. 296–322.

38. White JC, Sweet WH. *Pain and the Neurosurgeon. A 40-year experience.* Springfield, IL: Charles C. Thomas, 1969, pp. 123–256.

39. Dalessio DJ. Diagnosis and treatment of cranial neuralgias. *Med Clin North Am* 1991; 75: 605–15.

40. Fromm GH, Graff-Radford SB, Terrence CF, Sweet WH. Pretrigeminal neuralgia. *Neurology* 1990; 40: 1493–5.

41. Terrence CF, Gromm GH. Trigeminal neuralgia and other facial neuralgias. In: Olesen J, Tfelt-Hansen P, Welch KMA (eds). *The Headaches*. New York: Raven Press, 1993, pp. 773–86.

42. Zakrzewska JM. Trigeminal neuralgia. In: *Major Problems in Neurology*. London: W.B. Saunders Company, Ltd., 1995, pp. 108–55.

43. Zakrzewska JM. Trigeminal neuralgia. In: *Major Problems in Neurology*. London: W.B. Saunders Company, Ltd., 1995, pp. 157–70.

44. Dalessio DJ, Silberstein SD. Diagnosis and classification of headache. In: Dalessio DJ, Silberstein SD (eds). *Wolff's Headache and Other Head Pain (6th ed)*. New York: Oxford University Press, 1993, pp. 318.

45. Rushton JG, Stevens JC, Miller RH. Glossopharyngeal (Vagoglossopharyngeal) Neuralgia. *Arch Neurol* 1981; 38: 201–5.

46. Bruyn GW. Glossopharyngeal neuralgia. In: Vinken PJ, Bruyn GW, Klawans HL (eds). *Handbook of Clinical Neurology*. Amsterdam: Elsevier, 1985, pp. 459–73.

47. Kost RG, Straus SE. Postherpetic neuralgia—pathogenesis, treatment, and prevent. *N Engl J Med* 1996; 335: 32–42.

48. de Moragas JM, Kierland RR. The outcome of patients with herpes zoster. *Arch Dermatol* 1957; 75: 193–6.

49. Whitley RJ, Weiss H, Gnann J et al. The efficacy of steroid and acyclovir therapy of herpes zoster in the elderly. *J Invest Med* 1995; 43:Suppl 2: 252A (abstract).

50. Scelsa SN, Lipton RB, Sander H, Herskovitz S. Headache characteristics in hospitalized patients with Lyme disease. *Headache* 1995; 35: 125–30.

51. Pinaidi G, Scanlatp G. The chronic fatigue syndrome. A multifactorial approach and treatment possibilities. *Recent Progress in Medicine* 1990; 81: 773–7.

52. Das G. Pacemaker headaches. *Pace* 1984; 7: 802–7.

53. Moran JF. Headache following pacemaker implantation (Letter). *JAMA* 1985; 254: 1511–12.

54. Edmeads J. Headaches and head pains associated with diseases of the cervical spine. *Med Clin North Am* 1978; 62: 533–44.

55. Martin TJ, Soyka D. Ocular causes of headache. In: Olesen J, Tfelt-Hansen P, Welch KMA (eds). *The Headaches*. New York: Raven Press, Ltd., 1993, pp. 747–52.

56. Birt D. Headache and head pains associated with diseases of the ear, nose and throat. *Med Clin North Am* 1978; 62: 523–31.

57. Joseph DJ, Renner G. Head pain from diseases of the ear, nose and throat. *Neurol Clin* 1983; 1: 399–414.

58. Edmeads J. The headaches of ischemic cerebrovascular disease. *Headache* 1979; 19: 345–9.

59. Portenoy RK, Abissi CJ, Lipton RB, Berger AR, Mehler MR, Baglivo J, Solomon S. Headache in cerebrovascular disease. *Stroke* 1984; 25(6): 1009–12.

60. Fisher CM. Headache in cerebrovascular disease. In: Vinken PJ, Bruyn GW (eds). *Handbook of Clinical Neurology (Vol. 5)*. New York: Elsevier, 1968, pp. 124–58.

61. Leviton A, Caplan L, Salzmen E. Severe headaches after carotid endarterectomy. *Headache* 1975; 15: 207–10.

62. Leviton A. Post carotid-endarterectomy "hemicrania". *Headache* 1985; 15: 13–17.

63. Nishikawa S, Harada H, Takahashi K, Shimomura T. Clinical study on headache in patients with Parkinson's disease. *Clin Neurol Neurosurg* 1982; 22: 403–8.

64. Lorentz IT. A survey of headache in Parkinson's disease. *Cephalalgia* 1989; 9: 83–6.

65. Indo T, Takahashi A. Early morning headache of Parkinson's disease: a hitherto unrecognized symptom? *Headache* 1987; 27: 151–4.

66. Indaco A, Carrieri PB. Amitriptyline in the treatment of headache in patients with Parkinson's disease: a double-blind placebo controlled study. *Neurology* 1988; 38: 1720–2.

67. Raskin NH. *Headache (2nd ed)*. New York: Churchill-Livingstone, 1988.

68. Cull RE. Investigation of late-onset migraine. *Scot Med J* 1995; 40: 50–2.

69. Saper JR. Daily chronic headache. *Neurol Clin North Am* 1990; 8: 891–902.

70. Fisher CM. Late-life migraine accompaniments as a cause of unexplained transient ischemic attacks. *Can J Neurol Sci* 1980; 7: 9–17.

71. Fisher CM. Late-life migraine accompaniments — further experience. *Stroke* 1986; 17: 1033–42.

72. Silberstein SD, Merriam G. Sex hormones and headache. In: Goadsby P, Silberstein SD (eds). *Headache*. Newton MA: Butterworth Heinemann, 1977.

73. Goodman AG, Goodman LS, Gilman A (eds). *The Pharmacological Basis of Therapeutics (6th ed)*. New York: MacMallin, 1980, pp. 930–44.

74. *Physicians Desk References (44th ed)*. New Jersey: Medical Economics Publishing, 1990, pp. 1556–1957.

75. Galer B, Lipton R, Solomon S et al. Myocardial ischemia related to ergot alkaloids: a case report and literature review. *Headache* 1991; 31: 446–50.

76. Cassel C, Riesenberg D, Sorenson L, Walth J. *Geriatric Medicine*. New York: Springer-Verlag, 1990, pp. 184–211.

77. Schrier RW (ed.). *Geriatric Medicine*. Philadelphia: WB Saunders, 1990, pp. 91–103.

78. Silberstein SD, Lipton RB. Overview of diagnosis and treatment of migraine. *Neurology* 1994; 44(Suppl 7): S6–16.

79. Cassel C, Riesenberg D, Sorensen L, Walsh J. *Geriatric medicine*. New York: Springer-Verlag, 1990, pp. 66–77.

80. Alders EEA, Hentzen A, Tan CT. A community-based prevalence study on headache in Malaysia. *Headache* 1996; 36: 379–84.

81. Tomsak R. Ophthalmologic aspects of headache. *Med Clin North Am* 1991; 75: 693–706.

82. Raskin N. *Headache (2nd ed)*. New York: Churchill Livingstone, 1988, pp. 229–30.

83. Mokri B, Sundt T, Houser W. Spontaneous internal carotid dissection, hemicrania, and Horner's Syndrome. *Arch Neurol* 1979; 36: 677–80.

84. Kudrow L. Diagnosis and treatment of cluster headaches. *Med Clin North Am* 1991; 75: 579–94.

85. Mathew N. Advances in cluster headache. *Neurol Clin* 1990; 8: 867–90.

86. Solomon S, Lipton RL, Newman LC. Prophylactic therapy of cluster headaches. *Clin Neuropharm* 1991; 14: 116–30.

87. Raskin MN. The hypnic headache syndrome. *Headache* 1988; 28: 534–6.

88. Newman LC, Lipton RB, Solomon S. The hypnic headache syndrome. In: Rose FC (ed). *New Advances in Headache Research (2nd ed)*. Great Britain: Smith-Gordon, 1991, pp. 31–4.

89. Newman LC, Lipton RB, Solomon S. The hypnic headache syndrome. *Neurology* 1990; 40: 1904–5.

90 Goadsby PJ, Silberstein SD (eds). *Headache*. Boston: Butterworth–Heinemann, 1997.

Index